HANDBOOK OF
PSYCHIATRIC
CONSULTATION
WITH CHILDREN
AND YOUTH

Edited by
Norman R. Bernstein, M.D.
Department of Psychiatry
University of Illinois
Chicago, Illinois

and

James Sussex, M.D.
Department of Psychiatry
University of Miami
Miami, Florida

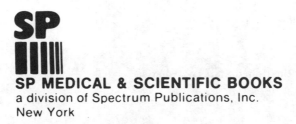

SP MEDICAL & SCIENTIFIC BOOKS
a division of Spectrum Publications, Inc.
New York

SPECTRUM PUBLICATIONS, INC.
175–20 Wexford Terrace
Jamaica, NY 11432

Library of Congress Cataloging in Publication Data
Main entry under title:

Handbook of psychiatric consultation with children and
 youth.

 Bibliography: p.
 Includes index.
 1. Child psychiatry. 2. Psychiatric consultation.
I. Bernstein, Norman R., 1927-   . II. Sussex, James.
[DNLM: 1. Consultants—Handbooks. 2. Mental dis-
orders—In infancy and childhood—Handbooks. 3. Referral
and consultation—Handbooks. QS 39 H236]
RJ499.H327   1984   618.92   84-3376
ISBN 0-89335-188-1

Printed in the United States of America

Dedicated to

Marilyn, Genya and Michael

Contributors

Robert S. Adams, M.D. • Psychiatrist-Director, The Child Guidance Clinic of Waterbury, Inc., Waterbury, Connecticut; Associate Clinical Professor, Yale Child Study Center, New Haven, Connecticut

Norman R. Bernstein, M.D. • Professor of Psychiatry, University of Illinois, Chicago, Illinois

John G. Clark, Jr., M.D. • Director, The American Facmily Foundation, Weston, Massachusetts; Assistant Clinical Professor, Harvard Medical School at Massachusetts General Hospital, Boston, Massachusetts

Raquel Cohen, M.D. • Associate Director of Child/Adolescent Division, and Associate Professor of Psychiatry, University of Miami School of Medicine, Miami, Florida

Donald D. Dunton, M.D. • Professor of Psychiatry, Columbia University, New York, New York

Philip DiMattia, Ph.D. • Principal Director of the Gaebler School, Waltham, Massachusetts; Assistant Professor of Special Education and Rehabilitation, Boston College, Chestnut Hill, Massachusetts

Norbert B. Enzer, M.D. • Associate Dean of Academic Affairs, and Professor of Psychiatry, Michigan State University College of Human Medicine, East Lansing, Michigan

Susan M. Fisher, M.D. • Lecturer and Consultant Psychiatrist, University of Chicago Pritzker School of Medicine, Chicago, Illinois

Donald S. Gair, M.D. • Professor and Chairman, Department of Child Psychiatry Boston University School of Medicine, Boston, Massachusetts; Superintendent, Gaebler Children's Center, Waltham, Massachusetts

Joseph M. Green, M.D. • Professor of Psychiatry and Director of Child Psychiatry, University of Wisconsin, Madison, Wisconsin

Thomas P. Hackett, M.D. • Professor of Psychiatry, Harvard Medical School, Boston, Massachusetts; Chief of Psychiattic Service, Massachusetts General Hospital, Boston, Massachusetts

Richmond Holder, M.D. • Director of Training, Adolescent Psychiatry, McLean Hospital, Belmont, Massachusetts; Instructor, Harvard Medical School, Boston, Massachusetts

Irving Hurwitz, Ph.D. • Professor of Educational Psychology, Boston College, Chestnut Hill, Massachusetts

Michael D. Lagone, Ph.D. • Director of Research, The American Family Foundation, Weston, Massachusetts

John F. McDermott, Jr., M.D. • Chief of Psychiatry, University of Hawaii at Monoa, Honolulu, Hawaii

Joseph D. Noshpitz, M.D. • Professor of Psychiatry, Department of Psychiatry, Children's Hospital, George Washington University, Washington, D.C.

Eva Poznanski, M.D. • Professor of Psychiatry, University of Illinois Health Sciences Center, Chicago, Illinois

Elizabeth Aub Reid, M.D. • Director of Training and Psychiatrist to Harvard University Health Service, Cambridge, Massachusetts; Assistant Clinical Professor, Tufts University, Medical School, Boston, Massachusetts; Instructor of Psychiatry, Harvard Medical School, Boston, Massachusetts

John B. Reinhart, M.D. • Professor of Psychiatry, University of Pittsburgh, Pittsburgh, Pennsylvania

William H. Sack, M.D. • Professor of Psychiatry and Chief of Child Psychiatry, University of Oregon, Portland, Oregon

Marshall D. Schechter, M.D. • Professor and Director, Division of Child and Adolescent Psychiatry, University of Pennsylvania, Philadelphia, Pennsylvania

James Sussex, M.D. • Professor and Chairman, Department of Psychiatry, University of Miami, Miami, Florida

George Tarjan, M.D. • Professor Emeritus of Psychiatry and Chief, Division of Child Psychiatry and Mental Retardation, University of California, Los Angeles; Past President, American Academy of Child Psychiatry, Washington, D.C.; President, American Psychiatric Association, Washington, D.C.

Hugh C. Thompson, M.D. • Professor of Community Medicine (Pediatrics), University of Arizona, Tucson, Arizona

Jack C. Westman, M.D. • Professor of Psychiatry, University of Wisconsin, Madison, Wisconsin

Virginia N. Wilking, M.D. • Former Director, Division of Child Psychiatry, Harlem Hospital Medical Center, New York, New York; Special Lecturer, College of Physicians and Surgeons, Columbia University, New York, New York

Lee H. Willer, M.D. • Associate Clinical Professor, Tufts University School of Medicine, Boston, Massachusetts

Herbert M. Woodcock, M.D. • Associate Professor of Psychiatry and Pediatrics, University of Oregon, Portland, Oregon

Henry H. Work, M.D. • Professor of Psychiatry, George Washington Medical School, Washington, D.C.; Deputy Director Emeritus, American Psychiatric Association, Washington, D.C.

Preface

I have spent the best part of the last quarter of a century working on the consultation service at the Massachusetts General Hospital. Much of my satisfaction has stemmed from working with nonpsychiatric physicians, especially in having them come to realize the value of psychological methods in the treatment of their patients. It has always been my belief that learning to understand the patient's mental life was as much a part of medicine as the taking of vital signs. To treat adequately, certainly to treat well, a physician must know something of his patient's thought processes. Teaching others the value of this knowledge is the first step in educating them to seek ways of learning it themselves. Rarely can this be done in the lecture hall. One can best pique curiosity by demonstrating worth, and that is done at the bedside or in whatever setting the consultation is carried out. Every consultation then carries an implicit imperative to attest its value. It can be covert teaching at its best. I have found the practice of consultation psychiatry satisfying and compelling enough to want to remain in it for at least another quarter of a century.

The consulting situations described in this excellent volume range through many settings, yet the core elements remain constant. Whether you are brought in to examine a frightened child in a pediatric intensive care unit or to talk with an anxious teenager in the ghetto, the consultant deals with nonpsychiatrists or nonphysicians who want an answer now and want it to work now. The consultant must learn another vocabulary. He must be able to translate his thinking into a nontechnical, understandable language. Often, the consultant must be able to persuade someone to do something he doesn't want to do. And much of this must be conducted in territory that is alien and unfriendly. I think that the role of psychiatric consultant requires of the candidate a need for excitement.

The authors assembled by Drs. Bernstein and Sussex are seasoned professionals who not only bear the mantle of authority, but bring to the reader a genuine sense of the action in their consultancies. These authors all share a trait that is a hallmark of the career consultant, a penchant for the practical. There is no time for lofty theorizing in the fast lane traffic described in these chapters.

There is a message to be learned for all psychiatric consultants in whatever setting they may practice from the recent evolution of the consultation/liaison movement in this country. Prior to the mid-1970s consultation psychiatry (and I include the concept of liaison in this heading) was practiced by a small band of individuals. We all knew each other by first name. Largely as the result of two forces, consultation psychiatry, in the last decade, has emerged as a subspecialty. The first of these forces is Public Law 94–484, Health Professions Education Assistance Act of 1976. This legislation emphasized the need to increase the number of primary care doctors—internists, family medicine practitioners, and pediatricians. It also recognized the necessity to include psychosocial skills in their training. It did so by insuring that federal money would be available to pay for their training. In this way, psychiatrists could receive salary support for teaching nonpsychiatric physicians. The second factor was the policy of the Psychiatric Education Branch of the National Institute of Mental Health (NIMH) which, starting in 1974, gave specific encouragement in the form of fellowship program support to the development of consultation liaison services in general hospitals. Not since 1934, when Alan Gregg advised the Rockefeller Foundation to provide start-up funds for five psychiatric programs to be started in general hospitals, has consultation psychiatry received such a boost.

The fickleness of federal funding now threatens to put the blight on these programs for psychiatric consultation. Without federal support will the consultation movement wither? Our fate is largely in the hands of third-party payers. Unfortunately, this puts us in lively competition with other medical and surgical specialties, where we are handicapped from the outset by being a time-based specialty. We are further disadvantaged because we lack sufficient evidence to show that our interventions are cost effective. While we can do little to alter the fact that time units constitute our basis for payment, we can and must devise research projects to demonstrate the cost benefit gains from consultation activities. This can be done. It should have been attended to long ago.

I would advise my fellow consultants, wherever they consult, to think of ways to prove that your efforts not only help patients, but save money for those who pay the bill.

THOMAS P. HACKETT, M.D.
Professor of Psychiatry
Harvard Medical School
Chief, Psychiatric Service
Massachusetts General Hospital

Contents

Acknowledgements

All of the myriad ideas and clinical experiences flowing into these chapters cannot be recalled. However, some antecedent events are clear. Robert Bragg, Director of Education and Training at the University of Miami and veteran consultant in Boston and Miami sparked this book. Lee Willer over the years has called out for more training in consultancy. John McDermott's efforts to define the roles and functions of child psychiatrists have abetted us. So have many teachers and colleagues. The late Lucy Jessner, once Director of Child Psychiatry at the Massachusetts General Hospital was a superb and stylish consultant. Stanley Cobb and Carl Binger enriched liaison work, as did Avery Weisman and Thomas Hackett. Each of the contributors has added to knowledge about consultation with children. Dana Farnsworth's splendid efforts in college mental health led the way, as did Gerald Caplan's community psychiatry efforts. Bill Lipowski clarified theory, as did Greta Bibring. Oliver Cope's dedication to surgical and psychiatric collaboration sustained this work. Susan Fisher and Ravindra Manek were very helpful in discussing cultural aspects of consultation. Experience on the Examinations for the American Board of Psychiatry and Neurology has helped to keep the image of clinical child psychiatry in focus.

Much gratitude is due Maryhelen Coughlin for typing and organizing the initial material. Jo Schuda helped go over the chapters and Roxanne Young pursued this work. Mary Winnicke helped peruse references in odd places. Above all, Fran Mysker typed, called, retyped and followed through on the myriads of details and contacts.

NORMAN R. BERNSTEIN, M.D.
JAMES SUSSEX, M.D.

Introduction

George Tarjan

Historically, the discipline of child psychiatry grew in the United States along two major routes. One followed the principles developed in the child guidance clinics and emphasized the interdisciplinary approach, which included the professions of child psychiatry, psychology, and social work. The other was based on psychoanalytic principles and focused primarily on practice carried out in single offices.

The establishment of the Committee on Certification in Child Psychiatry of the American Board of Psychiatry and Neurology in the late 1950s aimed to combine these two historical routes and thereby unify our concepts of child psychiatry. It is interesting to note, however, that during the last two decades a substantial trend in subspecialization began. Soon, groups became identified by their main interests of work with families, infants, adolescents, the mentally retarded and otherwise developmentally disabled patients, and physically handicapped children or those "entwined" with the legal system. In addition to direct care of children, consultation about individual patients and to institutions, hospitals, clinics, the schools, and the courts around child psychiatric principles became a major endeavor of many of our colleagues. Rapidly the field of consultation and liaison gained center stage in our specialty.

There is an ongoing debate concerning the size of our national deficit in the number of child psychiatrists. Some estimates suggest that we need three times as many as we have today, and others place the deficit at a lower figure. As president of the American Academy of Child Psychiatry, I suggested that it was high time to take stock of where we are, to identify trends in the field, and to plan for the future. Project Future of the academy began. Under the leadership of Irving Philips and Norbert Enzer, this work is now nearing completion (Philips et al., 1982). Consultation and liaison work gained a prominent position in the thinking of those who participated in the project.

Similar sentiments were expressed by John McDermott and his colleagues earlier in a document on the roles and functions of child psychiatrists. Their opinion was succinctly stated:

> The most frequent, nonclinical, or only indirectly clinical activities in which child psychiatrists engage probably relate to their role as consultants. While consultations are often made in response to a request to evaluate a particular child, or to help other professionals manage a particular child, they may also arise in a variety of situations in which the child psychiatrist is expected to undertake continued work with interdisciplinary teams or with institutions and agencies of varied types, where he will need to function in a liaison capacity to the agency or institution. In all such cases, the child psychiatrist must be able not only to assist other professionals to improve their understanding and skills in working with a particular child and with children generally, but also to advise on agency-wide policies and problems. Finally, the child psychiatrist may function as an expert resource to institutions and/or the community as a whole in suggesting ways to improve health care delivery in the field of child psychiatry, and in advising on long range planning of health care policies and facilities for children in general (McDermott, et al., 1976).

Training programs for child psychiatrists around the country are beginning to talk more about systematic education in consultancy, but much more needs to be done. We can all recall child psychiatrists who were pioneers in consultation, and skilled child advocates in many different settings. Most of these persons were highly gifted clinicians who learned primarily from their own successes and mistakes and who practiced more by intuition than as a consequence of formal learning. What is needed now is sound material on the realities of consultation and liaison work, focusing more on practical advice than on theory.

Major growth in our competence in consultation demands the availability of textbooks and reading materials that define the field of consultation, describe its current status, and advise on potential pitfalls. Despite the increasing numbers of excellent and authoritative texts in child psychiatry, an obvious gap remains in the literature on consultation. This volume by Norman Bernstein and James Sussex provides the type of practical insight needed today in this busy but inadequately charted region. The authors do not adhere in a doctrinaire way to any one ideology of consultation but offer a general eclectic philosophy. All of the authors see the consultant as a child advocate working to better the quality of life of children in each of the contexts of consultation. The emphasis is more on liaison than on single consultation, with attention to the complexities of the situation in which children are served and to the overt and covert relationships among children and their caretakers. The book is intentionally free of consultation theory, though it derives from psychodynamic and sociological principles. Even the first chapter on the consultant and the consultation experience is intermingled with a description of the characteristics of today's consulting child psychiatrists. In general, the book is focused on recounting the experiences and the issues faced by clinicians who have been out in the field for many years. It has the flavor of what really happens and how consultants feel about it. It explains how these modern pioneers work.

The book is a delight to read and has material for the adult and child psychiatrist as well as for pediatricians, teachers, special educators, parents, and all others committed to the welfare of children. Some chapters imply that the successful consultant must be a skillful politician, others emphasize the role as a medical ombudsman, but in none of them is the basic medical orientation overlooked. Even when special biomedical knowledge of the physician is not the most salient facet of the work, the medical orientation retains its centrality. This stance is particularly relevant today when the contrasting roles of child psychiatry, psychology, and education are frequently debated.

The message is clear. Consultants need to be competent in the clinical evaluation of children. They must first be good physicians and masters of their field. They also have to be able to move into the complex and often tricky realms of alien nonmedical situations. They have to be durable and calm in the face of conflicting approaches, oppositional perspectives, and eccentric or trendy styles of teaching and child mental health care. This volume gives samples of the experiences of many wise doctors in a personal vein that makes the material simple to absorb. The authors do not view consultation as a separate subspecialty of child psychiatry, but rather as varied applications of the skills and techniques that should be taught to all good clinicians. In this process the contributors persuasively fill in the road map to implementation.

Each of the sections of this book can be viewed as an independent essay on a particular area of consultancy. There is some overlap in coverage but it all leads to an artful mosaic. Adams contrasts consultation to a factory-town clinic with that given to a private school. The chapter on school consultation in the public elementary school by Willer discusses work with teachers. Holder describes work at private schools with faculty and students, while Reid discusses struggles with the administration. DiMattia focuses on the teacher's role in determining who should have psychiatric consultation. It is in this cross-cutting approach that supplementary facets of the consultancy issues in schools are examined, and the chapters support each other handily.

In addition to institutional approaches there is material on special settings such as Wilking's overview of emergency consultation and of her work in a ghetto, or the sections on mental retardation, psychosis, and depression by Work, Poznanski, and Gair, with each of the authors examining a particular disease or disorder. Thompson tells when pediatricians should refer. The traditional inpatient and outpatient child psychiatry roles are reviewed by Sack and Enzer, while Noshpitz gives an overview of problems in consultation with adolescents. Fisher and Hurwitz talk about a particular program in a treatment center for delinquent children. Westman examines family consultation, and Clark and Langone examine intervention strategies for consulting with cult victims. Cohen approaches the problems of consulting with refugees, and Green shows the problems of a rural clinical consultant. This overlapping approach explicates the complex tapestry of the field of consultation and shows the common denominators in the functions and roles of child psychiatrists. This point is made particularly clear in the complementary chapters of McDermott on divorce and custody and Schechter's on the child psychiatrist in court.

Here is a special book to be read, savored, and consulted. It is a guide for the beginning resident or fellow in child psychiatry, the experienced clinician, as well as for parents, pediatricians, social workers, psychologists, teachers, and all who mold the lives of children.

REFERENCES

McDermott JF, McGuire C, and Berner ES: Roles and functions of child psychiatrists (Committee on Certification in Child Psychiatry of the American Board of Psychiatry and Neurology, Inc: Evanston, IL) 1976.
Philips I, Enzer N, et al.: Project future of the Academy of Child Psychiatry (Preliminary report in press) 1982.

1

The Temperament and Preparation of the Consultant

Norman R. Bernstein and H. Donald Dunton

Advice must be judged by its results – Cicero

CONSULTATION

Lipowski (1974, 1975) defined medical consultation by psychiatrists as "the provision of expert advice on the diagnosis, management, and prevention of mental disorders by specially trained mental health professionals at the request of other health professionals and within the constraints of available knowledge and techniques." He believes the liaison psychiatrist acts as an interpreter and bridge builder between two conceptual domains and professional groups. Gerald Caplan (1970) wrote of mental health consultation in other settings as well, stating that consultation "is used to denote a process of interaction between two professional persons—the consultant who is a specialist, and the consultee, who involves the consultant's help in regard to a current work problem with which he is having some difficulty and which he has decided is within the other one's area of specialized competence. The work problem involves the management or treatment of one or more clients of the consultee, or the planning or implementation of a program to cater to such clients." Caplan distinguished other activities such as supervision and education and collaboration and noted some characteristics of mental health consultation:

1. The consultant has no administrative responsibility for the consultee's work or professional responsibility for the outcome of the patient's care.
2. The consultee is under no compulsion to accept the consultant's ideas or suggestions.
3. The basic relationship between the two is coordinate. There is no built-in hierarchical authority tension.
4. The coordinate relationship is fostered by the consultant's usually being a member of another profession and coming briefly into the consultee's area from the outside.
5. Consultation is usually given in a short series of interviews.
6. Consultation is expected to continue indefinitely.
7. A consultant has no predetermined body of information to impart. He responds only to the current work difficulty. The consultant does not seek to remedy other areas of inadequacy in the consultee. He expects other issues to be raised in further consultations.

The aim is to improve the consultee's job performance, not his sense of well-being. The consultant does not focus overtly on personal problems of the consultee and respects his privacy. Caplan described four types of consultations:

1. The client-centered case consultation.
2. Consultee-centered consultation.
3. Program-centered administrative consultation.
4. Consultee-centered administrative consultation focusing on programming and organization rather than on a particular patient.

Cohen-Cole et al. (1980) expanded on Caplan's formulation of the consulting role. They underscored the distinction between consultation and supervision. The *supervisory* relationship (e.g., attending/resident) is based on delegated authority and direct legal responsibility. The relationship is hierarchical, and the supervisor can require that the supervisee carry out certain actions. In the consultation relationship, neither party has authority over the other, and the consultee can accept, reject, or modify the consultant's recommendations. The consultant has no direct legal responsibility for the actions of the consultee.

Cohen-Cole and colleagues also underscored the difference between consultation and *referral* tasks. In the case of referral, partial or total responsibility for the care of a patient is transferred from one physician to another. Each physician is directly responsible to the patient, but not necessarily to each other. Each may make and carry through autonomous decisions about treatment. In consultation, on the other hand, primary responsibility for making decisions remains in the hands of the physician who requests the consultant's help. The consultant is responsible both to the patient and to the consultee. He is limited to making suggestions to the consultee and cannot make autonomous decisions about the patient's treatment.

In *psychotherapy*, the therapist elicits, clarifies, and modifies the patient's pattern of emotional or behavioral responses. The psychiatric consultant may similarly seek to clarify patterns of emotional responses in either the referring medical personnel or the patient, both of whom may affect the patient's adaptation. The consultant, however, generally limits such inquiries to the clarification and modification of *specific* disruptions in the professional relationship between the consultee and the patient. The consultant should not attempt to modify the consultee's general adaptation to life.

Many factors shape the consultation: the timing of the consultation in the course of the patient's hospitalization, the preparation of the patient, the nature of the primary physician-patient relationship, the consultee's covert expectations of the consultation, the patient's expectations of the consultation, group dynamics of the medical team or recent stress on the ward, the "fit" between consultant recommendations and the resources and attitudes of the consultee.

Child Psychiatry Consultation

McDermott (1976) in his study of the roles and functions of child psychiatrists stated:

> The most frequent nonclinical, or only indirectly clinical, activities in which child psychiatrists engage probably relate to their role as consultants. While consultations are often made in response to a request to evaluate a particular child, or to help other professionals manage a particular child, they may also arise in a variety of situations in which the child psychiatrist is expected to undertake continued work with interdisciplinary teams or with institutions and agencies of varied types, where he will need to function in a liaison capacity to the agency or institution. In all such cases, the child psychiatrist must be able not only to assist other professionals to improve their understandings and skills in working with a particular child and with children generally, but also to advise on agency-wide policies and problems. Finally, the child psychiatrist may function as an expert resource to institutions and/or the community as a whole in suggesting ways to improve health care delivery in the field of child psychiatry, and in advising on long range planning of health care policies and facilities for children in general.

McDermott stressed that the child psychiatrist consultant should "assist others to function better in their roles." McDermott et al. (1976, 1981) thought that a consultant should possess the following types of information:

1. Knowledge of the history, traditions, and organizations of other disciplines.
2. Knowledge of the operation of child-related institutions (i.e., the school system, classroom, hospital ward, residential treatment center).
3. Knowledge of institutional goals and constraints of the organization with which the consulting is done.
4. Knowledge of emotional reactions in adults who work with emotionally disturbed children and their families.
5. Knowledge of community and national resources for children and families.
6. Knowledge of the legal status and "rights of children" (e.g., custody and other laws relating to children and the institutions caring for them.
7. Knowledge of legal procedures in giving testimony.

Simmons (1981) described in contrast to some of the foregoing writers, that the child psychiatrist consultant often has to be the one who provides the therapy because in practical terms he is the most available and informed person. He also stressed that the consultant's responsibility is primarily to the *consultee*, not the patient, in this role. Langsley and Hollender (1982) reviewed the roles and functions of the adult psychiatrist in a form equally relevant for the child psychiatry consultant—he needs to be able to diagnose, prescribe, and develop a treatment or management plan.

While Krakowski (1972) and Guse (1978) argued whether the psychiatric consultant should know the specialty in which he is working or whether this is not a useful kind of information, it generally seems that doing good liaison work inevitably requires some sophistication about the setting, not just in the language used but in terms of the overall planning needed and the work style, rhythm, and time pressures on the people in the social system in which the psychiatrist is consulting.

Glickman (1980) stated that the liaison psychiatrist above all is a teacher. He teaches nonpsychiatric personnel methods of preventing emotional stress or treating patients with less advanced symptoms. Strain (1975) describes liaison psychiatry as a "pedagogic pursuit that attempts to teach medical caretakers about core issues in medical psychology . . . with the expectation that in time . . . other health care professionals will provide most of the psychological care of the patients themselves." Glickman said that "the liaison psychiatrist is like the fire inspector, while the psychiatric consultant is like the fire fighter." As the authors in this monograph are almost all psychiatric physicians, the medical role is an important aspect of consultation–liaison, making problems in some areas and facilitating in others. Some schoolteachers fear that physicians focus only on pathology, while some nurses defer to the authority of physicians regardless of their wisdom.

Pruzansky (1982), after 30 years of running a large interdisciplinary clinic for craniofacial deformities, said that he believed the kind of people who could do this work are people who are internally secure, confident of their knowledge of their own field, and interested in the details of the field in which they are collaborating. Greenhill (1970) concluded after decades of liaison work that the "liaison psychiatrist is some sort of twentieth-century medical masochist, half-deluded and saintly at the same time, teaching in the face of opposing values."

Light (1980) noted that the qualities thought to be admirable in a psychiatrist were intelligence, empathy, sense of humor, personal interest in others, and a capacity for growth. The psychiatrist should be a man of breadth and accomplishment who shows sincerity, honesty, and maturity. The Menninger Foundation engraved in stone the "Criteria of Emotional Maturity," which should characterize the psychiatrist:

The ability to deal constructively with reality.

The capacity to adapt to change.

A relative freedom from symptoms that are produced by tensions and anxieties.

The capacity to find more satisfaction in giving than receiving.

The capacity to relate to other people in a consistent manner with mutual satisfaction and helpfulness.

The capacity to sublimate, to direct one's instinctive hostile energy into creative and constructive outlets.

The capacity to love.

Menninger (1952) believed "that if a man is not all of these things by the time he has entered medical school, it is probably too late for him to acquire them. The psychiatrist as a person is more important than the psychiatrist as a technician or scientist. What he *is* has more effect upon his patients than anything he does."

This seems to be particularly true for the consultant. Park and Shapiro (1979) made the point that in finding a therapist, the patient should see someone who is "real," in other words, an emotionally accessible person. This quality seems to be important in the psychiatric consultant. Weisman (1978) advised consultants to assume a style in which they "learn to listen and observe . . . the wait-and-see technique of office therapy should be shunned."

Hendrick inveighed against the psychiatrist's being too conventional and complained that the profession was suffering from too many matter-of-fact, commonsensical, and well-adjusted individuals who were all-around, normal, and not too bright. He contrasted the pioneers in psychiatry, especially those in psychoanalysis, as introspective persons inclined to be studious and thoughtful, who were highly individualistic, and who limited their social life to clinical and theoretical discussions with colleagues. While one would not argue for dullness in consultants, they are less likely to fit this template than most psychiatrists. The creativity of the consultant is shown in the clinical area and is that of a social activist more than an innovative theoretician.

Consultation-Liaison Psychiatrists

Liaison functions involve continued work with a group—ward, clinic, school, or unit—over a period of time. When a physician goes into a school or on to a ward where he is attempting to do liaison work, most of the features of consultation need to shift. The consultant can usually get in and out quickly, while the liaison person must develop and sustain a relationship with the persons whose consultation request he is answering. He will get to know them. He should learn the overt and covert agendas, and he will develop a sense of the atmosphere and emotional quality of the ward or school in which he is working. On the other side, the staff with which he is working will get to know him. They will get beyond the professional persona. They will usually discern whether he smokes, drinks, jogs, or votes Republican. They will learn whether he is divorced or has children, whether his children are in trouble, whether he is readily available at the office, and whether he is skillful in phrasing problems. The liaison psychiatrist must enter the world of the group with whom he works (Adams, 1968, 1974).

While liaison and consultation overlap, with consultation seen as more brief, focused on a single, stated problem and liaison as more involved with the context of the clinical problem, consultation is used by most of the authors in this work to include liaison functions and style of operation—deriving from the French definition of *liaison* as linking, joining, or connecting. In many situations, traditional distaste and devaluation of the psychiatrist persist and the media shape many of the attitudes of professionals as well as lay people (1982). The psychiatrst must rely on his colleagues outside the consultation setting for most of his approval, although if he does not obtain some positive approval and support in the setting, consultation will not work either. The liaison psychiatrist does well to be articulate but not to be known as a "bull thrower." He has to be able to shift from the rhythm of office practice or psychiatric ward functioning to the rhythm of the institution in which he is working.

Light (1980) avers that psychiatrists and psychotherapists require insight into themselves, creativity, sublimated voyeurism, and a grasp of cultural implications and of the relativity of behavior. For the consultant, voyeurism may be nearer the surface, and creativity needs to be controlled to avoid the tendency toward vain and charismatic manipulations. Hackett (1982) has inveighed against the consultant as a "doctor in mufti, well-tailored and eager to convert his consultees, vainly trying to get them to meet with him." Hackett advised sticking to a sharply limited focus on the patient and donning the white coat. Strain (1977) maintained that "unless he is recognized as an ambassador . . . he will remain an ear-clutcher, a doctor-chaser, a patient-chaser, pleading to be heard."

Consultants vary greatly in style and presentation. The young consultant is more likely to try very hard to show what he can do, while some older ones radiate a manner that declares that they have "seen it all." This can evoke very different responses from their consultees. Some consultants are more "folksy" than others, and some are more willing to invest time sitting and having a cup of coffee with teachers, nurses, or colleagues, or are more ready to provide quick advice to people they meet in the corridors. This can mean referring the cook or the cleaning lady to a clinic, or talking about the husband of a teacher who wants help. This has to be done with caution as the information can be too skewed or meager for a sensible response, or the corridor questioners can be angered if the consultant wards them off too abruptly. In most situations the peripatetic consultant will gradually establish a preferred routine, whether a formal presentation, a written summary of the problem, or a casual chat in the dean's office is desired.

In some settings a male consultant may be more useful, as Beardsley (1982) described in his intensive care work with neonates, where the nurses are all women and the male physicians are rarely around. He found that the nurses took well to having an older male adviser to whom they could turn. Elizabeth Reid (1982) found that in the college setting, a professional woman had an advantage in being able to show maternal concern about students. Some consultants rely heavily on personal charm which is helpful when it works, and a painful embarrassment when it misfires. Being a purveyor of charm is hazardous when it keeps the consultant himself in the foreground instead of the professional problem. When it works it is a personal style; when it fails it is an affectation.

There is no doubt that the consultant often has to "sell" himself in a new environment, and his counsel is accepted because he is considered "such a sensible guy" or "a really practical person." The older man or woman can be ascribed wisdom, and at the same time be left out of the joking and teasing that are part of any working group. Joking is fine as long as the consultant likes the people involved, so that hostility or contempt does not slip out. Even Freud liked to tell stories to illustrate points. One young, woman consultant reported that she never got involved in power struggles with the male physicians and carefully avoided flirting. James Q. Simmons of UCLA (1982) said that the consultant must have the ability to break down the problem into its smaller parts, examine them analytically, and then reintegrate them in a form that makes sense to the consultee. Professionals who have a rigid format or a gimmick (either of conceptualization or language) that they try to apply in all situations are soon likely to annoy their hosts. Jargon is not helpful. The person who does liaison work is obviously someone who likes to get out of the office and move about in a different environment. He must be somewhat more extroverted than his suburban therapist colleagues. He certainly has to be better able to bear disapproval, criticism, and teasing as he does his extramural work. He has to be able to put himself in the shoes of his consultees and empathize with their frustrations about the problem being presented. He has to feel more like a doer while acting as a *teacher*. Nurses, physical therapists, occupational therapists, pastoral counselors, practical nurses, ward clerks, teachers, and volunteers all assert that they need a psychiatrist who seems natural, who is interested, and *who puts them at ease*: "He shouldn't give us the feeling he is analyzing us or every word we utter." Socializing at a staff party or similar functions may be required in small doses to make the staff comfortable with a "shrink." Some consultants manage to be friendly and still avoid all such activities.

One surgeon remarked that the consultant should provide "help, not advice. I need to be told what I should do, even if I don't agree with it. And it should be clear" (Parsons, 1982). Some schoolteachers stress the need for friendliness from their consultants and feel that too many doctors are status bound, superior, and pessimistic, seeing only the pathology in the problem and being needlessly concerned about disasters. In contrast, teachers have the experience that most things work out with time for the majority of children. Nurses in hospitals note that too many consultants are obviously residents in training themselves, and they prefer consultants who are self-assured enough to be able to ask questions and take information from the nurses without becoming too embarrassed or anxious. For some staff members there is concern that the consultant not be discouraging and that he be cheerful and active in his orientation, telling people precise programs to implement. Others feel that in the face of death and disaster, too much cheer is only frivolous and inappropriate. All seem to agree that the consultant must accept the affects of the consultee and the patient with great tolerance. One nurse noted that a psychiatrist came on a burn ward and, after seeing the horrendous injury, immediately remarked, "I wouldn't want to live if I were in his place." This was too close to what the staff felt and it failed to provide any chance for the staff to examine their own feelings.

LANGUAGE AND CULTURE

Effective consulting requires speaking plausibly and persuasively. If a foreign consultant is not facile in English he will have a considerable handicap. Foreign medical graduates (FMGs) often feel prejudice against them both for being psychiatrists and for being culturally or racially different. Chen (1981) writes that the FMG tends to be a listener who is cautious in order to avoid conflicts in interpersonal relationships. Without good verbal communication skills, their assessments of situations may also go awry. Teja and Akhtar (1981) specify problems when "slang, puns, slips-of-the-tongue, and metaphorical allusions go unnoticed. . . . American humor is hard to understand and impossible to create." For training directors to give residents handbooks of American slang is hardly an answer to this problem. Thorough language training is in order, as this is the key to knowing the society. While there is a body of writing on the differences between cultural perspectives of Korean, Japanese, Indian, Peruvian, and black patients and therapists, these subtleties are not often the center of consultation–liaison work. However, when they come up the most important thing is for the consultant to feel comfortable enough to stop and ask for an explanation of the culturally unclear material. Just as an American doctor might want to know how an Indian patient's prearranged marriage influences her when she complains of "lack of love" from her husband, a consultant from the Philippines can pursue questions about the significance of a third and fourth marriage in an American patient or attitudes toward work and breaking the law. Chen has written about the need for the FMG to develop "biculturalism," an ability to experience and comprehend his native society and the new one in which he is working. There is an analogous biculturalism for liaison workers. They need to move from the psychiatric milieu of their colleagues into the special subculture of the school or ward on which they are consulting. Both situations require that the consultant have a clear sense of self-identity as a psychiatrist and also as an individual. Most of the authors of this book had foreign teachers with interesting and sometimes impregnable central European accents, which served as an asset rather than a handicap. They felt no sense of cultural intimidation and assumed their extensive education and knowledge of language and literature gave them a clear sense of identity and confidence, even arrogance, about bringing truth to the "barbarian" Americans. They assumed basic mental mechanisms were universal and felt they had a mission to teach them. This contrasts greatly with what Chen reports of the more recent and generally Asian psychiatrist, describing him as "compliant, passive, and intimidated, with a thin veneer of submission to people in authority . . . a listener, cautious about making his position known so others won't disagree with him." For any liaison worker, it is vital to have resolved most of his personal problems of identity and to have achieved a level of personal and professional security that arms him to pursue diverse clinical encounters. The FMG needs enough skill to express himself automatically so that he is not exhausted by having always to work at translation and can use his energies for understanding the special situation confronting him. Then he can use his special cultural assets, such as the exceptional ease in developing an empathic relationship so evident in Latin American physicians, the calm and sympathetic acceptance of tragedy so basic to Indian physicians, or the Iranian FMGs' perceptiveness for nonverbal communication. The consultant must be able to identify with the basic human condition of his patients and his consultees and to explain them without self-consciousness.

The consultant should, then, embody some of the ideal traits of the good psychiatrist. The qualities that make a good therapist may be a disadvantage in the consultation–liaison world. Storr (1975) commented that a therapist is often concerned with "understanding persons rather than with abolishing symptoms." The "reluctance to take over," Storr advised for therapists, "to give orders, to seek immediate practical solutions to problems" is exactly what a consultant must attempt. These traits turn out to be unevenly and imperfectly supplied throughout the profession, but part of the spectrum of medical and action-oriented qualities is more necessary in consultation and liaison work. The problems of training for this are hardly resolved, although many different good consultants have emerged both with and without formal training. How is the good clinician converted into a skillful consultant? Goin and Goin (1981) declared that "The type of psychiatrist who will be most useful . . . is one whose life work is the understanding of the workings of the mind; a psychodynamically oriented psychiatrist." But this is not sufficient, and training generally has not been developed to transform the good therapist into a good consultant.

CONSULTANCY TRAINING FOR THE CHILD PSYCHIATRIST

The essentials of approved residencies (1974) state: "For all trainees, there should be experience in consultative work with children and adolescents on pediatric and other medical services. There should be opportunities for cooperative consultative work with child care agencies in the community." The training experience and evaluation of training were left to the discretion of the residency program.

Lipowski (1977) believed that "training of unique breadth and complexity is indispensible. Its two basic components are thorough medical training and acquisition of expert knowledge about man as a body–mind complex in social interaction. The core training should include exposure to all behavioral sciences and grounding in the broad range of therapeutic techniques available today. It should foster clear communication, diagnostic reasoning, and an open-minded scientific attitude." He felt that three months in full-time liaison work in the second or third year of training was necessary. Mendel (1966), in a survey of training of consultation in 202 centers, revealed that 75 percent offer training and 25 percent offer none. The method of training is primarily supervision. Only four percent evaluated the results of the consultation. The performance of the trainee is evaluated informally in 60 percent and formally in 30 percent. Twenty-five percent conduct formal lectures or seminars.

Schwab (1968) described a program with a basic format centered around seminars, lectures, clinical conferences, clinical experience, and supervision. The training program was evaluated in terms of its effectiveness, increase in number of consultations, earlier referrals, and fewer emergencies. Residents felt the training was valuable; case formulations were useful in other areas. There was increased flexibility in treatment approaches and opportunity for learning and self-development. Kanter et al. (1979) developed a psychiatric consultation record to aid in the training, to evaluate the impact of the teaching as well as the training program itself. The quality of progress of the residents' work could be rapidly assessed. Most authors (Adams, Mendel, Lipowski, LaVietes, Chess, and Jellinek) hardly referred to evaluations.

Auerbeck (1975) discussed the value and difficulty in consultancy teaching. He emphasized the debate over its value and the low motivation for psychiatrists to remain in the field. He stressed the importance for educators to give training the emphasis it deserves and the importance of role modeling. Guse et al. (1978) described teaching goals in four building blocks:

1. Awareness of psychosocial stresses as a predisposing initiating, and/or sustaining factors in physical illness.
2. Skills of acquiring relevant psychosocial data through a rapid but effective interview technique.
3. The capacity to relate and integrate psychosocial data to illness and make biopsychosocial assessments.
4. The ability to develop treatment play that includes biopsychosocial considerations.

Small et al. (1968) viewed training as primarily a supervisory experience: "The most useful educational purpose served by this program was in the identification of the kinds of behaviors which made for effective, well-recorded psychiatric consultation." The resident took part in a comparative study of patients referred for psychiatric hospitalization and obtained feedback from the referral sources.

Haupt et al. (1976–77) applied competency-based education to consultation–liaison psychiatry. The aim was to delineate the knowledge, skills, and attitudes required of a consultation–liaison psychiatrist and how to integrate these into training and practice. Behavioral objectives are presented as a focus for resident supervision and this application to a clinical situation with case examples covering core areas.

LaVietes and Chess (1979) described a training program in the manner in which a child psychiatrist works with schools. The training was centered primarily around observation and supervisions. Jellinek et al. (1981) addressed themselves specifically to a description of the organization of a child psychiatric consultation service and its functions. They described types of patients and services but said little about training.

Caplan's (1970) training program consists of a series of lectures, seminars, supervised field work, two to three months' full-time internship experience, and discussion of cases. Supervision is the crucial element. The evaluation of training centered around the trainees objectivity, knowledge, self-awareness, skill, and confidence. Most of the evaluation was concerned with the changes in the consultee, changes in numbers of referrals, changes in performance, and attitudes. In reference to children, the evaluation concerned the changes in the mental health of the students and increased tolerance of teachers.

DISCUSSION

Overall there has been a great increase in training, research, and practice of consultation–liaison psychiatry. There remains considerable difficulty in the teaching and practice because of funding, relationships to other departments, time, location, political and social pressures, and status. A relatively small proportion of the programs have organized protocols for training and evaluation. The basic model is supervision of clinical work and varying amounts of time devoted to lectures and seminars. Many institutions offer a good education experience focused on specific research projects.

In child psychiatry the majority of reports relate specific projects with schools, psychosocial pediatrics, collaboration with a variety of nonmedical staff, and communication of psychiatric concepts. It appears that many centers believe that an intensive consultation–liaison experience in one area over a short period of time can adequately teach the principles. Here again the evaluation focuses more on the consultee's and client's response and change rather than the trainee's. The primary method of teaching seems to be based on individual supervision.

The Committee on Certification in Child Psychiatry of the American Board of Psychiatry and Neurology has had the opportunity to see the end product of training. Often there is a wide discrepancy between what is on paper (for accreditation of a center) and what the trainee has actually experienced. As expected, the organization, teaching, learning, and evaluation depend on the leaders. When the director of child psychiatry and director of pediatrics have common goals and interests in liaison, the educational system works. No amount of curriculum reorganization, testing, evaluation, and research will be of much help without this. J. Apley said many years ago that the protracted courtship between pediatrics and child psychiatry should soon end in marriage—if only for the good of the children. This remains the goal in most spheres of consultation.

REFERENCES

Adams PL: *Primer of Child Psychotherapy* (Little, Brown and Co) 1974.

Adams PL: Techniques for pediatric consultation. *Handbook of Psychiatric Consultation*, Schwab, JJ (ed.) (Appleton-Century-Croft: New York) 1968, pp 107–123.

Auerback DB: Liaison psychiatry and education of the psychiatric resident. *Consultation-Liaison*, Pasonow, RO (ed.) (Grune and Stratton, Inc: New York) 1975, pp 277–284.

Beardsley W: (Personal communication: Cherry Hills, NJ) 1982.

Caplan G: *The Theory and Practice of Mental Health Consultation* (Basic Books, Inc) 1900, pp 330–352.

Chen R: *Foreign Medical Graduates in Psychiatry* (Human Sciences Press: New York) 1981.

Cohen-Cole SA, Haggarty J, and Raft D: Proposed objectives for residents in consultation psychiatry. *Task Force on Consultation-Liaison Objectives* (Association for Academic Psychiatry) 1980.

Glickman L: *Psychiatric Consultation in the General Hospital* (Marcel Dekker, Inc: New York) 1980.

Goin JM and Goin MK: *Changing the Body* (Williams and Wilkins: Baltimore) 1981.

Greenhill M: The development of liaison programs. *Psychiatric Medicine*, Usdin G (ed.) (Brunner/Mazel: New York) 1977, pp. 115–194.

Guse LH, Manne S, and Morgan M: An instrument for evaluating liaison teaching in the primary care setting *J Psych Educ* 2(2):215, 1978.

Hackett TP: Consultation held valid, liaison held invalid. *Clin Psych News*, p 36, Jan 1982.

Haupt JL, Weinstein HM, and Russel MP: *Int J Psych Med* 7(4):295–320, 1976–77.

Jellinek MS, Herzog DB, and Selter LF: A psychiatric consultation service for hospitalized children. *Liais Psych* 22(1):29–33, 1981.

Kantor SJ, Chiaranclinic I, and Heller SS: The use of the psychiatric consultation record for residency training. *Hosp Psych* 1(3):202–213, 1979.

Krakowski J: The process of consultation. *Psychosomatic Medicine: Its Clinical Applications*, Wittkower ED and Warners H (eds.) (Harper and Row: New York) 1977, pp 26–39.

Langsley D and Hollander M: The definition of a psychiatrist. *Am J Psych* 1: 82–85, Jan 1982.

LaVietes K and Chess S: A training program in school psychiatry. *J Acad Child Psych* 8(1):84–96, 1979.
Lipowski ZJ: Consultation–liaison psychiatry: Past, present and future. *Consultation-Liaison Psychiatry*, Pasnow RO (ed.) (Grune and Stratton: New York) 1975, pp 1–30.
Lipowski ZJ: Consultation-liaison psychiatry: An overview. *Am J Psych* 131 (6):623–630, 1974.
Lipowski ZJ, Lipsitt DR, and Whybrow PC: *Psychosomatic Medicine* (Oxford University Press: New York) 1977.
Light, D: *Becoming Psychiatrists* (WW Norton: New York) 1980, p 36.
McDermott J: (Personal communication: University of Hawaii) 1981.
McDermott JC, McGuire C, and Bener E: *Roles and Functions of Child Psychiatrists* (American Board Psychiatry and Neurology, Inc: Evanston, IL) 1976.
Menninger KA: What are the goals of psychiatric education? *Bulletin of the Menninger Clinic*, vol 16, pp 153–156, 1952.
Mendel WM: Psychiatric consultation experience. *Am J Psych* 123(2):150–155, 1966.
Park CC and Shapiro L: *You Are Not Alone* (Little Brown and Co: Boston) 1979.
Parsons R: (Personal communication: University of Chicago) 1982.
Pruzansky S: (Personal communication: University of Illinois) 1982.
Reid E: (Personal communication: Cherry Hills, NJ) 1982.
Schwab JJ: Consultation–liaison program. *Handbook of Psychiatric Consultation*, Schwab JJ (ed.) (Appleton-Century-Croft: New York 1968, pp 237–249.
Small JF, Foster LG, Small JG, and Goodman J: *Disease of the Nervous System* 29(12):817–823, 1968.
Simmons JE: Consultations. *Psychiatric Examination of Children* (Lea and Febiger: Philadelphia) 1981, pp 250–281.
Simmons JQ: (Personal communication: Cherry Hills, NJ) 1982.
Stacy J: Psychiatry given mixed image in cinema. *Amer Med News*, vol 25(12) March 26, 1982.
Storr A: *The Art of Psychotherapy* (Methuen: New York) 1979.
Strain JJ: Letter. *Am J Psych* 134:1050–1051, 1977.
Strain J and Grossman S: *Psychological Care of the Mentally Ill: A Primer in Liaison Psychiatry* (Appleton-Century-Croft: New York) 1975.
Teja J and Akhtar S: The psychosocial problems of FMG's with special reference to those in psychiatry. *Foreign Medical Graduates in Psychiatry*, Chen R (ed.) 1981, pp 321–335.
Weisman A: Coping with illness. *The Massachusetts General Hospital Handbook of General Hospital Psychiatry*, Hackett TP and Cassem NH (eds.) (CV Mosby: St. Louis, MO) 1978, pp 264–275.

The Consultant,
the Family, and Divorce

2

The Psychiatrist as a Consultant in Divorce and Custody

John F. McDermott, Jr.

INTRODUCTION

In the 1970s, a curious contradiction appeared. A study of child psychiatry training programs (McDermott et al., 1976) showed that forensic training was rarely included; preparing the child psychiatrist for work with the courts was a low priority. Yet at the same time, the rapidly accelerating divorce rate and custody disputes over children had caused family and juvenile court judges, as consumers of child psychiatric services, to list as their primary need the assistance of "experts" in custody determinations.

It is well known that almost one out of two marriages fail, and most of these involve children. Children of divorce constitute a large part of our clinical practice. But how many child psychiatrists are aware that these cases also constitute the largest single category of all civil matters handled by America's legal system (Weiss, 1976)? The determinations over custody of these children are crucial in shaping their personality development.

In this chapter the author will first consider the effects of divorce on children, the history of custody, changes and trends, and how the courts actually operate in the United States today. Next, the subject will turn to the child psychiatrist's role in divorce and custody cases, with specific consideration of the evaluation, the report to the court and courtroom testimony, along with suggestions and operating guidelines.

THE EFFECTS OF DIVORCE

Wallerstein and Kelly (1974–80) have described the effects of divorce on children at different developmental levels, from the early signs of depressive illness and developmental constriction in preschool children, to the depression and regression in school-age children, to the anger and bitterness in adolescents. Perhaps the most alarming finding is that half of the children they followed gave evidence of consolidated depressive behavior patterns after one year, combined with frequent school and peer difficulties. The postdivorce living arrangements that the court decides are crucial factors influencing these problems of adjustment. As Wallerstein and Kelly state: "The divorce *event* is not the central factor in determining the outcome for the child, but rather, the divorce process or chain of events set in motion by the separation." They have concluded from their follow-up studies that access to *both* parents is the single most important factor determining the outcome for children. This finding is critical to know for child psychiatrists working with these youngsters. But it also makes it critically important for child psychiatrists to become more involved in the judicial custody determination process itself. Child custody consultations should become a familiar skill; they are critical for the mental health of the nation's children. The psychiatrist's professional expertise is both wanted and needed.

HISTORY OF FAMILY LAW AND
CUSTODY DETERMINATION

It is useful to view custody from an historical perspective and to understand its evolution, the reasons for change in its practices, its present status, and future trends. Historically, perhaps the earliest and most vivid recorded case of custody determination is the biblical story in which King Solomon, confronted by two women both claiming to be the mother of an infant, threatened to cut the infant in half in order to give each woman an equal share. His keen clinical judgment was borne out when the real mother demonstrated her strong attachment by offering to give up the baby to the other woman. But that single common-sense test was lost in time. The most powerful influence became Roman law, under which the father had exclusive rights over his children. They were his property. He could sell them or even kill them. This notion of children as chattel or property carried over into English law where it prevailed until the fourteenth century (Derdeyn, 1976; Westman, 1975), Gradually, instead of simple property, children began to be viewed as petlike animals or incomplete humans—the early precursor of our developmental perspective. By the sixteenth century, children began to be seen as unique individuals in their own right, individuals worthy of affection. But because the father's financial position made him more capable of supporting children than the mother, his automatic right to custody was not questioned.

By the eighteenth century, the notion of custody began to be broadened to involve not only *rights* but *responsibilities* for the care of children. The concept of *parens patriae*—a responsibility to protect helpless children—evolved. The court now could consider alternatives for infants (children under the age of seven). The idea of the mother as a custodian came into being—the so-called Tender Years Doctrine, and United States law being based on English law, it became a blanket rule in the United States that mothers were better suited to care for children than fathers. The standard had changed from financial to emotional or, more correctly, moral. It was moving toward the interests of the child, but parental rights were still predominant. They had simply shifted from the father to the mother. There was one clause however. The mother had to be deemed a fit parent. And "fitness" was interpreted in a moral sense—usually religious—rather than as emotional capacity for parenting.

The "best interests of the child" standard evolved in this century as the courts began to take more responsibility for the welfare of children. It was formalized in 1925 by Judge Cardozo who stated that the court "acts as *parens patriae* to do what is best for the interests of the child." Today, society has moved even further away from the era of parental rights to the era of the best interests of the child, which has become the single most important test in custody determinations. The Tender Years Doctrine is rapidly disappearing but fitness and unfitness in modified form will undoubtedly remain as important secondary criteria inextricably related to the "best interests of the child."

The "best interests of the child" sounds as if it is the ideal test. But because it remains so vague, it often becomes meaningless. Actually, it is not a test at all, but a general principle that can be used or misused. Its application is so variable that many believe it leaves the decision to the judge's own discretion and bias. For example, in America's best-known, contested custody case, shown in the Academy Award winning movie "Kramer vs. Kramer," the Tender Years Doctrine was actually quoted by the judge as representing the best interests of the child.

Frustrated with this problem, Watson (1969) suggested methods for determining the psychological best interests of a child who is the focus of a custody dispute. Goldstein, Freud, and Solnit (1973) suggested that identification of the "psychological parent" was the most important consideration. But difficulty doing just that led Goldstein, Freud, and Solnit to suggest "the least detrimental alternative" as the best solution to maintaining continuity in the child's life—a speedy decision.

Meanwhile, some states had developed specific child-oriented criteria for determining custody. Michigan's Child Custody Act of 1970 defined the best interests of the child as meaning the sum total of ten clearly stated factors, including "the love, affection, and other emotional ties existing between the competing parties and the child," to be used in determining a decision (Benedek, 1972). The federal Uniform Marriage and Divorce Act of 1971 has been adopted in several states and has influenced legislation in many others. Its criteria for awarding child custody include:

1. The wishes of the parents
2. The wishes of the child
3. The relationship of the child with his parent or parents, his siblings, and other persons
4. The child's adjustment to his home, school, and community
5. The mental and physical health of all individulals involved

So while mental health professionals and courts alike have been frustrated in implementing the "best interests" concept, criteria are being developed to move it forward. In general, they include the emotional attachment between the child and competing parties, the capacity and commitment of each competing party to provide continuity in the child's development, and the "reasonable preference" of the child.

FACTORS GENERALLY CONSIDERED BY
COURTS IN DECISION MAKING

In actual practice, the courts find it easier to consider concrete physical living arrangements than emotional ties. One study (McDermott, 1978) of the actual workings of a family court assessed sixty-four consecutive cases of contested custody and the criteria emphasized by the court in its determination. A broad range of factors was considered. However, the *deciding* factors which were emphasized in the final decision-making were four: 1) *the caretaking arrangements* (the physical care each parent could provide), 2) *the parenting skills and commitment* (past and present involvement in taking care of the children and ability to provide emotional support and understanding) 3) *the child's wishes* (primarily a casual evaluation of the child's declarations and interpersonal relationships with the significant individuals—parents, siblings, relatives and babysitters), and 4) *the child's adjustment* (a general assessment of the child's functioning). The data on which these judgments were based, except for care-taking arrangements, were difficult to obtain and of uncertain validity. It was concluded that in order to facilitate the intention of the court to consider the best interests of the child, the child psychiatrist's willingness to become involved is essential. The court may be able to assess the immediate physical and emotional needs of the child and the fitness of the parents as measured by character and reputation. But the longitudinal developmental needs of the child, and how they relate to the more subtle aspects of the parent-child attachment, are best evaluated and presented by a trained child psychiatrist.

PRESENT ALTERNATIVES FOR CUSTODY ASSIGNMENT

In making an assessment, the child psychiatrist must work within the alternative options used by the court. The most common custody decision has traditionally been to award custody to one parent and visitation rights to the other. Visitation periods, weekly or annually, are generally specified by the court. Almost all custody awards were to the mother because of presumed closer emotional ties to the youngster and more time available to be with him. Fathers rarely contested this. Occasionally, the court awarded each parent one or more children in a split or divided custody, but this has generally been frowned upon by psychiatrists because it disrupts the sibling bond at a time when the parental bond also is altered.

During the past decade, the number of divorcing parents has increased dramatically. At the same time, blurring of parental roles—mothers working and fathers sharing the nurturing responsibilities of child-rearing—has significantly increased the number of contested custody cases. A slight increase of awards to fathers has occurred, but the most common arrangement remains the traditional one—custody to mother and visitation rights to father.

Recently, settlements called "joint custodies" have become more and more common. The initiative in awarding joint custody has not come from the courts but from parents themselves. There are two basic versions of joint custody—legal and physical. Joint legal custody means continued, shared financial responsibility and decision-making by the divorced parents for the children. It does not necessarily mean alternating residence. Joint physical custody means shared residence; that is, the children live with *each* parent. They can alternate residences on an equal-time basis or any time variation is possible. Often families experiment with different living arrangements until they find one that fits best for everyone.

Joint custody is controversial, but increasingly accepted by the courts. It is now a real option. The child psychiatrist should be aware of its advantages and limitations (Benedek and Benedek, 1979). For example, if both parents are physically and psychologically capable of good parenting, providing love, and making appropriate decisions for the child, joint custody may be a real consideration. But they must also share a capacity for mutual cooperation and similar childrearing values. If there is not a part of each parent that is not hostile toward the other, a part that can come together with the other to co-operate over child care, joint custody is probably unrealistic. Or, if joint custody is simply used as a device for maintaining equality so that nobody wins and no-body loses, it is unlikely to work. Parents must understand the concept, be able to focus on the child's best interests together, and be able to cooperate with each other in this one crucial area.

THE CHILD PSYCHIATRIST'S ASSESSMENT

Perhaps the most important question to keep in mind when working with custody cases is "What does the court want?" Usually, the court wants as-sistance in choosing between competing parties to determine who will be the custodial parent for the child, that is who will be primary and who will be sec-ondary in the child's life thereafter. The court needs specific data that relates to each involved individual—mother, father, and child—as well as their inter-relationships with each other. Thus, the psychiatric assessment uses the basic elements of any good child and family evaluation. But the court's special focus means that some modifications are needed. This section will consider these spe-cific aspects of child custody work—the referral, the evaluation itself, and the report.

Referral

The most common referral mechanism in custody disputes is for the child psychiatrist to be contacted by an individual parent or by his or her attorney. This involves the psychiatrist directly in the adversarial process. Of course, the child psychiatrist should avoid becoming a biased advocate for the parent as the parent's lawyer is. The lawyer's job and the child psychiatrist's job are complete-ly different, but it is often difficult for the child psychiatrist to focus on the best interests of the child when working for one of the parents. Lewis (1974) has described the danger, in an adversary proceeding, of losing one's "scientific detachment." He feels it is exceedingly rare not to slant the presentation to the court in favor of the hiring parent, yet most are unaware of this underlying motivation.

More importantly, evaluation based on information from one parent is only partial information, since the other parent usually does not agree to be interviewed. This compromises the assessment because alternative family subsystems for the youngster cannot be adequately compared and this makes a recommendation hazardous. Any recommendation should be limited to the competence of the parent seen; *no* statements should be made regarding the other parent whom the psychiatrist has not seen.

The next most common mechanism by which the child psychiatrist is involved in custody evaluation is when both parents, or the attorneys of both parents, or the court itself, designate a single psychiatrist as the consultant. Indeed, many child psychiatrists now refuse to accept the first or "adversarial" involvement and insist on the latter, that is that both parents and their lawyers agree on a single psychiatric comprehensive evaluation, even though each knows that the recommendation may favor the other. This arrangement offers the best opportunity for a complete psychiatric evaluation in the best interests of the child. Of course, all parties should be aware that the psychiatrist's role is to attempt to make a recommendation that fits the child's needs best, but that the final decision will be made by the court. And the family should be informed that a report will be submitted and, therefore, that what they disclose cannot be held confidential.

The Evaluation

A complete evaluation includes an interview with each parent and the child or children separately, then with each parent and child together. Psychological tests may be ordered for any of the individuals evaluated. While the usual personal history and mental status evaluation of each party may be important, as well as the family's psychodynamics, the single most important question to address is the nature and quality of each parent–child attachment and the degree of competence of each parent to fulfill the child's needs. This will provide the information pertinent to the custody question, the one the court must answer.

The Interview with the Parents

During the interview with each parent, the psychiatrist should consider which of them seems to have the best understanding of the child's (not the parent's) needs, the child's strengths and weaknesses, and his or her developmental level. The more personal and intimate the description of a child, the child's likes and dislikes, worries and fears, the closer the attachment is likely to be. Another measure of the degree of psychological parenting can be sought by asking the parent about a realistic plan for the future in the event he or she gains custody.

Mr. and Mrs. Anderson had agreed to a single psychiatric evaluation and had even paid for ten hours of consultation in advance because they suggested that payment should be independent of who "won or lost." Each wanted the custody decision to be the best one for their eight-year-old son Billy, although each wanted custody of him. The parents were interviewed separately, each for one to two hours. Mrs. Anderson could describe Billy as clearly as a photograph. She talked of his best friends, what they liked to do together for fun, Billy's allowance and chores. She knew his likes and dislikes in school. She had made plans to continue to live in the same old neighborhood, getting a smaller apartment but one that had plenty of room for Billy and his toys. She would return to her old job teaching school. The next day, Mr. Anderson was seen. He, on the other hand, seemed flustered by questions about Billy. He didn't know Billy's birthday. When asked about school, he simply said, "He doesn't work hard enough in school," but wasn't even certain which grade Billy was in. Plans for the future were vague except that he planned to move away for a better job. His difficulty handling the divorce and facing his friends afterward preoccupied him. He felt that Billy would be better off with a "fresh start" elsewhere and had no sense that friendships, neighborhood, school, and sameness of surroundings might be important to an eight-year-old boy whose world was breaking up.

This example provided clear information for assessing the relative parenting skills and attitudes of each parent and for comparing their emotional attachment to the child.

Joint Interview with Both Parents

Sometimes the psychiatrist may want to see the parents together. This should only be done after individual interviews suggest such a joint meeting would be useful and they agree to it. If they do, it may be possible to mediate some of their differences around custody. The marriage has ended, but their role as the children's mother and father has not. But the marriage can be reviewed first in order to search out these roles. For example, you might structure the interview by indicating you wish to hear a history of the marriage from each parent, from its beginning to the end. Each will be given a turn to talk as much time as he or she wants and is not to be interrupted by the other.

Often this structured approach is the first time each has listened to the other's story without the usual interruptions and arguments. It is designed to *avoid* the negative entanglements—the same ones that may be *encouraged* for reenactment in couples or marriage therapy. It may then allow you to shift from their old marital relationship to the continuing parental role, and to help shape a more businesslike approach to the needs of the children. If both parents are able to do this—that is, a part of each of them has been relatively undisturbed by the divorce process and remains a parent who can continue to collaborate with the other around a plan of ongoing child care—then they may wish to consider joint custody. If not, the psychiatrist has made another comparison between them as alternative parents in this joint interview. It has provided additional information as to which parent would be the best primary custodian for the child and would be most tolerant and flexible in allowing visitation by the other.

The Clarks had two children. They had been living separately since Mrs. C. moved out. After the child psychiatrist had seen them separately, she suggested they meet together. They agreed. Each gave his or her own version of the history of the marriage. Mrs. Clark seemed preoccupied with who cared for the children and who didn't. When asked to step back and consider the youngsters, Mrs. C. took the opportunity to scold her husband about his lack of interest in the children and pointed out that the man she was living with was their favorite new daddy, "They love him, they tell us so every Sunday when they visit us. He'll make them a good daddy, and I can tell you they really needed one." Mr. Clark was visibly hurt and became quiet and sullen. When the psychiatrist pointed out how Mrs. C. had attacked him in his role as a parent and how hurt and angry he looked, Mrs. C. answered, "Well, it's true," and repeated the story of how she cross-examined the children about who they loved the most. But she showed little feeling for the children themselves, using them mainly to attack her husband. Mr. C., while admitting that he had been a poor husband, talked of his life with the children directly—how the give-and-take of having to care for them had given him a chance to really become a parent. It was clear that he had a conflict-free role as parent while his wife was principally determined to prove that she and her boyfriend were the "good" parents and that her former husband was the "bad" one.

The Interview with the Child

The interview with the child (or children) alone should contain the basic elements of any good child psychiatric interview. Play materials or a playroom should be available as well as an office setting. After asking the child what he or she understands about coming for the appointment, the psychiatrist should explain that he or she has been asked to help the judge make a decision about where the child will live. Although this might be frightening and confusing to the child, many children go through it and the psychiatrist's job is to help determine what is best for the youngster. The interview should be directed to find out as much as possible about family life, what the youngster does with each and both of the parents, where attachments and identifications lie. A variation of the usual house–tree–person drawing might involve asking an older youngster to draw his or her family doing something. The evaluation gathers data about the youngster's thoughts, fantasies, feelings and behavioral responses to the divorce, defensive maneuvers to deal with the hurt, and the parental behaviors which seem to facilitate or block adaption (Kelly and Wallerstein, 1977). The consultant should not be reluctant to ask the youngster about the divorce, what he or she has been told, and what his or her own ideas are about the reasons for the divorce. Preschool children usually have little or no understanding and may be paralyzed, regressed, or helpless. School-aged children and adolescents have personalized versions of the divorce, often accompanied by depression and/or anger and bitterness toward both or one parent whom they may blame for the divorce.

Many courts do not consider the child's consciously verbalized preference before "the age of reason'" seven in some cases, ten or twelve in others. After that they may give it consideration or, after age fourteen, even assign it a deciding role. This follows the child's own mental developmental capacity to understand what is happening to him or her. But it doesn't consider emotional factors that are more subtle. Indeed, it is usually very difficult for a child to verbalize the wish to live with one parent, when both want him or her, because of the loyalty conflict, the fear of making one parent angry and losing that parent's love. Some older children make their preferences quite clear, a realistic assessment of one parent's capacity to meet their needs as opposed to the other's deficiencies. But this actually may not be a realistic approach at all because of the adolescent tendency to divide, to see one parent as all good and one as all bad. So clinical judgment must be used to separate fact from fantasy. In any event, the youngster can be asked about preference in the interview but should never be *forced* to make a choice. It is not only harmful but unnecessary. The main question to be answered by the child psychiatrist in a custody evaluation is the degree and nature of the *attachment* to one parent compared with the other. It includes the child's preference but goes beyond it. And it can be determined without asking the child to make a direct choice between them. Here is an example of how it can be done.

Sally was seven. So far the evaluation showed a sad little girl who had difficulty using play materials, who seemed frightened and regressed. She cried as she answered that her best friend was her cat. It was clear that Sally's reaction to the divorce went beyond family relationships and could be seen in her withdrawal in the neighborhood and at school. The child psychiatrist asked her about things she did with each parent but wanted to avoid direct questions about preference. Yet, the assessment had to be made. So Sally was asked to draw a map of her family, a circle for everybody on a piece of paper. Three circles—Sally, mommy, and her brother—were clustered together; one was apart. That was Daddy. Next they went to the table where the dolls and puppets and cars lay next to the dollhouse.

"Sally, let's pretend everybody in this family is going on a trip together. Here, let's use this car. And here's a mommy, daddy, and two kids. Good. That's the way. Put them in a car. Oh, oh, it looks like there isn't enough room for everybody. Somebody has to stay home."

"No, I want them all to go. I'll get them in."

"Sally, let's just pretend somebody has to stay home. Who will it be if we had to?"

"The daddy. He's too big. And, besides, he doesn't like to go on trips."

The Parent-Child Interview

As the last example shows, the child psychiatrist is expert at interpreting and understanding the child's inner world. But there is another critical dimension—the interactional one between each potential custodial parent and the child. If we consider that in divorce the family as a nuclear system has broken down and the custody decision by the court will in effect create a new family subsystem—mother and children or father and children—an attempt to evaluate these alternative subsystems is crucial. So it is important to see the youngsters with each parent separately, and sometimes with grandparents, stepparents, or others who will be major caretakers in the child's life too, to match capacities with needs and to gain a preview of their actual functioning. The psychiatrist might wish to observe their interaction around a familiar object: a game or a toy they bring to the office themselves or find in the playroom. Of course, it is recognized that relationships are fluid and changing during this time of stress and that parents will try to be on their best behavior. But youngsters will generally force the most natural and usual behavior from parents. The psychiatrist can assess the child's "attachment behavior" toward each parent in such dimensions as degree of comfort, initiative, spontaneity, fantasy expression, range of feelings, and separation behavior. The parents' attachment to the child can be measured by such criteria as physical closeness, empathy, and sensitivity to meeting the child at his or her own level, the parent's capacity to guide, comfort, and discipline, intellectual stimulation offered to the child, facilitation of emotional expression and spontaneity, patience, encouragement, and acceptance. In any event, the psychiatrist should be certain to observe specific concrete examples and record them. The court is interested in evidence—observational data, not just conclusions. Here is a case example:

Mr. and Mrs. Gordon were both anxious to obtain custody of their two children, Gail, 6, and Tommy, 4. Both father and mother seemed interested in their youngsters' welfare in separate interviews. Mr. Gordon wanted reconciliation but Mrs. Gordon was not interested in renewing the marriage and was enthusiastically restructuring her life to provide a new home for the children. First, Mrs. Gordon was seen with the two children and asked to play with them for a few minutes. She chose blocks and they built a house with a tower together. She seemed to push them a little beyond their capacity: "Come on, build it together, kids. Gail, let's see if you can remember what our house looks like and make one like it."

But when the children became frustrated, she was sympathetic and helped them out of the problem she had set up for them. Tommy seemed to be having the most fun and the mother laughed as he knocked down the tower. The next day Mr. Gordon was seen with the two children. He ignored all the play materials in the room. He recalled all the "good times we all used to have together" in a sorrowful voice. Gail and Tommy wanted to explore the room, but he took them on his lap and kept recalling old times. "Remember how we used to go shopping, and I'd let you push the cart?" He did this until their more spontaneous ideas were extinguished and Gail sat sadly quiet while daddy fussed with her hair and cuddled her. Tommy cried and tried to get away. The psychiatrist noted the father's depression and loneliness, his inability to accept the divorce, and his regressive rather than progressive pull on the children. The comparison of the two parent-children interactions made a significant impact on the court because in every other part of the evaluation, no major difference could be found between the two parents, their motivation and competence. Mr. Gordon showed his own need for the children, to ward off his depression, only when observed with them.

The Report: General Considerations

A written report on the evaluation is usually submitted to the court and/or the appropriate attorney(s). It contains the consultant's findings, organized to fit the needs of the court. It is the court that has the responsibility to arrive at a decision regarding custody and visitation. The report can be a powerful influence in that decision, however. If it is well organized, containing "evidence," that is direct observations and quotes rather than simply hearsay, theory, or conclusions, it will impress the court and may be the single most significant factor in the outcome of the hearing. It should be clearly written without psychiatric terms. Such jargon represents professional shorthand for complicated concepts but is not appropriate to present to lay persons. Even a clinical term, such as "depression," should be descriptively illustrated by observed behavior. The findings should provide an outline that leads naturally and logically to a practical, sensible recommendation. In preparing the report, the psychiatrist should begin the process by reviewing all the notes taken during the interviews, sifting through this larger body of data in order to select and organize the more significant pieces of the puzzle which will fit together into a precise form. This, then, will lead to a specific formulation and recommendation that will allow a judge to make the best decision for the child.

Reference to psychiatric theory and literature, citing divorce and custody studies to support findings and opinions, is perfectly acceptable. However, remaining abstract and relying on general guidelines from the literature instead of using them as supporting the particulars of the consultant's case will quickly be noted by the judge and attorneys and will detract from the impact the report could have on the decision.

How to Write a Report

The introduction of the report should clearly state the reason for and sources of referral by the court, one of the contesting parties, guardian *ad litem*, or social agency, and the specific questions raised regarding custody, visitation, or termination of parental rights. These are the questions to be addressed in the body of the report and answered at the end to the best of the consultant's ability. A general formulation, as sound as it may be psychodynamically, is not enough. Record *all* sources of information used in the evaluation, such as pediatric and other medical records, teacher and school records, and everyone seen as part of the evaluation. Strange as it may seem, it is extremely important to the court that the dates and lengths of time of every contact with or about the child and parents be recorded. This should include telephone calls and conferences as well as interviews.

Next, in the body of the report, state your most significant findings. Move from the general to the specific. Recount pertinent family history and then describe each parent. Always the focus should be on the parent's motivation and capacity for custody, the assessment of each parent as a functioning adult and parent. It should be based on factual history which relates to his or her actual functioning, as well as on preparation for the caretaking role and the practicality of arrangements. The assessment of parenting skills should include statements, based on observations whenever possible, of the parent's ability to foster age-appropriate behaviors in the child, guiding the child toward independence and individuality and stimulating the child emotionally and intellectually. Point out, using examples and quotations wherever possible, how each parent seems oriented toward the child's needs and whether one or both seem to want custody out of spite toward the other parent or perhaps to prove his or her own adequacy. This means describing each parent's reaction to the divorce, attitude toward the other parent, and particularly, attitude toward visitation.

Of course, in describing each parent as a potential custodian, appropriate information about work experience, previous marital history, relationships with others, any difficulty with the law, alcohol and drug use should be included. Physical or mental illness that would influence custodial capacity should also be mentioned. Include psychiatric diagnoses and previous hospitalizations where pertinent, but be aware of the implications. They should bear directly on parental capacity as a parent. A psychiatric diagnosis *does not* automatically disqualify a person from parental adequacy. The report should make clear whether the individual is in therapy and/or is controlled through medication. State whether or not, in your opinion, the psychiatric condition impairs the ability to respond to the child. If you believe it does, describe how. Again, examples are important.

After a history of the family and an assessment of each parent, give a summary of your evaluation of the child or children and of any psychological testing you may have obtained. As with the parents, a mental-status format can be used, but special attention should be paid to the child's adjustment to the divorce, including his or her attitudes toward and relationships with each parent. The child's preference should be considered carefully, both in direct and indirect expression in play, not simply stated as a fact to be taken at face value.

You may wish to describe parent-child interactions you observed which point out differential attachment and relationship factors, as with the example of Mr. and Mrs. Gordon. In this way, you can compare some of the potential strengths and weaknesses of alternative custody arrangements. The court will particularly appreciate a discussion of the several possible alternative dispositions—the way in which the psychological factors you have described in parents and child might be expressed in various custody arrangements. Always be careful not to try too hard to predict the future. All you can give is a calculated guess from what you have actually observed.

Finally, your considered opinion about the case may appear in the form of a recommendation at the end of the report. You may or may not choose to make one. But once again, if you do, it must be backed up by a sequence of data and evidence that leads inevitably to your conclusion and recommendation. Perhaps the most important caution is *never* to make a recommendation if only one of the contesting parties has been seen. You can state your opinion of the competence of the parent you evaluated. But a recommendation in his or her favor is inappropriate as the other parent must be considered an alternative. Their competence is relative to each other. Even if you have evaluated the entire family, you may not wish to make a firm recommendation but rather to discuss the strengths and weaknesses of various alternatives. Or you may wish to state that both parents are competent.

After finishing the report, you may wish to offer an interpretative interview to the parent(s). If you are the only expert and have a recommendation in favor of one parent as the custodian, the parent who is not chosen will naturally feel angry and disappointed. But you should not avoid a clear recommendation in favor of one if it seems a significant advantage to the child's future development. Sometimes you may wish to discuss the report with the youngster(s), particularly older children, so they will not be surprised by your recommendation. Of course, if joint custody is likely, the practical aspects of this can be discussed, such as continuity of living arrangements, expense involved, and division of responsibility for decision making regarding the child. The psychiatrist can also be helpful by educating the parents about the advantages of flexible visitation and the potential pitfalls involved in sole custody with specified visitation periods.

THE HEARING–YOUR TESTIMONY

You will be expected to testify at the custody hearing. A report is rarely, if ever, accepted by itself unless the author is available for testimony to explain and defend the interpretation of the data in the report. Occasionally, you may be called upon as an expert to testify *without* having submitted a report. Even if you do not need to prepare a report, it is a good idea to have an outline of one on paper or in your mind. It provides a sound framework for testimony. If you have prepared a report that reflects a comprehensive evaluation of parents and children, and have carefully evaluated your information, you have done the major preparation for the hearing.

If you have been asked to testify by one of the attorneys, be sure to arrange to have that attorney prepare you in advance (Adams, 1980). Point out that it is to the attorney's advantage to rehearse the testimony so that you will be a better witness. It will also be helpful because most attorneys have only a superficial knowledge of psychological principles and child development. You should know the questions the attorney will ask and what questions you may be asked on cross-examination.

Your personal testimony is to help the judge in making a decision. You must be able to verbally communicate and defend your findings and recommendations from the report. The attorney for the parent *not* recommended for custody will most likely attack your report point by point. The weight given to your opinion is related not only to the completeness and objectivity of your report but also to how you conduct yourself in court. Since you are an "expert" witness, you can state opinions, not just facts, a privilege which an ordinary witness is not allowed. But do not abuse this privilege. Give evidence, observations and data, which support your conclusions. And of course, never be afraid to say, "I don't know." The greatest danger to your credibility is to appear to be clearly biased—an advocate for one of the parents—rather than one who seeks the best interests of the child.

The time of your appearance may be arranged for your convenience. That is a double-edged sword. You will probably only be asked to be in court during the time of your own testimony so that you will not hear what others say. So be aware that the judge will have much more information than you have because he or she heard testimony from other sources. And there may have been events and changes since the evaluation that might make you modify your recommendation.

When you go to court, you will first be sworn in. Then you will take the witness stand and give your name, address, occupation, and the background necessary to qualify you as an expert witness. It is helpful to give a resumé in advance to the attorney qualifying you, and also to bring one to court to help the court's stenographer.

If you were appointed as the sole expert by the court, you may still be involved in the adversarial process. Even though you see yourself as an independent, objective witness, your recommendation creates disappointment in one of the parents. And the cross-examination will reflect it. So be prepared to have your opinion challenged. That is the attorney's job. Do not take it as a personal attack and respond inappropriately. If you do not feel comfortable in this, the adversarial legal setting, custody cases are not for you. Admittedly, the adversarial system is a poor one in which to insure the best interests of the child. But it is the one which society presently relies on in family as well as criminal law with the justification that a presentation of all evidence and points of view can lead to the best decision. After several cases, you will probably feel less and less intimidated when your opinion is challenged. And with good reports and sensible testimony you can help to soften the harmful effects of the adversarial process on children and parents.

The following describes the adversarial court procedures. If you are engaged by one attorney or parent, the first or direct examination will be conducted by that attorney. It will focus on your report and be structured in such a way as to help you develop your points. Prepare an outline or a flow sheet which gives you at a glance the dates, times, and people interviewed. This is very important to have at your fingertips since it may have been several months since the evaluation, and this factual information is extremely important in the legal system.

Next, cross-exaimination by the other parent's attorney gives you the chance to defend your opinion. If your recommendations for custody have gone against his client, he will of course try to discredit your report and testimony. He will try to find weaknesses, inconsistencies, and contradictions. He may question your facts, your opinions, and your theoretical framework. Perhaps examples of both a well handled and a poorly handled cross-examination will illustrate.

(Dr. Wilson has been sworn in as a fully trained child psychiatrist. She has recommended custody to the father after having seen both parents and the two children in a comprehensive evaluation. The attorney for a disappointed mother was cross-examining. Here are excerpts from the testimony.)

Dr. W.: I have had two years of specialized training in general psychiatry and two years in child psychiatry since I obtained my medical degree.

Attorney: How much experience have you had with cases like this one?

Dr. W.: This is my fourth.

Attorney: Did you receive a fee for your opinion?

Dr. W.: I received the usual fee that I charge by the hour for my services. The fee was for my time and has nothing to do with my opinion.

Attorney: In your report you seem, like many psychiatrists, to ignore religion. The mother in this case is a religious person. She has moral values that the father does not seem to have. Yet, you are recommending custody to him. Why?

Dr. W.: The mother's devotion and absorption in a particular religious sect seemed to me largely responsible for the marital conflict and the ensuing divorce. She has strong fundamentalist religious beliefs which she insists the youngsters accept. She takes them with her several evenings a week on her missionary work and talks to them about God most of the time she spends with them. I observed this in my contacts with the family. I do not feel she is in touch with the children's own needs because she is overwhelmed by such strong religious pressures from inside.

Attorney: Has this damaged the children?

Dr. W.: I find no evidence that it has. In fact, the youngsters were able to break through the almost constant discussion of religion and express their own ideas.

Attorney: Then could you be wrong in predicting that it might be damaging to them?

Dr. W.: Of course I can be wrong. But I am not predicting damage. I am recommending the father as more sensitive to the children's best interests.

Attorney: Do you have any religious beliefs yourself, doctor?

(Pause.   Dr. Wilson looks toward the other attorney who objects and the judge sustains this.)

Attorney: I noticed that your report states that the youngsters have a need for a "single psychological parent." Why is that?

Dr. W.:   Because of the intense disagreements between the mother and father over childrearing, the contradictions that come from this, and thus the need for stability and predictability in the children's lives.

Attorney: Is there any authority for this?

Dr. W.:   Yes, this is a commonly accepted principle—it is described in the book *Beyond the Best Interests of the Child* by Professors Goldstein, Solnit, and Freud. They have advocated this principle.

Attorney: Do you always apply it?

Dr. W.:   No, but in this case it would appear to be appropriate because the parents cannot agree. And this may account for the confusion I found in the youngsters about who was right, the father or mother. They are becoming withdrawn and isolated from friends, they told me, and their school performance is declining, which I found out from their teachers. This seems to be their way of showing they cannot deal very well with this problem. They can't solve it by themselves.

Attorney: But doctor, isn't there other literature? Isn't the opinion you quoted about single psychological parent a controversial one? Don't other experts disagree?

Dr. W.:   Yes.

Attorney: Isn't shared custody a better solution?

Dr. W.:   Well in this case, I feel that the need for stability and permanence for these youngsters is the most important consideration. Divorce shouldn't become a way of life for them. A new family needs to be formed as soon as possible, one in which they can feel secure. It's true that recent research by Wallerstein and Kelly, published in a book called *Surviving the Breakup*, point out that children fare much better after a divorce when they have continuous and easy access to both parents, that visitation should be flexible and open. But in this case, I feel that visitation should be limited because of the constant fighting between the parents over the children. The youngsters need stability, they need to know exactly what is happening to them and who is who in their lives.

Attorney: But what if these parents wanted joint custody? Shouldn't we try to promote joint custody these days because it *lessens* many of the problems you described that are created by divorce? What about the fighting over visitation when one parent has sole custody?

Dr. W.: Joint custody is being used more and more by parents who can agree and share the same values in childrearing. But it can't be imposed on parents who have fundamental differences.

Attorney: But let me pose my question another way, doctor. Isn't it best for children to have *both* parents share responsibility for them? Doesn't it reduce the incidence of kidnapping by the parent who is unhappy with limited visitation and may decide to run away with the children? Just answer yes or no.

(Dr. Wilson turns to the judge and asks if she may give full reply in the interest of providing the most complete information to the court. The judge nods.)

Dr. W.: You are posing a hypothetical question. You have introduced new information and changed the circumstances. I can only go back to *this* case; and in this case, the parents could not agree to work together on any aspects of their children's life and joint custody is impractical.

Attorney: Thank you, doctor; that is all.

Here is a different case and result.

(Dr. Jackson has been sworn in. During his credentialing, he mentioned that he was certified "board eligible in psychiatry." In his report, he recommended custody of the two children to the father but had not examined the mother. The attorney for the disappointed mother was cross examining. Here are excerpts from the testimony.

Attorney: Doctor, what does "board eligible" mean?

Dr. J.:   It means I am eligible to be considered a board-certified specialist in psychiatry.

Attotney: Have you taken the examination?

Dr. J.:   Yes.

Attorney: Did you pass it?

Dr. J.:   No.

Attorney: How many times did you take it?

Dr. J.:   Three.

Attorney: Doctor, are you receiving a fee for your opinion?

Dr. J.:   Of course I am; do you expect me to work for free?

Attorney: How many cases involving contested custody have you handled before?

Dr. J.:   I don't remember.

Attorney: You don't remember?

Dr. J.:   Well, maybe a dozen or two dozen. Why is that important?

Attorney: Doctor, you recommended that custody be given to the father, but you have not seen the mother, is that correct?

Dr. J.:   Yes, but she had a diagnosis of schizophrenia, made a few years ago.

Attorney: You have not examined her, yet you recommend the father over her, and now you suggest that a diagnosis by itself should disqualify her. Why is that?

Dr. J.:   Because the illness she had is a narcissistic disorder. There are ego, and probably superego, deficits. It is the most severe of the mental illnesses.

Attorney: Just what do those terms mean?

Dr. J.: Her defenses are primitive. She can't adequately function as a mother.

Attorney: How do you know that this relates to her ability to function as a mother?

Dr. J.: Just look in any textbook.

Attorney: Doctor, you mean that you are referring this problem to a textbook? Which one? And what about this case, this situation?

Dr. J.: Anyone will tell you the same thing I am telling you. And I trained for years to diagnose and treat mental illness. I know what schizophrenia means.

Attorney: Doctor, what if I told you that there have been a number of people, including hospital personnel, who can testify that this mother has been observed over and over again to behave appropriately with her children, to be warm and supportive with them? And what if I told you those same individuals found the father to be cold and impatient with them?

Dr. J.: I would say you were making that up, you have added new information which is not true.

Attorney: But what if I could produce these witnesses and they testified to this?

Dr. J.: I refuse to answer. You are badgering me and harrassing me. Lawyers disagree about things too, don't they?

Attorney: That's all the questions I have for now, doctor.

As you can see, there are many ploys and attempts to provoke. But there are also techniques the psychiatrist can use to deal with these. The main point is not to take the harrassments personally and get angry. For example, if the attorney asks you how many custody cases you have been involved in (especially if he suspects you are a beginner), always be prepared to give an approximate number in a matter-of-fact fashion. Do not let the question rattle your confidence, as it is intended to do. It has no bearing on your report or credibility. Your report stands on its own and your behavior in court will either strengthen or weaken it.

You may or may not wish to bring your notes from the interviews themselves, organized so you can refer to them during testimony. If you have brought them to court, an attorney may ask to see them. If your notes are legible to him, he may ask you why certain details you considered irrelevant were omitted from the report. It is simply a way of trying to discredit your report. Simply answer that it would be impossible to include every detail without making the report too lengthy, that you have considered to be the most significant data which led to your conclusion (Adams, 1980). Attorneys often ask your opinion as to at what age the child's preference becomes important and how much weight should be given to it. They may ask if a child can manipulate and tease parents via changing declarations of preference. Answer questions such as these very carefully, qualifying your answer with the specific data in the case, noting that situations vary considerably, and admitting the possibility that you could be wrong. If you are asked a question in an area not related to your expertise, you may respond that it is a matter for the court to decide since it is a legal rather than a psychiatric issue.

Finally, second or "redirect" examination is an opportunity for either attorney to come back to earlier issues and for you to amplify your answers if you have been cut short during cross-examination. It is a time for tying up loose ends, for closing off, for restating your main position and the evidence for it. Always remember—you are the advocate for the child's best interests.

SOME SPECIAL PROBLEMS AND PITFALLS

Nothing is more discrediting to the profession than an array of conflicting testimony by psychiatrists representing opposing parties, each presenting such a different picture that it is hard to tell they are even talking about the same parent or child. If you know another psychiatrist is involved in the case, try to find out what he or she has found and how he or she arrived at a conclusion. It is best to work *with* your colleagues rather than against them. Do not be afraid to try to confer with another psychiatrist, even if the attorneys discourage it. Of course, the best solution is to avoid this problem entirely, to have *both* parents accept you as the psychiatrist for the case. You can do a more complete job that way; the whole family, rather than pieces of it, can be evaluated. The single psychiatrist can actually work with the family during the evaluation to mediate and to enhance the child's best interests. Realistically, to refuse to take any cases unless both parties accept you will reduce your custody work to a very small practice. But your principles will be intact.

A word about a different kind of involvement in custody disputes. You may be subpoenaed to testify at a custody hearing because you have previously treated one of the parents or one of the children. Try to give only the barest essentials, the length and period of time you saw the parent or child as a patient, a general statement about the type of treatment given, the progress or lack of progress and the diagnosis, if necessary. Be prepared to answer regarding any direct evidence or opinion you might have regarding the parenting ability of your adult patient. If you are required to testify while you are therapist for the child, discuss it openly with the child in advance. You must do your best to prevent your therapeutic alliance with the child from being compromised by disclosing his or her fears, wishes, and anxieties which were private property, shared only with you in your therapeutic role.

CONCLUSION

To become an expert in custody work, you must be able to communicate well with youngsters and parents, to view problems from both developmental and interpersonal frameworks, and to communicate effectively with those not trained in psychiatry. You will need to develop skill in combining 1) a complete psychiatric evaluation that is 2) oriented to the specific problem of custody and the court's needs with 3) the ability to write a concise and comprehensive report and 4) the ability to articulate it well. If this has not been part of your formal training, sit in on a custody hearing that you are not involved in and ask other psychiatrists to give you reactions to their experiences.

The era of the custodial rights of parents, which shifted from father to mother, is over. We are now in the era of the rights of the child. But we are in a transition period and a partial vacuum exists. Longstanding assumptions and rules-of-thumb have been discarded. There is an increasing awareness by the courts that the best interests of the child must be more specifically defined. They are aware that these interests relate to a determination of the child's emotional and developmental status and needs and that these, in turn, can be related to an assessment of the competence of each parent. Courts are also aware that predictions can be made about the operational success of potential new subfamilies and environments which the court shapes by its decisions. Because of this, it is likely that the courts will increasingly call upon child psychiatrists to help them with these difficult decisions. As Derdeyn (1976) points out, the child psychiatrist's role as child-development consultant to the court will be subject to further development and definition.

This provides a unique opportunity for the profession. Now is the time for child psychiatry to actively participate in what is best for children. We have been invited by society, as represented by its most powerful agent—the court—to play a key role in shaping child development. Our training programs must directly address this problem and prepare child psychiatrists for it. Otherwise, we will continue to be ill-equipped for involvement in the legal system, and we will continue to be viewed as a group of professionals who "avoid going to court at all costs." In the 1980s, the cost of noninvolvement is too great.

REFERENCES

Abarbanel A: Shared parenting after separation and divorce: A study of joint custody. *Am J Orthopsych* 49(2):320–329, 1979.

Adams E: (Personal communication) 1980.

Benedek EP: Child custody laws: Their psychiatric implications. *Am J Psych* 129(3):326–328, September 1972.

Benedek EP and Benedek RS: New child custody laws: Making them do what they say. *Am J Orthopsych* 42(5):825–834, 1972.

Benedek EP and Benedek RS: Joint custody: Solution or illusion. *Am J Psych* 136(12):1540–1544, 1979.

Benedek RS and Benedek EP: Postdivorce visitation: A child's right. *J Am Acad Child Psych* 16(2):256–271, 1977.

Derdeyn AP: A consideration of legal issues in child custody contests: Implications for change. *Arch Gen Psych* 33:165–171, 1976.

Derdeyn AP: Child custody consultation. *Am J Orthopsych* 45:791–801, 1975.

Derdeyn AP: Child custody contests in historical perspective. *Am J Psych* 133: 1369–1376, Dec 1976.

Goldstein J, Freud A, and Solnit AJ: *Beyond the Best Interests of the Child* (Free Press: New York) 1973.

Kelly J and Wallerstein J: The effects of parental divorce: Experiences of the child in early latency. *Am J Orthopsych* 46(1):20–32, 1976.

Kelly J and Wallerstein J: Brief interventions with children in divorcing families. *Am J Orthopsych* 47(1):23–39, 1977.

Lewis M: The latency child in a custody conflict. *J Am Acad Child Psych* 13 (4):635–647, 1974.

McDermott JF, McGuire C, and Berner E: *Roles and Functions of Child Psychiatrists* (American Board of Psychiatry and Neurology, Inc) 1976.

McDermott JF, Tseng WS, et al.: Child custody decision making: The search for improvement. *J Am Acad Child Psych* 17(1):103–116, 1978.

Miller, D: Joint custody. *Family Law Quarterly*, vol 23, no. 3, Fall 1979.

Wallerstein, J and Kelly J: The effects of parental divorce: The adolescent experience. *The Child in His Family: Children at Psychiatric Risk*, vol 3, Anthony EJ and Koupernik C (eds.) (Wiley and Sons: New York) 1974.

Wallerstein J and Kelly J: The effects of parental divorce: The experiences of the preschool child. *J Am Acad Child Psych* 14(4):600–616, 1975.

Wallerstein J and Kelly J: The effects of parental divorce: Experiences of the child in later latency. *Am J Orthopsych* 46(2):256–269, 1976.

Wallerstein J and Kelly J: Divorce counseling: A community service for families in the midst of divorce. *Am J Orthopsych* 47(1):4–22, 1977.

Wallerstein J and Kelly J: Divorce and children. *Basic Handbook of Child Psychiatry*, vol 4, Noshpitz JD et al. (eds.) (Basic Books: New York) 1979.

Wallerstein J and Kelly J: *Surviving the Breakup: How Children and Parents Cope with Divorce* (Basic Books: New York) 1980.

Watson AS: The children of Armageddon: Problems of custody following divorce. *Syracuse Law Review* 21:55–86, 1969.

Weiss RS: The emotional impacts of marital separation. *J Soc Iss* 32(1):135–145, 1976.

Westman JC: Guidelines for determining the psychological best interests of children. *Readings in Law and Psychiatry*, Allen RC (ed.) (Johns Hopkins Press: Baltimore, MD) 1975.

3

The Child Psychiatrist in Consultation within the Legal System

Marshall D. Schechter

CONSULTATION TO THE COURT

Understanding the Judge

It was a cold and blustery day in March. My colleague, an individual certified in child psychiatry, had already finished eighteen hours of testimony. He said the parent's counsel, the District Attorney's office, and the attorney for the children presented him with difficult questions, but it was the judge who gave him the greatest trouble. As my colleague's last day of testimony ended, he stated that he would never take another case that required a court appearance.

It was a case of homocide. The parents had already been convicted and were about to be released back into the community. A daughter aged 13 and a son aged 7 were both living in the same foster home. The latter child had been in treatment with my colleague, and I had been asked to do an evaluation of the daughter.

Being forewarned, I did not become overwhelmed by the bombardment of questions from the three attorneys and the judge. It became evident that this case was to be a precedent for others involving child abuse and homicide. The

---

judge wanted to be sure that evidence uncovered on direct and cross examination would be allowed into the record.

At the end of the first day of testifying, the judge pointed a finger at me and told me to report back to court at one o'clock the following afternoon. He would brook no excuses. If excuses were made concerning emergencies or care of other patients, he indicated I would probably be found in contempt.

Thereafter at the appointed time, I appeared in court and waited outside the judge's chambers. This trial was being conducted "in camera," and as I waited to be called by the bailiff, there was a flurry of activity in the hallway. People were running rapidly back and forth down the hallway, including the judge. On the third pass by the waiting area, the judge pointed at me and stated, "You're a doctor; follow me." A woman had collapsed on the steps of the court house and the judge felt that I might give aid to the victim. While running, I suggested that perhaps I was the wrong kind of physician. But the judge was obviously deaf to my excuses.

Arriving on the court house steps, indeed we found a prostrate woman without pulse or breath. I instructed the bailiff to do mouth-to-mouth resuscitation while I instituted cardiac pressure. We were thus occupied, kneeling on the cold pavement with the winds whipping about us, for at least twenty minutes before the ambulance arrived. By the time it arrived I was able to detect a pulse, and clearly there was breathing, albeit shallow.

The bailiff and I returned to the waiting area. Shortly after that the bailiff announced that the judge and various attorneys were ready for my continued testimony.

The questions from all three of the attorneys were presented in the same derogatory and hostile fashion as they had been the day before. However, this time, the judge held up his hand to the attorneys and turned to explain to me the nature of the attorneys' questions. During three hours of examination the judge continued to do this, interposing himself between the lawyers and me and interpreting, in a kindly fashion, the intent and meaning of the questions if there was any ambiguity.

At the end of the day, the judge turned to the court reporter and indicated that what he was about to say was to be off the record. He then turned to me and thanked me profusely for saving the woman's life.

From that point on, this judge, who had been most hostile to all mental health workers, would call me into consultation on cases before his bench. These subsequent cases were all done "in camera" or by phone without my having to go to court to testify. The effect of our conversations became clearly evident in the decisions this judge handed down. After developing mutual respect, there were increasing opportunities to appreciate each other's point of view, leading to more satisfactory solutions of psycho-social problems.

It is necessary to understand the attitudes and perspective of the court. Decisions are influenced by a multiplicity of circumstances, including interpretations of the law by, and the biases of, each judge sitting on the bench. It is incumbent upon the child psychiatric consultant to prepare a report which takes into account the idiosyncrasies of the specific judge before whom the case is to be tried.

In those instances where the consultant has been informed about the judge's viewpoints, either through the attorney or by being given prior testimony before this judge, the report can sometimes be prepared accordingly. In no way does this suggest any skewing of the report away from the consultant's fundamental beliefs. Rather, it implies that the report and its emphasis has to reflect knowledge of the judge's opinions in order for the judge to weigh the evidence it contains. Even after following this suggestion, it may be impossible to take into account all of the variables that can influence a judge's moods and decisions. This was illustrated by the following case.

It was a hotly contested custody case. Parents who were physicians were on opposing sides. The mother's attorney asked for psychiatric evaluations of all of the people involved. This included not only the father of the children, his wife, and their small child, but also the mother, her new husband, and the three minor children aged 8, 11, and 14. The judge agreed with this recommendation and ordered the evaluation. The fact that I was appointed by the court to perform this service in no way preempted opposing counsel from having additional evaluations performed.

The parents had been divorced for approximately four years. The father signed a custodial agreement at the time permitting the mother to be the custodian for all three children. Following the divorce decree there were innumerable court requests by the father to change the custody, to change the visitation, to change the child support, to modify vacation periods with the children, and so forth. The current trial was the fifth court appearance in that calendar year that had involved the judge sitting on the bench. At this particular time, the father was asserting that the two older children, should be in his custody while the younger child should remain with the mother but with increased, more liberal visitation rights for him. As I viewed the situation, it seemed to me that the father was a permissive parent who potentially could create increased anxiety in the fourteen-year-old, especially because of his laxity in manner and his encouragement of a number of instinctual discharges. I felt that the mother was a more stable and competent individual who, like the father, had the best interests of her children at heart. I saw neither parent as potentially extremely harmful, although I saw the father's home situation as possibly more difficult than the mother's living circumstance. I presented all of this at the trial.

Another psychiatrist was called in by the father. This psychiatrist had only seen the father and the three children, and had not visited with either of the spouses or with the mother. Based on the information given to him by the father, the opposing psychiatrist went so far as to conclude that the children's mother was an obsessive compulsive—with a depressive character severely in need of treatment. This led the psychiatrist to recommend that the father have custody for all three of the children.

The mother's attorney, one of the outstanding matrimonial lawyers in the state who had actually helped to write the code for the legislature concerning divorce and custody, skillfully demonstrated the inappropriateness of the other psychiatrist's testimony. He objected to the statements concerning the children's mother when the psychiatrist admitted he had not seen her and was basing his conclusions on the father's testimony. The judge, however, permitted the psychiatrist's remarks to remain in the record because the psychiatrist, as an expert, could make judgments on hypothetical as well as real cases. The trial lasted approximately five days. The children were called into chambers to testify as to their desires which reflected, in the main, the recommendations which I had presented to the court previously.

Everyone, including the attorney for the father, was very surprised when on the last day of the hearings the judge awarded the older two children to the father, keeping the younger child with the mother. This was contrary to what had been presented as in the best interest of the children. When asked subsequently about his rationale, the judge indicated he felt that any ruling contrary to the father's position would be contested by the father. The judge believed that the father would continue to bring the case back into court time and again until he won his point. The judge stated that what was in the best interests of the children was clearly to reach a conclusion which would stop the battle between the parents over the children. This judge went against the Tender Years Doctrine which characteristically in the past had given custody to mothers. In effect, because of pressures the judge felt from the father, his decision was an attempt to protect the children in favor of the father. Excellent preparation of the case by the mother's counsel, designed to play to the knowledge of the judge's personality and past decisions, obviously was not effective because of a variable that had not been considered: the probability of continued pressure from the father and the effects on the children as predicted by the judge.

Sometimes to give the court a sense of what is going on with the children, a judge may appoint a child psychiatrist as an expert witness to oversee the total situation and to submit a report directly to the court. In effect a judge appoints the expert as *amicus curiae* or "friend of the court." Such testimony is prepared subject to cross-examination or to be used at the discretion of the court. In most jurisdictions, attorneys, and judges alike prefer that the adversarial system be maintained even when the psychiatrist is appointed as friend of the court. This is believed to be the best way to tease out significant facts. Because of this, courts tend to ask child psychiatrists or other mental health workers for opinions based on knowledge of the people in their own community who might also be able to render an unbiased appraisal of the familial dynamics and, therefore, a judgment as to what would be in the best interests of the children.

Many jurists and their colleagues practicing law do not have a clear understanding of the differences between a general psychiatrist and a child psychiatrist or even between a psychologist and a school psychologist. It behooves members of the child psychiatry discipline to help the court understand the differences among the various mental health professionals and how each of them can best serve the court. It is vital that the child psychiatrist doing consultation for a court be as precise as possible in making recommendations based upon observable data. It helps to include references from the literature that may clarify for the court how a child psychiatrist arrives at the decisions concerning the children. This enables the court to appreciate the depth of consideration that has gone into the report.

The judge may elect to meet with the appointed *amicus* to go over the report in detail for fullest understanding. The judge will determine whether the information should be shared with opposing attorneys and, if so, at what point the material might be subject to cross-examination. It cannot be emphasized enough the extent to which decisions about what happens to people within the legal system are determined entirely by judges. The consultant must remember that his or her opinions can be entirely disregarded if the court so desires. In no way do judges assign to others their responsibility for making the decisions concerning the people who appear before them. A child psychiatrist who is asked to take on the function of an *amicus curiae* may easily assume that the power of decision-making is in his or her hands. It is not.

One of the primary roles of the child psychiatrist is to educate the court and other members of the legal profession when in the position of an *amicus curiae* or when appearing on behalf of one of the litigants. The consultant's job is to give the legal system an understanding and appreciation of the basic needs of the children and of how, within the framework of the environment in which they are living, these needs can best be met.

The separation between the parents had occurred five years before. The divorce occurred some three years ago. At the time of the appointment of the child psychiatrist as an amicus curiae, *the children were a twelve-year-old girl and a nine-year-old boy. There had been repeated conflict between the girl and her mother. The child complained continuously to her father with whom she had liberal visitation rights. Following one very major upset, the girl decided that* she would remain with her father regardless of the custodial agreements assigned by the courts to her mother. The father insisted that the girl confront her mother with some of their differences, which the child did. The mother agreed that, because of the intensity of the child's feelings, the girl could remain with the father without changing legally the custody agreement. With this shift to the father, the girl's grades improved markedly as did her difficulties in falling asleep.

After some six months with the girl remaining with the father and visiting with her mother on every other weekend, the younger child decided that he too wanted to live with the father. This was a severe narcissistic blow for the mother. She consulted her attorney to see whether she could, in effect, regain the custody that she seemed to have lost de facto to the father of the children.

The court, hearing of this matter with its complications and the burdens that seemingly were placed upon the children, elected to appoint me as an amicus curiae to investigate the total situation. I obtained all of the school records of both of the children as well as their medical records. I was able to interview the mother, the father, and the woman who lived with him.

I discovered that the mother worked full-time and was attempting to establish herself as an independent entrepreneur. She was actually home with the children no more than one and one-half hours per night. She was often quite exhausted by her day's activities. At the end of the day she was frequently too tired to prepare dinners or to prevent the fatigue from being expressed as irritability toward the children. She was a most attractive woman who had many opportunities for dating but she kept these at a minimum to preserve as much time as she could for her children. As we talked, the mother became increasingly aware of her resentment toward the children for inhibiting her social life.

The father on the contrary had a very stable job situation which permitted him to have breakfast with the children and to be home with regularity every night. The woman with whom he was living had a four-year-old son. She was unemployed but brought into the living arrangement through child support and alimony an equal amount to support of the home that they had jointly just purchased. Both of the children felt extremely comfortable with the father who was much more liberal and non-punative than the mother. They both admired and showed considerable affection for the woman with whom their father was living. They had met her family, forming a close relationship with a number of the members of that group.

In preparing the report for the courts I was able to detail the importance of stable relationships within the home as an important feature in the rearing of children. I also was able to indicate the importance to female children around the girl's age of having a significant male to complement her femininity in terms of future identifications. The importance of the father for the young male was emphasized as well. I presented the neutral data of the school reports that *indicated a significant increase in academic production once the change to living with the father had taken place. This material was of great help not only to the court but to the mother herself in considering relinquishment.*

The judges and the attorneys on both sides recognized the importance of the remarks of neutral observers from school and the importance of the developmental states of both of the children in determining the custodial parent. With psychiatric consultation, a court should be able to gain a clearer picture of the home environments of both parents and an understanding of the home that would provide the greatest amount of security and comfort—physical, material, and psychological.

I think the opportunity to function with the authority of the court enables the consultant to delve into areas which ordinarily would be denied him because of the privacy that most people attach to their feelings. The consultant has the appearance of authority; hence, most people feel they're "under oath" and required to be as honest as possible in talking to someone who represents the court.

Individual litigants will present their lives and relationships in as favorable a light as possible. And they will develop stories about the other litigants that show them in the worst possible light. Part of the function of the court-appointed consultant is to discriminate among these different postures that people assume.

Under no circumstances is it up to the consultant to be the determiner of the truth. This is the responsibility of the court. Often the psychiatric consultant must make the difficult decision to oppose the litigant's wishes or even the wishes of the children. At such times preserving the best interests of the children at their developmental stages is the primary guiding principle.

In the last case cited, the judge made his determination in favor of the mother without calling the psychiatrist to court for testimony and cross-examination. But as noted earlier, in many instances the *amicus curiae* may be subjected to cross-examination—a procedure which many psychiatrists find uncomfortable. It is often difficult for physicians, functioning in systems where they are not acting as the final arbiter of the best interests of their patients, to have their views questioned and dissected. This, however, is the primary mode used by the legal system to arrive at an understanding of the cases presented in court. Therefore, it must be expected in the vast majority of instances even though one may feel protected under the rubric of the appointment as a friend of the court.

One's report as noted in all the subsequent illustrations must be made in the simplest of language. The usual descriptive terminology that we use in our profession should be omitted. The statements must be simple and concise as well as definitive. It must be recognized that the report will be subject to scrutiny possibly by the adversarial attorneys and potentially by an appellate court.

CONSULTANT TO DEFENDANT OR PLAINTIFF

Relationship to Client

When the consultant is retained for evaluation by one side in a custody dispute, in most cases the client is referred by a physician or attorney. In these instances or when the client comes independently, it is important that the child psychiatrist describes his role clearly. He should state his function as that of understanding the entire situation and acting primarily as an advocate for the children. It should be understood that this means that the evaluation and the report may or may not be utilized by the attorney. The attorney will decide whether the report is of value to the client (the parent) whom he is serving. The primary concern of the child psychiatrist is to represent the children's needs, regardless of the positions taken by the adult parties.

Many forensic psychiatrists determine together with attorneys and parents the approximate amount of time that will be needed for the evaluation and that will be spent appearing in court. This is decided during the initial contact. Using this kind of approximation, many forensic psychiatrists charge people in advance for the evaluation period. This may seem crude or calculating. Yet it serves a significant purpose. The opinions rendered by the consulting psychiatrist can often be viewed and accepted as neutral and unbiased—and they can, in fact, be made so—because he is not pressured to make a favorable report in order to get paid.

Regardless of the circumstances it is best to try to appreciate and understand the other side's position. At times, certainly with custody cases, it is imperative to see the other parent or significant others before rendering an opinion. However, even in accident cases or in criminal cases, it is of value to consult the records or the other parties directly involved in order to get as clear a picture as possible of the circumstances before writing a report.

In defining one's relationship with the client, the consultant must also state that anything discussed with the client may have to be revealed in court. The psychiatrist may be subpoenaed by the other party and cross-examined. The psychiatrist may be doing an evaluation ordered by the court for which the parties are paying. There are times when the doctor–patient relationship is maintained inviolate but this is rare because of state laws governing revelation of material germane to a court trial. There should be a discussion of fees with the attorney, as well as the client, either immediately when one is called or during the very first consultative hour. A schedule of payments should be determined early on in consultation with the client and/or attorney.

After hearing the story presented by the attorney and/or client, the consultant must decide whether he is the appropriate party to undertake the study requested. It is often impressive to the courts when, during cross-examination, the consultant indicates the kind and number of cases the consultant has refused or for which he would have rendered an opposing position. The consultant needs to protect against the impression that he offers services as a hired gun. In order to prevent this, it is important to demonstrate impartiality in selecting cases as well as in rendering opinions. This particular position will be recognized and respected by attorneys and judges alike. This kind of professionalism can lead to increased referrals.

The case focused on a three-year-old girl whose parents had divorced when she was two. The apparent father had maintained an active involvement with the child, visiting on weekends and in the evenings during the week. The mother revealed at the time of the divorce that her former husband in fact was not the father of the child. She intended to marry the biological father of the child as soon as it was legally possible. This she did. A blood test was done to prove her current husband's paternity of the child. The mother and her attorney sought to have me testify that the visitations of the former husband should be disallowed because he was not biologically related to this child.

I consistently refused to enter into this case. I told both the mother and her attorney that I considered the former husband the "psychological" parent of this child. I stressed that my report might conclude that the former spouse should retain his ongoing visitation privileges. The attorney decided not to arrange an evaluation.

I received a call from an attorney stating that he wished my help because of my interest in adoption. He was representing the adoptive parents. The child was placed with the couple at five days of age. This was a placement by a third-party agency. The relinquishment papers had not been signed by the birth mother. The child was with the prospective adoptive parents for four months when the birth mother filed suit to recover the baby. The birth mother was a nineteen-year-old woman. Even the attorney of the adoptive parents acknowledged that she had been pressured into giving up her child for adoption.

I was offered an extraordinary fee approximately quadruple of my usual charge. The attorney was rather shocked when, in the one-hour phone conversation I had with him, I indicated that I would support the position that the child potentially would be better off with the birth family than she would be with an adoptive family (assuming stability of the birth mother at this point in time and in the future). I discussed a number of my own studies to help the attorney understand why I was unwilling to take the case on behalf of the adopters.

Relationship to Attorney

An attorney in any case has the responsibility for representing his client to the best of his ability. The employment of a consultant child psychiatrist is an attempt to give his client the best possible opportunity to win the case. It is incumbent on the child psychiatrist to confer with the attorney either by phone or in person to hear the attorney's views on the case. The attorney should outline how the case is to be presented. The attorney should also explain the merits of both sides of the case.

The last is an important consideration. As the consultant listens to the history and weighs the developmental factors, he should review all the possible recommendations and positions he could take in the case. This will help the psychiatrist understand and prepare for what may be presented in court by the other side to oppose the position taken by the client whose side you have chosen to support. It is helpful to ask the attorney and others what the other side may say in an effort to negate your testimony.

The consultant should demand complete candor from the attorney and the client and realize it may not be forthcoming. Issues which could be presented as a surprise in court could seriously damage the attorney's case and undermine the consultant's position in the matter.

The attorney takes responsibility for the development of the case, using the advice of the consultant as a guideline. By anticipating together what the opposition may present, the consultant can help the attorney strengthen his case.

The attorney not only should explain the general structure by which the case will be conducted in court, but also should help the consultant understand the rules of evidence that apply in the particular jurisdiction where the case is tried. He should review with the consultant the kinds and direction of the questions he will be asking the consultant during testimony. If counsel does not initiate preparation of the consultant, the consultant should raise this issue and request this information.

The attorney also serves as the liaison for the client and the consultant. Any questions the consultant has concerning the client's actions and attitudes should be discussed beforehand with the client's attorney. This is especially true when findings that derive from the evaluation of the children conflict with the consultant's first impressions of the case.

It is the responsibility of the consultant to inform the attorney of significant literature which may be presented by opposing counsel or by a psychiatrist for the other side. The consultant should discuss the meaning of the literature with the attorney. In this way, the consultant can prepare the attorney for the psychiatric opinions which opposing counsel may use to refute the consultant's recommendations.

Each of the fifty states has its own family law. This is a state's right guaranteed by the Constitution. Over the years, state legislatures and state supreme or appellate courts have determined the laws, procedures, and rules of evidence for cases involving children, especially in regard to custody. The child psychiatrist participating in cases in different jurisdictions should be aware of differences in the statutes, precedents and regulations. Attorneys should explain the laws and rules of evidence when the consultant accepts a case in a jurisdiction which is new to him.

It is in the interest of the attorney and his client to inform the consultant of any of the judge's idiosyncrasies. The attorney should specify areas to be avoided so as not to open up detrimental areas for cross-examination. The advice of counsel should go even so far as to include the particular records that might be of value in court. This would obviously include any materials which the lawyer feels might be of a confidential nature undermining the main thrust of his case or not germane to the central issues. It is often very helpful for the psychiatric consultant to be present during major portions of the trial if other expert witnesses from the mental health field are testifying for the opposition. The consultant then can function as an aide in developing questions or clarifying issues, particularly on cross-examination.

He can be of major help as well in defining the limitations of opposing witnesses with regard to the qualifications and areas of expertise.

This was a case of a custody hearing brought by the father to change the custody which had been established some seven years before for three children: a boy aged 9, a girl aged 13, and a girl aged 16. The divorce had been without acrimony. But the father, who lived quite a distance from the mother, felt that his children were being deprived of his paternal input on a regular basis, although relatively liberal visitation had been agreed upon originally. At the request of the mother's counsel I was asked to interview her and the children. I also requested the opportunity to interview the father, his new wife, and their young child. This latter request was denied by the father through his attorney.

During the evaluation process it was discovered that the eldest daughter suffered from juvenile diabetes and that the other two children had a series of depressions following the father's announcement that he was instituting new custody hearings. All three of the children were extraordinarily bright and verbal and all three had independently written down the pros and cons of changing custody, with a heavy loading of positives favoring the custody of their mother. The vast majority of the details dealt not only with their affection for their mother, but also the fact that their school was very close to their house. All three of the children were occupied in extra-curricular activities and enjoyed their friends in their neighborhood. They all expressed the feeling that they were saddened by their father's action which they saw as impulsive and totally unnecessary. As a result, they harbored negative feelings toward him, which they had not experienced markedly before.

The attorney for the father, knowing that the mother had asked me to evaluate the situation, had asked another psychiatrist to do an evaluation of the father and his family. The psychiatrist was a general psychiatrist who was not board certified and had no specific training in child psychiatry. He met for about twenty minutes with the father and his wife, but did not meet their two-year-old child. He did not make a request to meet with the mother and the three children involved in the custody action. The major portion of this psychiatrist's income was derived from being utilized in forensic matters. Among attorneys he was known as a psychiatric whore.

I pointed out to the mother's attorney the lack of qualifications and lack of adequate investigation methods used by this psychiatrist to arrive at his opinion. The attorney, through the help I offered, was able to direct many of his questions to this psychiatrist to reveal that this consultant was a hired gun. When it was brought out by cross-examination that the psychiatrist did not even request to see the mother and the children and was only answering questions on a hypothetical basis, the judge incredulously asked whether this slipshod approach was common practice within our field or just peculiar to this individual who was testifying.

Illustrative of the sharing process between the attorney and the psychiatric consultant, the attorney told me that the judge's own daughter had juvenile diabetes. During the trial process, the father indicated that he wanted to be much stricter with his eldest daughter, who was not watching her urinary sugar as closely as he wished. The judge permitted the mother's attorney to ask me what might be the results of increased pressure on an adolescent who had juvenile diabetes. He also asked if the girl might be antagonistic toward her father for instituting the custody suit and potentially winning this suit. When I spoke about my experience with adolescent diabetes, I could see the judge's confirmatory nod on a number of occasions. He had lived through the tightrope situation for parents with adolescents who suffer from diabetes.

The case also highlighted the need of the attorney and the client to be open and candid with the consultant. Prior to the trial I asked the attorney and the client what the other side might bring up to support their case. They talked about the involvement that the mother had with another man. Although unmarried, they had formed a very close and affectionate living arrangement for a number of years. It was not clear whether marriage might be the outcome of their relationship. When it came up on cross-examination, I already knew the circumstances. I had insisted on meeting the gentleman. I was able to testify that I had queried the children about their feelings toward his man, and found them to be positive.

When there is another mental health worker involved on a case, especially a colleague whom one knows well, there is a tendency to discuss the merits of both sides. In general, I am in favor of this kind of discussion. However, I think this discussion has to be approved by the attorney whose side the consultant represents.

Even more to the point, but certainly a problem at times, is the tendency of opposing counsel or even other litigants to involve you in conversations about a case. Such discussion should not be held unless it has met the approval of the counsel on your side. The attorney may feel that conversations with the other parties and their counsel could lead to a revelation of his own case strategy. The consultant should be cautious and work closely with the attorney.

DEVELOPMENTAL PRINCIPLES IN EVALUATING CHILDREN

In almost all instances the role of the consulting child psychiatrist can best be described as bringing to the courts a greater understanding and sensitivity to the needs of children. The primary mission is the potential betterment of a child's position.

In almost every case of divorce, there is acrimony and vitriol between the parents, both of whom have suffered severe narcissistic injuries because of the divorce. Children, in effect, become pawns. Custody of children, like property rights, determines the emotional wealth of the parent who gains it. Unfortunately, children usually are not able to recognize the more subtle forms of behavior which define the parents' relationships with each other. There are many cases where the children's needs are completely ignored; the parents only seem concerned about victory over one another.

The children in cases like this are the primary losers. Such children need the strength that can be given them after a thorough investigation and recommendations addressing their developmental state. The need to evaluate developmental states is particularly important with children suffering accidental injuries or physical or psychical abuse.

Often these children carry with them wounds from the circumstances that brought their custody case into court. Having these memories stirred up again and again through repeated court experience serves to revive unpleasant memories for the children. Often this tends to fixate them at a particular level of development. With children who have elements of retardation and/or psychosis, the delays in development often place them into an entirely different developmental stage than other children of their chronological age. It is the developmental age which I feel should determine how the courts adjudicate cases involving children.

In all circumstances, children must be seen as needing a qualified neutral individual to speak for them. The consultant must urge their placement in systems of care which are responsive to their developmental needs.

In order to present a developmental profile of the child it is necessary to use various tests. When psychological test batteries and neuropsychological testing are used, it is quite likely that the courts will insist that the administering psychologist be present to testify rather than rely merely on the consultant child psychiatrist to interpret the results. With medically oriented tests—such as a neurological, electroencephalogram, evoked potential, and computerized tomography—the results can be integrated into the clinical picture by the consultant child psychiatrist.

Of inestimable value is the collection of information from neutral sources such as school records, medical records, birth, and pregnancy records. Even baby books, still photographs, and movies of the children at various ages can be used. The correlation of life events, such as the separation of parents, with lowered school grades, behavioral disturbances, or emotional symptomatology as indicated by neutral sources graphically illustrates the intrapsychic impact of the circumstances on the child.

It is incumbent on the child psychiatrist to evaluate the totality of options available for custody and/or visitations. During the investigative process, with regard to custody, the child psychiatrist should particularly note the following areas for consideration and possible comment.

1. The capacity of each setting to maintain proper intergenerational boundaries
2. The gender linked role divisions
3. The communication patterns within each family
4. The stability of familial and/or significant other relationships
5. The friendships of each parent outside of the home
6. The stability of each parent: mental, physical, and financial
7. The possible history of physical abuse and/or sexual exploitation of the children
8. The willingness of the parent to permit visits with the noncustodial parent

The child psychiatrist needs sufficient time to develop information about the case to decide if he would be willing and able to undertake a total investigation and appear as an expert witness. This requires education of the court and our legal colleagues, since often they call a few days before a court hearing to request a psychiatric opinion. The consultant should stand firm in refusing to do a rush job.

ACCIDENTS

In the case of traumatic events occurring during the early years of life, it is impossible to predict all of the possible outcome variables. Yet this is precisely what the court is expecting a consultant to do with reasonable certainty. The court wants this prediction so that decisions can be made about the effects of future trauma and the monetary cost of relief in the settlement of the accident case.

Often the evaluator is in a more difficult position than the treating psychiatrist. The treating psychiatrist has more definitive information about the evolution and meaning of traumatic events to the individual child. More times than not, the treating physician, if indeed there is any at all, will object to going to court and testifying. It is incumbent on the examining doctor to make a determination about the amount of injury a child has sustained and what its potential meaning in the future could be.

When the child was two-and-a-half years old, she and her mother went to a roadside vegetable stand to purchase fresh corn. As the mother was purchasing produce, the owner's police dog jumped out from behind the counter and almost totally bit off the nose of this child. The mother held the nose in place while she rushed the child to the hospital. The nose was sewn back on.

Plastic surgery was done three times afterward in the child's third and fourth year. Each time the child showed extreme anxiety. Immediately after the injury, the child developed pavor nocturnus, *awakening in fear and playing out the scene of being attacked by the dog. It was for this latter syndrome that the child was originally brought for possible treatment as well as possible court consultation. The owners of the dog had admitted their guilt and responsibility for not having the dog tied adequately. The case was to go to trial to determine actual damages as well as anticipated damages into the future.*

There was a direct correlation between the attack by the dog and the symptom of sleep disturbance. As this connection became conscious, the withdrawn and immature child became more outgoing and concerned about social relationships. At age six, when first seen, she was considered to have a learning disability. As the treatment progressed the learning problems seemed to lessen and then disappear. She began getting top grades in all subjects during her second and third year of treatment.

Trial was set in the county where the accident had occurred. I conferred with the girl's counsel to understand his direction in the development of the case and the questions he would address to me. I made some suggestions about questions I felt could be of help within his courtroom probing of the needs of this child. I had indicated that with plastic surgery during adolescence and the growth of the nose, the scar would probably need revision at least once and maybe two or three more times. We anticipated that in adolescence the scarring, which already she felt sensitive about, would probably become the focus of her attention and would lead to the feeling of being unattractive. Based upon the cost of her treatment to date and the anticipated recurrence difficulties around the time of puberty, a cost was projected for subsequent necessary treatment. The attorney used this projection to determine the financial award from the insurance company.

At the trial the judge sustained every single objection by the opposing counsel. It was clear that the opposing lawyer was a personal friend of the judge; they were from the same county and same law schools. It was also clear that the judge looked with disfavor upon the child's attorney who came from a large metropolitan area. During the trial the judge repeatedly admonished the witnesses for the child to be brief in their answers but he permitted the witnesses for the defense much greater latitude, over the objections of the child's attorney.

This was a jury trial. I had already engaged the eyes of two of the jurors who seemed sympathetic to this child's plight. I felt relatively comfortable about what would be asked in cross-examination. The opposing counsel began asking about my qualifications, but stopped short when the child's attorney gave him a copy of my curriculum vitae. *He then acknowledged that I was qualified. He began asking me what I charged for sessions with the child. He wanted to know what charges I had made for the time I had seen the parents and the attorney preparatory to the trial. He tried to suggest that perhaps the attorney had fed me not only the questions he was to ask but also the answers I was to give. With the question about my fees, there was a definite reaction of surprise from some members of the jury about the extent of the fees. The attorney tried to claim that this was beyond my usual fee. I was not permitted to ask the attorney how much he charged.*

Next there was an admission of guilt by the owners of the dog. The instructions by the judge to the jury included a statement that the insurance rates of many people might go up if the award was too high. The jury came back with a verdict in favor of the child but the award was far lower than the amount anticipated by the child's attorney. Many things within the record could probably have been the basis for an appeal. However, it was felt by the child's attorney that the chances were that the award would not be significantly increased by an appeal. He also was concerned about the turmoil the child would go through during the process of a retrial.

In some courts it is a relatively new concept to look not only at the loss of physical function at the time of the accident, but also at the potential for long-range emotional suffering of a child and possibly of parents. The courts are called upon to consider the likelihood that the impact of severe trauma on the developmental process in childhood will affect later development. This is the kind of thinking that the child psychiatric consultant can detail because he recognizes the deviations in development that can occur with traumatic events. Courts and jurors alike are able to empathize with physical and emotional suffering as it affects not only a child but also the functioning of a total family.

CHILD ABUSE

Ordinarily when the child psychiatrist is presented with cases in which physical abuse or sexual exploitation has occurred, he is required to evaluate the effects of the abuse on the child, including the potential for later problems. In most instances of physical abuse, it is the pediatrician or the abuse team in a pediatric setting that intervenes. Evidence of multiple fractures and/or bruises in various stages of healing is presented. However, in sexual exploitation there usually are no such signs demonstrating misuse of the child. A child psychiatrist can be of great help to the court by defining the exploitation situation and the potentially damaging effect on the child's future.

The classical cases are those involving a female whose median age is eight-and-a-half. The offending male is usually a father, step-father, older brother or first cousin, all of whom who are well known to the child. The relationship generally begins as part of mutual affection which leads to fondling and then direct sexual contact. Because the relationship is most often an affectionate one, physical bruising does not occur. Most of the time the sexual involvement has gone on for a long period of time, and therefore genital injury is not likely to be seen.

Most often when the child abuse team hears of sexual exploitation, there is an immediate move to take the child out of the home or to remove the offending male. This is despite a tendency by the courts to reunite families that have been disrupted by violence. Our society, however, still objects vehemently to the sexual abuser and institutes criminal charges. Therefore in most of the instances in which ongoing therapy is recommended, it most likely does not occur. The charged male fears that what he would reveal in therapy would be brought up in court and used against him.

A four-year-old girl was brought to me by a social worker from a child abuse team. She was the third of three girls in the family. The mother involved all three of the children in sexual activities with various men. Charges were brought against one of these men after the oldest daughter, aged eight years, had broken down in school, crying uncontrollably that somebody had hurt her and she could not get sympathy or treatment from her mother. All three of the children had gonococcal infections which were treated adequately with antibiotics. The three children were removed from their mother's care and placed in a foster home.

I was asked to evaluate the four-year-old to see whether she had been involved sexually and, if so, to what extent. There had been some questions about the eight-year-old's story since it was felt that she might have fabricated some elements of the sexual exploitation out of jealousy of her mother and anger with her for leaving their putative father.

On first meeting, the four-year-old proferred me her hand without any signs of anxiety or concern as she left the social worker. Her face was expressionless. She looked depressed and was apathetic. Once in my office and presented with toys appropriate to her age, she didn't pick up any of them. Instead she rubbed her body against my leg and stroked my thigh as she looked into my eyes with a blank expression.

I discovered that indeed this child had been subjected to various kinds of sexual involvements since she was two years old. The only contact that she could make comfortably with adult males was that of offering herself as a sexual object.

It was recommended that she be placed in a foster home with other children, and with a foster mother and father who could withstand the sadness that the child demonstrated because of the lack of adequate human relationships in the past. It was also felt that the foster family would need considerable counseling, especially the foster father, who would be subjected to the same kind of treatment that I had during the first visit with the child. In that initial visit and two subsequent ones, the child described some of the activities that occurred when she was in the custody of her mother.

The court accepted the recommendation, relieving the mother of her rights. Criminal suit was brought against the offending male. This child, as well as the other two children, pointed him out as the person with whom they had the greatest amount of sexual contact. The judge of the family court was amazed at the language that all three children used. The testimony of the four-year-old child, primarily, was used to convict the offender and to place the mother on probation.

At the suggestion of the child psychiatric consultant, the court assigned the guardianship to the welfare department allowing supervised visits with the mother. Reevaluation was to take place every six months to determine whether or not the children were adequately cared for and the mother rehabilitated.

DELINQUENCY

Since the time of August Aichorn, delinquent behaviors have been understood by dissecting intrapsychic conflicts. Such conflicts are part of the common pathway for disorders that have resulted in offense to parents and/or society generally. Increasingly the treatment related to delinquency has been submerged to the more direct approach of a punishment befitting the crimes.

The child psychiatrist called for consultation can offer the court alternative ways of looking at those cases where the potential for remediation is considerable. In most penal institutions for youngsters or adults, what is learned best seems to be how to be a better criminal. It is up to the child psychiatric consultant to underscore the forces which may convert a minor into delinquent activities.

The young man was about fifteen when he moved from a rural to an urban area. He was slow although certainly not retarded. He was tall, heavy, and powerfully built. Because of his slowness and lack of awareness, he was frequently the butt of many jokes and cruel pranks. He joined a group of boys who were involved at first in petty thievery. During a break into an appliance store, he was caught. The referral came from his attorney. Both his mother and the attorney felt that something else was going on inside of this young man that warranted an investigation to explain behaviors that were certainly foreign to his mother.

When seen by the child psychiatrist, the aura of depression was present. The boy explained his participation in the gang's activities and described how anxiety overwhelmed him each time he participated, much as a preceding anxiety, then a feeling of elation once an activity is successfully accomplished. It was evident that this young man was acting out of fear rather than because of some distortions in his identification or superego formation. The treatment needed was psychiatric in nature. To further create anxiety by locking him up would not only be antitherapeutic but would lead him to greater delinquencies. External controls were needed for a period of time, but the internal need was to express the fears that he was peripherally aware of. The recommendation was made to the court to place him in a residential treatment center. The court accepted the recommendation.

PSYCHOSES

Children and adolescents often come to the attention of child psychiatrists because of some bizarre activity or delinquent action. Underlying many of these actions is a thought disorder that has gone undetected. The courts may find it very difficult to recognize the signs of psychotic thinking. The child psychiatric consultant will be aware of the subtle differences in thinking that represent this major mental disorder and can offer opinions to the courts as well as requests for definitive treatment.

The problem of the sixteen-year-old boy came to the attention of the child psychiatrist because of his truancy from school at exactly the same time every day. Although everyone indicated he was an isolated character with no friends, he seemed to create no disturbance. No one felt there was anything terribly bizarre about him. However, when questioned by the child psychiatrist who was preparing a report to the school authorities, the young man admitted that he left school because there was a bakery truck that passed the school at exactly the same time every day. The emblem on this particular bakery truck was that of the sun. The young man described its emanations as giving him power that drew him as a magnetic force to follow this truck throughout its entire route after it left the school area. The delusions of the absorption of power into his body were part of primary and secondary Schneiderian symptomatology characteristic of major psychosis.

It was discovered that there were a large number of schizophrenics in this young man's family. The history showed that he became increasingly isolated and withdrawn beginning with the second grade. School records indicated that several times during the third anf fifth years teachers commented about his mutism. Nothing was done about the symptoms of isolation or lack of communication. He was passed on from grade to grade partly because he did attend to some of his work but also because he was a large boy and school authorities felt it would be socially inappropriate to keep him back, even though his accomplishments were not up to the expected level.

The parents refused to believe that there was anything amiss with their child. Only when the school insisted on ongoing treatment did the parents admit their awareness of the disturbances this young man had had for many years.

As treatment was being arranged, two boys identified as perpetual bullies harrassed the patient as he was attempting to follow the bakery truck. The young man went into a frenzy and injured both of his attackers. This then brought the boy into court. By that time he was blatantly delusional with hallucinations, auditory and visual. He was committed to an institution on the recommendation of the child psychiatrist. By then a dossier of all of this boy's prior symptomatology had been developed, which was accepted gratefully by the court.

LAWS APPLICABLE TO CHILDREN

In most states the laws dealing with children are considerably different from those dealing with adults. States do recognize children's rights but each state exercises its prerogative within the structure of its own family law. Again, it is incumbent on the judges in the *amicus* cases and the attorneys in the adversarial cases to alert the consultant to the state's laws that are applicable to children and to tell how these statutes may affect the development of any particular case.

There has been a greater awareness of children's needs in recent years. But some aspects of state law should require a weighing of parental rights against children's rights. Often we see children treated as chattel. This brings into sharp focus the role of the child psychiatric consultant. The courts, attorneys, and clients seeking relief through the legal process need the input of a child psychiatrist as a child advocate.

In summary, the child psychiatric consultant to the court system is well advised to follow these guidelines:

1. Be entirely objective and impartial.
2. Avoid referring to the personalities of litigants, their counsel, or expert witnesses.
3. Charge fees that are commensurate with time and effort and with the usual professional charges of the consultant.
4. Answer questions clearly, firmly, simply, and definitively in language a layman can understand, and do not volunteer extraneous information or comments.
5. Help counsel define the role the expert will play in the trial, including specific points he will attempt to clarify.
6. Be aware of current literature and major treatises on the subject of the trial and show a special knowledge of the question before the court, not merely general experience in the field.
7. Be prepared to have one's qualifications, theories, publications, previous court testimony, and even personal life questioned during cross-examination.
8. Avoid inserting oneself into a case by communicating with opposing parties, counsel, or expert witnesses and avoid any public comment, especially to the news media. This point can be modified if there is an agreement by attorneys from both sides.
9. Be prepared for hypothetical questions besides questions directly related to the case being tried.
10. Be aware that the major objectives in *cross-examination* are:

    a. to question the expert's qualifications.
    b. to show a basis for bias, such as an exceptional fee.
    c. to challenge an opinion because it was improperly derived, such as using another's observation, perhaps a subordinate's, rather than directly observing the patient.
    d. to discredit the factual basis of the expert's opinion.
    e. to establish facts favorable to the opposing counsel's side through admission by the expert.

11. Be certain that testimony may be given in terms of probable causal relationship to trial case and "reasonable medical certainty."
12. Be advised by counsel about rules of evidence.
13. Be prepared to keep cool, while adhering to one's opinions developed as a result of professional training and experience. Also realize that if you can't stand the heat, it may be best to stay out of the kitchen.

It is unfortunate that a review of training programs in child psychiatry throughout this country shows that little effort is made to prepare trainees to function as expert witnesses and to expose trainees to actual experience in court. The child psychiatrist is in a unique position to protect children by serving as their advocate, to teach the legal profession something about the developmental process, and to articulate the needs that children have at various points of their development. Child psychiatry has a unique responsibility to explain the effect of various different forces—positive and negative—on the development of children's personalities. The profession has a special body of knowledge concerning psychological and cognitive development. It is up to us to help the legal system to be more responsive to the needs of children.

It is unfortunate, too, that professionals in the other mental health disciplines—including general and forensic psychiatry—are not acquainted with some of the developmental approaches inherent in child psychiatry training. With this knowledge, they too, could better serve as advocates for children.

BIBLIOGRAPHY

Benedek EP and Benedek RS: Child custody laws: Their psychiatric implications. *Am J Psych* 129:326–328.

Berman G: Family disruption and its effects. *Psychological Problems of the Child and His Family* (Stinehauer PD and Ray-Grant Macmillan: Canada) 1977, pp 371–382.

Cooke G: *The Role of the Forensic Psychologist* (Thomas: Springfield, IL) 1980.

Derdyn AP: Child custody contests in historical perspective. *Am J Psych* 133: 1369–1376.

Diagnostic and Statistical Manual of Mental Disorders (3rd edition DSM III) (American Psychiatric Association) 1980.

DiLeo JH: *Child Development-Analysis and Synthesis* (Brunner/Mazel: New York), 1977.

Escalona SK and Heider GM: *Predictions and Outcome* (Basic Books: New York) 1959.

Frankenburg WK et al.: Revised Denver developmental screening test. *J Pediactr* 79:988, 1971.

Freud A: *Normality and Pathology in Childhood* (International Universities Press: New York) 1965.

Goldstein J, Freud A, and Solnit A: *Before the Best Interests of the Child* (The Free Press: New York) 1979.

Goldstein J, Freud A, and Solnit A: *Beyond the Best Interests of the Child* (The Free Press: New York) 1973.

Goodman J and Sours J: *The Child Mental Status Examination* (Basic Books: New York) 1967.

Group for the Advancement of Psychiatry: *Divorce, Child Custody, and the Family* (Mental Health Materials Center, vol 10, no. 106, Nov 1980.

Lynn, DB: *The Father: His Role in Child Development* (Brooks/Cole: Monterey, CA) 1974.

McDermott JF, Char WFJ, et al.: The concept of child advocacy. *Am J Psych* 130:1203-1206.

McDermott JF, McGuire C, and Berner E: *Roles and Functions of Child Psychiatrists* (American Board of Psychiatry and Neurology, Inc) 1976.

Mundy J: The use of projective techniques with children. *Manual of Child Psychopathology*, Wolman BB (ed.) (McGraw-Hill: New York) 1972, pp. 791-819.

Robin AI and McKinney JP: Intelligence tests and childhood psychopathology. *Manual of Child Psychopathology*, Wolman BB (ed.) McGraw-Hill: New York) 1972, pp. 767-790.

Sadoff R: *Forensic Psychiatry—A Practical Guide for Lawyers and Psychiatrists* (Thomas: Springfield, IL) 1975.

Senn MJE and Solnit AJ: *Problems in Child Behavior and Development* (Lee and Feberger: Philadelphia) 1968.

Slovenko R: *Psychiatry and Law* (Little Brown and Co: Boston) 1974.

Thomas A and Chess S: *Temperament and Development* (Brunner/Mazel: New York) 1977.

Wallerstein JS and Kelly JB: The effects of parental divorce: Experiences of the preschool child. *J Amer Acad Child Psych* 14:600-616, 1975.

4

Family Assessment

Jack C. Westman

This chapter is devoted to the family diagnostic process and classifying of family disturbances as a basis for formulating treatment. Customary psychiatric diagnosis does not take into account critical family dynamic factors which play a key role in the psychopathology of individuals (Howells, 1975; Westman, 1979). Even more to the point is the fact that a family member identified as a psychiatric patient may be only an indicator of family distress or more disturbed individuals in the family. Furthermore, when insightful members of a family do seek help, devoting attention to them solely may leave sicker members of the family unrecognized.

Family diagnosis permits an expanded understanding of individual psychopathology and should be distinguished from family therapy which implies a clinical process intended to modify the family and its subsystems (Brown, 1980a). The growing evidence is that family and marital therapy may offer more effective treatment outcomes than individual therapy under many circumstances (Gurman and Kniskern, 1978; Schechter and Lief, 1980).

A family can be defined as a group living together and consisting of more than one generation with individuals who are economically dependent on others. For our purposes, however, the most important dependent elements are emotional and social in nature. Most families consist of two parents and dependent children in the nuclear·form. There has been a trend toward smaller families, and one in five contemporary families has a single parent. Families also may include more than two generations and biologically unrelated persons.

Families may be encountered occasionally through self-referral for help with family problems. More typically the referral is of a family member. It is important, therefore, to bear in mind the responsibility of the clinician to initiate involvement of families in the diagnostic process when single members are the identified patients. Mobilization and motivation of families are frequently needed. Friction between families and child-caring systems, such as schools, courts, and health-care workers, may also result in referral of families for assessment.

At the time of the consultation, families may be in the process of disintegration. They also may be reconstituting so that the request for help already signifies constructive change. In either case, the diagnostic process may stimulate introspection and self-evaluation that in themselves have considerable therapeutic potential.

In evaluating the assets and deficits of families, care must be taken to consider the cultural and socioeconomic context in which the family lives. When values of the clinician do not coincide with those of the family, the important issue is whether or not the family is competently functioning in its own social milieu. Clinicians should be aware of racism, sexism, elitism, and agism as possible factors in their judgments. Each family should be viewed against the down-to-earth reality of the American household, not against romanticized, ideal images of families. Rather than a haven of peace and tranquility, healthy families strike a balance between the antagonism and love characteristic of intimate relationships. Conflict and change are inherent in social life. The family is a resilient institution and is now, as it always has been, in a state of flux (Skolnick, 1980).

METHODS OF FAMILY ASSESSMENT

Methods for assessing families include interviews, history-taking, testing, observation of shared tasks, home visits, and collaboration with other professionals. If the office is not equipped for children, simple expressive materials should be made available, such as paper and crayons, modeling clay, and dart guns. The aim is to obtain information about family interactions, family themes and individual perceptions of the family and other family members. These perceptions often are more important than objective facts which may be similar in both pathological and nonpathological families.

The most revealing diagnostic interview of a family is one that includes interactions with the entire family, subsystems within the family and individuals alone. The initial phase of a family interview includes an introduction of the clinician and a general invitation to speak. It is centered on the question of why the family has come for help. Valuable information can be gained from the way the family accommodates to the surroundings, particularly the seating arrangement and the ways in which parents respond to the children (Stierlin, 1980).

As the diagnostic interview progresses, observation of all of the family members together reveals verbal and nonverbal interaction patterns. The stressful aspects of the interview often highlight disturbances in these areas. For example, in one family interview only the mother spoke. The father and four children were silent, and even when asked to comment, replied that they had nothing to say. The nonverbal signs of resentment were obvious, however.

Much valuable information is lost if the diagnostic interview is limited to the entire family as a group. Revealing information can be obtained by interviewing the parents and siblings separately. Members of the same generation may be hesitant to speak freely in the presence of another generation. Access to personal feelings, perceptions, and fantasies can be gained through individual interviews.

As is the case in all diagnostic efforts, the more time available, the more refined the assessment. Under brief consultation circumstances, however, a period of several hours can be used to conduct the interviews, ordinarily beginning and concluding with the family together. While waiting members of the family can be asked to make drawings and fill out questionnaires. With children, the Draw-A-Person and family drawing are useful. For adults, the Lewis Parental Relationship Questionnaire permits the rapid accumulation of personal information on the marriage (Lewis, 1979). The entire experience with the family from the first to the last moments of contact is a rich source of informal, unstructured interactional information.

There are a number of projective tests and tasks that have been designed to facilitate assessment of family interactions. Depending upon the examiner's interest, those can be employed and are particularly applicable in clinical research. The Rorschach and Thematic Apperception Tests can be used profitably as stimuli to elucidate transactional patterns, particularly with families who are difficult to interview (Stierlin, 1980).

The data drawn from the diagnostic process should include background information, which also may be provided by referral sources, the perceptions each member has of the family and its members, metacommunications, information of interpersonal relationships and coalitions within the family, the state of the marriage, and the detection of individual psychopathology and scapegoating patterns.

At the conclusion of the diagnostic process, meeting with the family together is a useful means of closure and sharing impressions.

The Smiths were seen because their ten-year-old son Tom was severely underachieving in school. The family consisted of an accountant father, a homemaking mother, a fourteen-year-old daughter, Susan, the ten-year-old identified patient, an eight-year-old daughter, Jane, and a four-year-old son, Billy. They arrived late for the appointment because Tom procrastinated in getting ready. When seen together, the mother and Tom sat closely next to each other on the sofa. The father sat opposite them apart from Susan and Billy. The clinician explained the diagnostic process and asked for ideas about why the family had come to the clinic. The mother did the talking and the others sat glumly. As the interview progressed, Billy took up a dart gun and precipitated anxious warnings to not point it at people from the mother and father. Although the mother spoke the most, the content of her complaints suggested that the father wielded the power in the family.

When seen together without the children, the parents divulged their belief that Tom's birth trauma had produced brain damage. They described their marriage as satisfactory. When Susan, Jane, and Billy were seen together, they rapidly engaged with the play materials appropriate to their ages. They agreed that Tom was lazy and that he had no friends in school. Susan pointed out that no one wanted to play with him because he always had to have his own way. Billy blurted out that his daddy didn't love his mommy. They all agreed that they were afraid their parents would get a divorce.

When seen alone, Tom revealed his depressed, hopeless feelings, although he denied having difficulty with school work and felt that the other kids were against him.

When seen alone, the mother acknowledged frustration with her husband's coldness and explosive temper. When seen alone, the father revealed his frustration with work pressures and acknowledged that he had long since lost sexual interest in his wife.

Tom's family drawing placed him in a remote corner and numerous erasures were involved in his drawing of his father. His Draw-A-Person was a vaguely identified girl.

At the conclusion of the interviews, the clinician shared his impression of the problems in the family and that they played a role in Tom's school difficulties. Mrs. Smith embraced the suggestion of family therapy; however, Mr. Smith did not comment. When asked, Tom said that he did not need a psychiatrist. Both parents did agree to return for further discussion of treatment possibilities.

CONTENT OF FAMILY ASSESSMENT

Since Ackerman's pioneering work with families, we have learned to recognize that the family is a carrier of elements predisposing both to mental illness and mental health (Ackerman, 1958). Degrees of success or failure of adaptation in the paired family roles of husband and wife, father and mother, parent and child, child and sibling bear directly on the question of staying well or getting sick. Despite distortions of their individual personalities, parents may interact in such a way as to create emotionally healthy children. At the same time, relatively healthy individual parents may interact pathologically and may adversely affect their children.

The major areas of emphasis in assessing a family are control, communication, individuation, coping patterns, and the progress of both the family in its developmental cycle and of each individual's personal development.

Control

The most important issue in any group, particularly the family, is the overt and covert distribution of power. In most families power over its members largely resides within the family unit, although disorganized families lack internal control measures and find themselves brought under external sources of control, such as courts and social agencies. The need that dependent children have for structure ordinarily is met by adults who provide limit setting. In healthy families the power usually is shared by the parents who cooperate in maintaining the stability and goal directedness of the family. In assessing this dimension the role of each family member in the power structure should be determined. The Smith father dominated the family.

Another measure of the family control system is the presence or absence of conflicts. When overt, the conflicts are obvious in the form of arguments and fighting. When covert, more subtle manipulative maneuvers should be sought. The passive–aggressive child Tom wielded covert power over the Smith family, as illustrated by their late arrival because of his procrastination.

Another indication of the effectiveness of a family's control system is reflected in the loyalty shown toward the family and other members by individuals in the family. The loyalty may be based upon fear and be fragile, or it may be based upon respect and affection and be enduring (van der Veen, 1971, 1974). In the Smith family, the children feared their father and the possibility of parental divorce.

Communication Patterns

Communication patterns in families are both verbal and nonverbal. Because communication depends upon both the sender and the receiver of messages the amount of talking in a family is less important than the reception the spoken word receives. In pathological communication family members may tune out the words flowing from a particular person. The way speech is used is also of great importance. Critical, complaining, and sarcastic expressions strongly influence whether or not and how verbal messages are received. Mrs. Smiths' complaining words were tuned out by her husband and children, but the father's occasional remarks registered.

The nonverbal communications in families are the most important indicators of underlying attitudes, power patterns, feelings and perceptions. Mrs. Smith conveyed her infantalization of Tom through her cuddling behavior. Mr. Smith's demeanor and physical distance in the office conveyed his emotional distance from the family. The release of the children's behavior and speech apart from their parents revealed their uneasiness when with their parents.

A particular form of communication found in a variety of troubled families is the *double bind*. This relational patterns consists of conflicting verbal and nonverbal messages, which cannot be acknowledged or resolved, occurring in a situation from which the receiver cannot escape (Satir, 1972, 1975). In their families, schizophrenic persons sometimes have been persistently exposed to distortions of meanings and paralogical reasoning which undermine reality testing (Lidz, 1973).

Individuation of Family Members

As a child-rearing and personal support system, the family promotes the individuation of its dependent members and the self-realization of all of its members. The family both meets dependency needs and fosters the autonomy of its individual members.

The development of personal autonomy and self-esteem depends upon a family atmosphere in which members are valued by each other, in which empathy prevails, in which there is genuineness of emotional expression, and in which mutual regard and acceptance is assumed. The level of ego development of each family member influences the degree to which that person contributes to or impedes the individuality of other family members.

The quantitative closeness of family members in shared activities can be readily assessed by inquiring about them. The more critical quality of family relationships is reflected in the degree of intimacy shared among family members. Both the amount of time spent together with other family members and the pleasurable quality of that time are relevant. Particular care should be devoted to assessing whether a family's togetherness is squelching or promoting individuation. *Pseudomutuality* as described by Wynne is an example of smothering closeness (Wynne, 1958).

Individuation further depends upon the freedom of family members to express their feelings. Under circumstances in which all or certain kinds of emotions cannot be expressed, family members cannot learn how to identify, accept and manage their feelings. The relations among family members call forth hostile emotions almost as readily as love. Brothers and sisters, parents and children are mutually dependent and find themselves in opposition to or in competition with one another. Both repressed hatred and lust may underlie pathological symptoms. The primitive emotions that undergird family life have long been apparent to psychoanalytic writers (Flugel, 1921; Grotjahn, 1960). In the Smith family, only the father was permitted to express anger directly. Mrs. Smith and Tom were obliged to resort go passive-aggressive behavior.

Coping Ability

The coping abilities of a family depend most heavily upon the responsible adult members. The most obvious forms of coping are directed toward the practical economic and social problems of life in modern society. Each family casts an image of relative competency in the neighborhood and community. The family helps each member meet the ever proliferating existential and material challenges that each faces in adapting to the world outside of the family. Although often related, coping ability in the affairs of the world may not reflect coping ability within the family.

A family's ability to resolve its internal problems is reflected in family decision making, such as in child rearing, and the ability to recognize and address sources of tension and dissatisfaction in family members. The family's excessive use of defense mechanisms, such as denial, projection, and displacement, obfuscates open, intelligible communication, and results in faulty decision making.

The values held by a family also influence its coping ability. A family low in ambition does not place a high value upon achievement by either the adults or children. Another factor is whether or not the family's values are compatible with dominant social values. In addition, the relative absence of articulated values within a family results in few guidelines along which decisions can be made. Contemporary families tend to be characterized by a lack of, rather than an excess of, values as in past generations.

The presence of obtrusive psychopathology in any of the family members, such as recurring depressions, alcoholism, chronic or recurring psychoses, impulse disorders, and sociopathy, influences the coping ability of the family even though it may be a product of family dynamics.

The ability to manage stress in the form of change or loss further reflects a family's coping ability. Disruption of a marriage imposes the stress of divorce and rearrangement on many families. Job and neighborhood changes can also be sources of stress.

The Smith family possessed the ability to cope successfully with external affairs. However, the failure to acknowledge internal strain led to impaired communication and counterproductive decision making in child rearing. Still, the family took the step of seeking help, indicating a desire to improve its internal situation.

Developmental State of the Family

All of the foregoing factors influence how a family progresses through its life-cycle and meets its developmental tasks (Brown, 1980b). The initial developmental task of a marriage is to successfully manage disengagement from each family of origin and reorder commitments to old friends, social activities, and career involvements. Elements of this task may not have been accomplished effectively in marriages of long duration (Martin, 1976).

Each partner in a marriage brings to it an individual unwritten contract, a set of expectations and promises, both conscious and unconscious. These individuual contracts may be modified during the marriage but will remain separate unless the two partners are fortunate enough to arrive at a single contract with professional help (Sager, 1976).

A second developmental task is to create an affectionate, empathic marital relationship in which ensuing children can prosper in the ambience of loving caretaking. The Smith family was foundering in this task. During the adolescence and young adulthood of the children, the developmental task is to sustain integrated family life in the face of intergenerational values, communication, and dependency conflicts. Under optimal circumstances, mutual validation of each family member as a lovable and valued person is achieved.

CLASSIFICATION OF FAMILIES

At this time there is no systematic classification of family pathology. There are a number of descriptive approaches to family disorders of which the one suggested by Lewis is useful for our purposes (Lewis, 1979).

Lewis describes the healthy family as one in which all of the family members are relatively free from individual psychopathology and the family ambience promotes the autonomy and self-actualization of its members. Seldom seen in clinical settings, healthy families vary immensely in their surface appearances, reflecting the interests and personalities of their members. They have in common, however, power invested in the parents, open, intelligible communication, individuating members, resilient coping ability and successful engagement with the stage-appropriate developmental tasks.

Faltering families are those in which there is dissatisfaction in the marriage, but the children may be doing well. Typically there is a failure of intimacy in the marriage with an unhappy wife and a distant husband. Coalitions evolve outside of the family with parents of origin, friends, and lovers. The parents are not disabled by emotional symptoms, but their unhappiness makes the future uncertain. Communication in the family may be open and clear, however, and the family may cope well.

Lewis refers to three kinds of troubled families: the dominated, the conflicted, and the chaotic. Dominated families are troubled families in which one parent wields the power. Some dominated families have a relatively stable structure with little open conflict, whereas others are in open strife with attempts to rebel, undercut, and maneuver against the heavy-handed control of the dominant member. There is diminished closeness in the family but clear communication. There is a strong tendency to avoid individual responsibility in these families. Often the family selects a scapegoat. The open expression of feelings is suppressed. These families are so rigidly controlled that there is insufficient flexibility to deal effectively with change and loss. Achieving autonomy is difficult for family members who may leave at an early age or cling dependently to the powerful parent. Dominated families often produce one or more psychiatric patients. The Smiths are an example of such a family.

Conflicted families present a very different pattern than dominated families and are characterized by a power struggle and warfare between the parents. Manipulation results throughout the family, often in shifting coalitions. Intimacy is absent in the marriage. Anger is freely expressed, but other feelings like affection and sadness are not. The values in these families tend to be intensely competitive. Communications are usually clear, but efficiency in problem solving is diminished because disagreements become escalating counterattacks between the parents. These families produce psychiatric patients such as children with serious conduct disorders and adults who develop midlife depressions.

Chaotic families involve either a fused relationship between the parents, so that neither functions as an individual, or an emotional divorce with little interaction between the parents. These families are often severely disorganized and isolated from the outside world. They may appear bizarre to others. There often are coalitions with the grandparents. The family lacks structure and control with weakness resulting from parental impotence. Communication is confused and family members experience pain and misery. Chaotic families have difficulty dealing with any change, particularly the advancing ages of their children. These families discourage individuality and independence. They produce chronic, severe mental illness.

DISPOSITION

Ideally, diagnosis leads to the formulation of a treatment plan. Too often psychiatric diagnosis confirms the existence of a problem but does not yield a specific therapeutic approach. Family diagnosis usually falls short of the ideal as well, but it can identify critical issues for therapeutic emphasis. To complicate the matter further, the family may not be motivated to accept help. Since families often lodge their concerns upon a single, identified patient, the other family members may not be disposed to see themselves as part of that patient's problem and certainly not as the focus of therapy. Ferreting out the family's expectations of the clinic is an important step toward assessing their motivation for change.

Lewis's classification of families provides guidelines for the nature and extent of therapeutic interventions. In most instances family therapy in some form is warranted. However, other modalities may be useful as well. For faltering families, the marital relationship is the most important focus. Marriage counseling or conjoint marital couple therapy may be useful.

Because dominated families involve both family and individual pathology, intensive family therapy may be used to prepare the way for concurrent or later individual psychotherapy for symptomatic family members.

Conflicted families usually require intensive family therapy in addition to consultation to other systems such as the schools, social services, and law enforcement agencies.

Chaotic families are the most difficult to engage in family therapy because their views of reality are not congruent with their social milieu. Hospitalization, medication, and consultation to other agencies may be necessary in order to provide a foundation for family therapy. Particular attention to parent–child units may also be necessary in order to address separation–individuation issues.

Once family disorder has been identified, the diagnostic process is not complete unless efforts are made to involve the family in treatment. The clinician should be sensitive to the misunderstanding, hesitation, and fear in family members as they approach help. Furthermore, each family member's level of sophistication about psychological problems and openness to using a mental health resource may vary. At the least, education of the powerful members of the family is required so that an intellectual understanding of the reasons for working with the family can be achieved. Explanation appropriate to the ages of other family members also is needed, so they can understand why they are receiving clinical attention. This step is often omitted with resulting misunderstanding of and understandable resistance to the therapeutic enterprise. Just as a patient deserves and needs an explanation of the nature and treatment of a physical illness, family members need a cognitive understanding of why they are assuming patient roles. Helping parents to recognize and discuss their perplexity and guilt is a particularly useful early step.

Mr. and Mrs. Smith were seen at a second interview. The clinician anticipated resistance from both parents and Tom, although Mrs. Smith had indicated agreement that there was a family problem. The interview was focused on the marriage, Mrs. Smith's infantalization of Tom and Mr. Smith's distance from the children. The parents acknowledged tension in their marriage. However, each

*blamed the other for it. Mr. Smith agreed that his wife would not allow Tom to
grow up, and Mrs. Smith agreed that the father was too busy to pay attention
to his family. They both agreed that something had to be done about Tom.
The leverage for motivating this family was their recognition of the need for
other members of the family to change. The parents accepted the recommendation of intensive family therapy to be followed by individual psychotherapy
for Tom.*

Troubled families are the most likely to lack insight and even the strength
to engage in therapy. The defensive maneuvers of manipulative families may be
so extreme that "hooking" the family may depend upon equally skillful maneuvering by the clinician or the external pressure of agencies such as the schools
and the courts. If given a choice, many of these families would either drop out
of view or limit their involvement to supporting treatment of the identified
patient. Pathological families erect powerful resistances to change and skillfully fend off intruders. Their denial and projection are particularly difficult
to handle. Several authors have written in greater detail about engaging families
(Minuchin, 1974; Westman, 1964; Wynne, 1965; and Zuk, 1971).

A delicate issue in motivating families for treatment is how to separate the
clinician's responsibility to assist the family from the family's responsibility for
change. This is a problem especially when other agencies are involved with the
family. For example, a pitfall in working with school difficulties is that both the
school and the parents may look to the clinician for answers about a child. In
these circumstances the clinician must carefully keep the child and the family
in the position of responsibility for intersystem negotiations. Unsuccessful
management of this issue can make the clinician a scapegoat.

The essential discrimination to be made is the level of therapeutic focus.
For some family therapists, the tendency is to treat all family problems at the
family level. For the child psychiatrist, the tendency is to draw upon all appropriate and available resources. For example, a family with an alcoholic might be
advised to join Alcoholics Anonymous in conjunction with family therapy.
Another example would be combining family therapy with medication to
ameliorate a child's attention deficit.

The range of interventions available to families is considerable. The health,
mental health, social service, pastoral care, and educational systems all deal
extensively with family problems. The field of marriage counseling has specifically focused on one aspect of the family, and family service agencies handle
all aspects of the family. Furthermore, self-help groups such as Alcoholics
Anonymous, Parents Without Partners, and Parents Anonymous are available
in most communities.

The actual recommendations made depend upon the interests and skills
of the clinician and the resources available in a specific community. A single

practitioner may well be able to provide all levels of service: educational, counseling, medication, and psychotherapy. When this is not the case, referral to resources specializing in each area may be advisable.

The fit between clinical resource and family is critical (Brown, 1980a). Ethnic and cultural factors may overwhelm psychological issues. Every clinical resource sets some limit on the range of factors it can work with in both diagnosis and therapy. These limits evolve out of the history peculiar to a given clinical setting, the training backgrounds of the professionals working in it, the socioeconomic surroundings and the nature of the social pressures playing upon it.

SUMMARY

This chapter has dealt with consultation to families through evaluating their assets and liabilities and identifying key areas for therapeutic intervention. Diagnostic methods were described for evaluating families on the basis of their control, communication, individuation, and coping patterns, in addition to their progress in mastering the developmental tasks of the family life-cycle.

The classification scheme devised by Lewis was used to conceptualize families. The characteristics of healthy, faltering, dominated, conflicted, and chaotic families were outlined.

Guidelines for therapeutic emphasis were suggested, based upon the characteristics of families. Special attention was devoted to the problem of motivating families and engaging them in treatment. The range of treatment possibilities was then described in the context of available community resources.

REFERENCES

Ackerman NW: *The Psychodynamics of Family Life* (Basic Books: New York) 1958.

Brown SL: Family interviewing as a basis for clinical management. *The Family: Evolution and Treatment*, Hofling C and Lewis J (eds.) (Brunner/Mazel: New York) 1980a.

Brown SL: Developmental cycle of families. *The Challenge of Family Therapy*, Christ A and Flomenhart D (eds.) (Plenum Press: New York) 1980b.

Flugel JC: *The Psychoanalytic Study of the Family* (The Hogarth Press, Ltd: London) 1921.

Grotjahn M: *Psychoanalysis and the Family Neurosis* (WW Norton and Co: New York) 1960.

Gurman AS and Kniskern DP: Research in marital and family therapy: Progress, perspective and prospect. *Handbook of Psychotherapy and Behavior*

Change, 2nd ed., Garfield SL and Bergin AE (eds.) (Wiley: New York) 1978.

Howells JG: *Principles of Family Psychiatry* (Brunner/Mazel: New York) 1975.

Lewis JM: *How's Your Family?* (Brunner/Mazel: New York) 1979.

Lidz T: *The Origin and Treatment of Schizophrenic Disorders* (Basic Books: New York) 1973.

Martin PA: *A Marital Therapy Manual* (Brunner/Mazel: New York) 1976.

Minuchin S: *Families and Family Therapy* (Harvard University Press: Cambridge, MA) 1974.

Sager CJ: *Marriage Contracts and Couple Therapy* (Brunner/Mazel: New York) 1976.

Satir V: *Peoplemaking* (Science and Behavior Books: Palo Alto, CA) 1972.

Satir V, Stachowiak J, and Taschman H: *Helping Families to Change* (Jason Aronson: New York) 1975.

Schechter MD and Lief HI: Indications and contraindications for family and marital therapy: An illustrative case. *The Family: Evolution and Treatment*, Hofling CK and Lewis JM (eds.) (Brunner/Mazel: New York) 1980.

Skolnick A: The American family: The paradox of perfection. *Wils Quart* 4: 113-121, 1980.

Stierlin H, Rucker-Embden I, Wetzel N, and Wirsching M: *The First Interview with the Family* (Brunner/Mazel: New York) 1980.

Swift WJ: Family availability for the working alliance. *J Child Psych* 20:810-821, 1981.

van der Veen F and Novak AL: Perceived parental attitudes and family concepts of disturbed adolescents, normal siblings, and normal control. *Fam Process* 10:327-343, 1971.

van der Veen F and Novak AL: The family concept of the disturbed child. *Am J Orthopsych* 44:763-772, 1974.

Westman JC: Communication between the family and the psychiatric clinic. *International Psychiatry Clinics*, vol 1 no. 1, Carek DJ (ed.) (Little, Brown and Co: Boston, MA) 1964.

Westman JC: *Child Advocacy* (Free Press: New York) 1979.

Wynne L: Pseudomutuality in family relationships of schizophrenics. *Psychiatry* 21:205-220, 1958.

Wynne LC: Some indications and contraindications for exploratory family therapy. *Intensive Family Therapy*, Boszormenyi-Nagy I and Framo JL (eds.) (Hoeber Medical Division, Harper and Row: New York) 1965.

Zuk GH: *Family Therapy: A Triadic-Based Approach* (Behavioral Publications: New York) 1971.

5

Consultation for Adolescents

Joseph D. Noshpitz

The experienced interviewer who is preparing for an initial contact with an adolescent is ready for the unexpected. He will be surprised only if the work turns out to be straightforward, positive, or easy; he anticipates that things will go that way about one time in five. More often, he will be working delicately with a patient who presents special problems. In many cases he will be mustering his resources to try as best he can to cope with hostility, arrogance, seduction, negativism, nonresponsiveness, or open defiance.

This clinical reality underlies all considerations of how to go about consulting with adolescents. There is an inherent unpredictability, a quicksilver quality in the shifting, unstable relationship, which mirrors the uncertainty and mutability of adolescence itself. It lends a certain quality of venturesomeness to the adolescent interview, of high excitement, of mettlesomeness. It is always a test of skills and the practitioner does his work in an ambience of gladiators meeting in an arena.

It is often precisely because of this uncertainty and the special character of adolescent development that psychiatric consultation is resorted to. It is worth taking a moment to consider the kinds of settings that utilize such consultation and what they seek. In fact, the agencies that most frequently request help with adolescents are highly diverse. They include a host of treatment agencies, the many arms of the juvenile justice system, and the full-range of educational settings. From time to time, other agencies connected with young workers, the military, and with housing have also been heard from. Each has its own concerns and the essence of consultation is of course to discover (or to help one's client discover) a question to which it is possible to provide a significant answer, one for which the answer will make a difference.

There is, of course, a tremendous variety of queries raised. In treatment settings the matter of diagnosis and disposition is central. Underlying this situation are a number of issues that provide endless grounds for uncertainty and lead to repeated referral. One question is: When are we dealing with adolescence and when with psychopathology? For better or worse, there is much that adolescents do that falls into a kind of misty area somewhere between the two. Two youngsters park one night, things go farther than either one had intended, and the girl is pregnant. Adolescence? Psychopathology? A police raid at a high school involves a series of spot searches at check points and nabs a youth with a marijuana cigarette in his pocket. A group of adolescents goes swimming in an off-limits abandoned quarry. Someone is hurt. Some of these things involve violations of law. Do they therefore imply psychopathology on the part of those involved? Is risk taking pathological? In one way or another, the inherent nature of the adolescent process brings the youth into areas that may all too readily challenge convention, abrogate custom, expose someone to danger and, to some extent, violate law.

A second group of questions has to do with the unfolding capacities of youth at different levels of development. A transportation agency wants to know at what age youths may safely be employed to drive a school bus. A civil rights group asks when youngsters can make their own decisions about treatment for VD or abortion without informing their parents. Judges wonder at what age it makes sense to remand a youth to adult court. There is no end to the varieties of concerns that arise in connection with the transition out of childhood and into adulthood. While a psychiatric consultant may not have all the answers, he is not at all surprised to have many of these questions posed to him.

It is fair to say, however, that the bulk of his experience is likely to fall within the realm of the clinical or the near clinical. He will be consultant to an outpatient clinic, a residential treatment center, a family agency, a setting for unwed mothers, a public school, a group home or halfway house, and the like. He will work with other mental health professionals, with child-care workers, with school teachers, with nurses, and sometimes with probation officers or police, and he will try to sort out issues of diagnosis and psychopathology and offer recommendations about interventional modes. Above all, he will try to make sense of adolescent developmental events, and to defuse some of the reactive resentment these bumptious and turbulent youngsters can provoke in adult bosoms. For surely Anna Freud's trenchant observation some decades ago continues to hold implications for us today. In a discourse on adolescence, she noted that many thorough and successful analyses which explored the Oedipus complex in great depth did not delve into pubertal material to any meaningful extent and left this sector of development virtually unanalyzed. Similarly, many adults who otherwise display well-balanced and well-integrated personalities nonetheless have little capacity to empathize with the feelings and the struggles of the adolescents about them. They find the behavior of these young people foreign, incomprehensible and dismaying. If the adults are asked, they say they are sure that they themselves never felt or acted in so outlandish a fashion. They have little or no recall of their own experiences during this phase and feel totally at odds with the egotism, the risk taking, the disrespect (to the point of effrontery), and the sexual exhibitionism they perceive in the young.

The consultant's task all too often involves an effort at coping with such alienation and an attempt to bridge the gap between these different sectors of the developmental spectrum. Not infrequently the undertaking is a thankless one, with the indignant adult and the rebellious youth damning him equally as the apologist for the one or the defender of the other. Nevertheless, it is important work.

Within the treatment agency, however, the effort takes on a different case. Here the problem is less one of coping with alienation and more a matter of distilling the underlying meaning of adolescent behavior. This is basic to any rational attempt at intervention. Here indeed the consultant comes into his own. For this is the realm for which he is uniquely well prepared and where he can be of maximum help.

It is with this in mind that the subsequent material has been assembled. The author is currently a consultant to several agencies and has selected some samples of his experience, with one of them serving as the raw material for this presentation. The details are actually drawn from the content of two consultative visits, with data culled from notes taken during the ongoing consultative interactions.

The consultation takes place in a red granite building that was designed to approach as closely as possible the style of a postmedieval castle. There is always a sense of incongruity coming here, to this formidable fortress-like structure that for so many years has provided a haven for women, especially young women, with problematic pregnancies. Its threshold is like a gateway to another time, another ethos—a huge doorway that opens onto high corridors, tall, windowed rooms and echoing passageways. In its earliest days this was the private residence of a single family. These portals opened only for the proud and the wealthy, the best families, the scions of the mighty. And then, in the fullness of time, the building was bequeathed to the Florence Crittenton Home for unwed mothers and they became the entranceway to a residence where pregnant girls lived, a hospital where they were delivered, and a nursery where their babies were cared for until it was time to leave. For nearly seventy years this function prevailed; the task was one of saving and serving and bringing succor to those in need.

In time it went beyond the charity of good people and became a social agency. A great many of the clients who came here were young—teenagers—or women barely out of adolescence. They were in hiding, the agency offered them haven, concealment, a fictitious address. The Boston Florence Crittenton Home routed its mail through the Washington branch, which in turn used the Boston agency to misdirect attention from its local clients.

Then the 1960s came and the revolution in American morals. No longer did one need to conceal pregnancy, a girl could simply stay at home, have her baby and little would be said. Or, by the end of the 1960s, a girl did not have to have a baby at all; abortion was freely available. A revolution indeed, and an imposing challenge to an agency that had for so long striven to protect a special group of the helpless and the victimized, a group that seemed about to disappear.

And so the Barrett program was designed and added to the Crittenton Home. This new arrangement involved a redistribution of space. There had been three floors that served as dormitories and housed pregnant girls. As the applications for service fell off, one dormitory was emptied and merged into a new entity, a residential treatment center for emotionally disturbed teenage girls who were *not* pregnant. This was a radical change, far more deep than anyone had dreamed. The new element that was now introduced was no longer a welfare agency for rescuing and giving succor to the unfortunate. Now it was a treatment service that had come into being, one that marched to a different drum. Different criteria for admission were set, a whole new staffing pattern designed, a novel approach to interactions between staff and clients set up. And for almost a decade, the two kinds of service existed side-by-side under the same roof, with innumerable tensions and disparities shaping their everyday work.

Something of the difference in their essential character is perhaps best illustrated through an anecdote. On one occasion a medical student assigned to the Crittenton program had come away in a state of dazed disbelief. "I was sitting in on this group session for pregnant girls that the social worker leads and one of the girls said, 'Gee I had an interesting dream last night. . . .' But before she could begin to tell it, the worker interrupted with, 'We don't discuss dreams in this group. Now who has any other problems' I thought you mental health people always liked dreams," he added in genuine puzzlement. He had to learn that there was a very real difference between welfare work for teenagers where the idea was to find practical solutions for concrete problems, and therapeutic work where the goal was healing through self-understanding, conflict resolution, and insight.

Indeed, consultation to this two-phasic agency had been a fascinating and complex business. The Crittenton staff and the Barrett staff alternated each week in presenting a case for evaluation and disposition. All of us sat together in a large circle in the antique drawing room of the castle: the teachers, the nurses, the caseworkers, the child-care workers, the cleaning ladies, sometimes the cooks. Most of those present were women, but sometimes there would be a male recreation worker, or a male teacher, and we would review the story of the particular girl under discussion.

The Crittenton cases would be rich with detail about the girls's behavior in residence, her way of relating to peers in the dormitory or in groups, and what she did during her meetings with the social worker. The Barrett cases would involve extensive case records from the past; there would sometimes be a developmental history, court records, agency contracts, psychological tests. The Crittenton workers would be concerned about the girl keeping the child or its placement for adoption, and how to prevent the recurrence of out-of-wedlock pregnancy; the Barrett staff would be worried about drugs, running away, violence, theft, manipulation, homosexuality, and general bad acting.

But times were changing steadily and the girls referred for care with the problem of pregnancy grew fewer in number and more disturbed in character. Presently the only ones who came were either those in a considerable degree of emotional turmoil or those in desperate straits because they had nowhere to go or perhaps most common of all, those with both problems. The questions about management with the pregnant girls were not significantly different from those raised with the girls admitted to the residential treatment program, and as personnel changed and new directors came, the two programs became one, the welfare style of work dropped out, and the therapeutic mode prevailed.

This took place through a series of stepwise changes rather than all at once, but each change moved the agency a little further. First, the hospital wing was closed and the girls sent to established local hospitals for their delivery. Next the wall between the two programs was dissolved. Pregnancy was still grounds for admission, but the pregnant and nonpregnant girls were now housed together in the same dormitories. Finally, the former hospital area was converted into an intensively supervised short stay unit for girls who were going through an episode of extreme emotional upset, perhaps in immediate danger of running away. The goal for everyone was long-term treatment. Pregnant girls could leave after delivery if they so desired, but every effort was made to encourage them to stay for at least a year, whether or not they decided to keep their babies. For pregnant girls who did agree to stay, the baby was placed with an agency in temporary welfare status and visited by the mother.

Throughout, I had been working with the agency as a consultant, first to the Crittenton Home, then to the "separate but equal" Crittenton Home and Barrett Treatment Program, and finally to the new unified Crittenton Barrett Program. At first I was invited for a two-hour case conference once a week. Then, as the program grew ever more therapeutic, the weekly visit was extended to half a day. During all this time my function varied widely. The original case conference format was punctuated periodically by my giving a didactic lecture; I would talk about child development, about violence, about homosexuality, or runaways. Then as I began to come for a half day a week, there would be requests to use the time for staff problems, for overall questions of where the agency was going, and what now needed to be done.

The late 1960s and early 1970s were truly a time of cultural tornado, and nowhere did the winds blow with greater force than in those aspects of the culture that touched directly on the lives of adolescents. The schools were the obvious sites to be swept by the great storms of the time, but the community agency in its own quieter way went through tribulations no less volcanic and unsettling. Nor have the reverberations died down completely. Indeed, by every reasonable measure they are likely to be with us for a good many years to come. The battles over abortion, over education, over parental involvement in adolescent decisions, over the age at which youth may drink, drive, marry, or be held sexually responsible—all these are among a host of ongoing issues that will not vanish tomorrow. And the staff of the youth-serving agency must tie themselves to the mast and ride the waves as best they can.

Here then was one of my major functions during these years, to help my client staffs meet their times, to try as best I could to interpret the crises of the young, and to help the grownups cope with the collapsing values of their day and go on when everything that made any sense had turned strange and lost direction. In our day it is a central task of consultation to recognize how cultural change is tormenting to culture bearers such as parents and therapists and caseworkers when the message they have learned can no longer be the message they can teach, and when treasured values give way, sometimes to the impact of new scientific advance, sometime to the scythe of shrillness and expediency. It is at such moments that clinical values come into their own as well as the principle of nonintrusion of one's own values into those of one's client, of accepting the client where he is, wherever he is, and working from there, of bringing the client a measure of peace through help in self-understanding. These become the holdfasts that the consultant can come back to again and again.

The pressures to evade these tasks, to drop this line of approach entirely and go the route of simple behavioral management or of some doctrinaire ideology—"since everyone here is a victim of a sick society we must forget the individual and focus our efforts on community organization"—were considerable. In discussing cases the number of theories that might be introduced, particularly by some militant member of the team, is legion, and the sense of an orderly balance in the way cases were to be approached was again and again open to challenge. Such ideological rifts, when they are acute enough and involve enough staff members, can sometimes wreck an agency. Certainly they can immobilize it for extended periods as each case conference and each clinical discussion are converted into a battleground, an arena for painful confrontation, and a site for the deepening of differences rather than for the resolution of conflicts and tensions. Hence the role of the consultant under such circumstances can become a key issue, one that unlocks pent up expression but one that moderates it as well. More conservative members who feel baffled and beleagured can be given the right of access to the exchange, the dominance of one subgroup or another can be blunted and balanced, and the hysterical edge of crisis and inflammatory denunciation can be balanced and moderated. The consultant can stand as an island of common sense solidity in the midst of the squall. Most important of all, he can continue his measured statement of clinical values as a factor not to be leapt over, not to be gainsaid, and not to be cancelled out by other issues, however novel and exciting. It is not always a part of such consultative work; when it does arise, however, it is an essential function.

A second level of consultative input arises in an area so obvious and so banal that it scarcely bears stating. The consultant is the voice of child development. Now of all the skills to take for granted in our expectations of a professional staff, surely, it seems, a thoroughgoing knowledge of child development would be a basic given, especially for a staff dealing with a population comprised exclusively of adolescents; they would certainly know adolescence in breadth and in depth.

Curiously enough this is seldom true. It is not that much isn't known; it is rather that major blind spots seem again and again to crop up, to block the appreciation by certain professionals or by a whole staff of the developmental elements in a particular clinical picture. Indeed, it is probably fair to say that one's right to be a consultant in the first place arises from the combination of training, experience, and self-awareness that allows the consultant fewer such scotomata than are borne by his clients. This is, of course, aided and abetted by his social role; he knows he is *supposed* to see things others do not; he thinks that way and approaches issues with that in mind. Richard Cohen comments that the great contribution a consultant makes is often that he is more complete, more exhaustive in his survey of the clinical situation than anyone else. In this way he discerns important factors that others have missed.

I would add to that that among the commonest and certainly most important such factors are those connected with developmental issues. In a sense this is curious and merits a certain amount of speculation in and of itself. It is important to note that developmental data are not like other information. The simple grasp of such knowledge implies a level of self-mastery, of encounter with and resolution of one's own early experiences. Paradoxically, some measure of the necessary capacity can be innate rather than learned. The kind of awareness of another person's developmental level and needs that makes for good interventional work can be a function of talent, of inborn ego capacities, of art rather than science. The "natural" child-care worker, the individual who knows where children are and how they should best be addressed, is a common presence in residential work; all of us have encountered the phenomenon and all of us value it. But precious as it is, it is not a form of communicable knowledge. The "natural" usually cannot tell other staff members how he does what he does. He or she does not have an inner map of what the child is all about; he simply does what comes naturally. For most staff members the more cognitive kind of apprehension is vital. They can approach questions about what to say and what to do when the patient says or does such and such. They can respond to a child's behavior in constructive ways when they have a clear picture of how the patient operates, what vectors press upon him, and how he is likely to respond to these pressures.

It is precisely here that a knowledge of child development occupies a peculiar centrality. There is no other theory of behavior that is nearly so comprehensive; no alternative array of formulations covers the same territory; the grasp of the levels of normal development implies an in-depth comprehension of the roots of behavior.

But even when the data have been learned and learned well, they do not of necessity lend themselves to ready translation into a better grasp of a given clinical picture. The little girl of five whose mother has a psychotic break may live quietly with her father during the ensuing grade school years and then explode into a wild pattern of running away, shoplifting, and promiscuity at age twelve. The staff recognizes the adolescent problem and the fact that the incestuous tensions of living with father are a contributory factor. The consultant brings in the developmental dimension and describes the Oedipal origins of the criminal from a-sense-of-guilt type of dynamics; this sheds light on an essential element in the case. Everyone present was aware of this theoretically; it remained for the senior and most experienced member to make the connection between the infantile neurosis, the theoretical formulation, and the clinical data.

Finally, a third function of the consultant is to work with many levels of the staff at once, and to fully utilize his role as an interpreter of administration to clinicians and to child workers, and vice versa back up the line. An action of administration may smack of arrogance or heedlessness and when the consultant arrives, he encounters the staff's accumulated outrage and injury. It may fall to him, then, to caution the staff to wait to find out the facts of the case in more depth, to recall similar instances where equally troublesome things were handled successfully and, in general, to try to cool down the situation. If he meets with the administrator, he can tactfully raise the matter as an issue requiring clarification. The consultant speaks always on the side of good communication, on the side of problem resolution through adroit management rather than powerful confrontation.

To illustrate these points in somewhat greater detail, the ensuing material will offer an account of the actual experiences and exchanges of a consultative day. Although the sequence of events covers four hours, no attempt will be made to depict everything that happens; instead, certain bits of conversation will be extracted from the overall experience to illustrate something of the nature of consultative interaction.

By way of outline, the day begins with a meeting between the consultant and a group of clinical staff where any staff member may bring up whatever is on his or her mind. Usually case management issues are raised but administrative matters often come up, as well. There are sometimes abreactive responses to current difficulties. This lasts for an hour, and at the end of this meeting, the three caseworkers continue to sit with the consultant for psychotherapy supervision. They take turns presenting, there is usually a verbatim account given of a therapy session. The supervisory experience can be quite an intense experience for consultant and supervisee. It is also (and perhaps for that reason) fragile. The consultant then moves over to the administrative area and meets with the executive director and the clinical coordinator for an hour. Finally, he returns to the clinical side of the building to conduct an in-depth case conference or to give a didactic lecture.

Let us begin with our example.

On a given Thursday, the staff and consultant meet in a newly refurbished office at 9:00 A.M. The nurse is present, as are the social workers and some of the child-care workers. Sometimes teachers show up; usually they don't get to this meeting. In any case, as the staff members assemble, someone begins to talk, often about a recent news event or an unusual movie, or perhaps about some new change in the setting itself such as new construction. Often some pleasantries are exchanged, and a transient jocularity may appear to help relieve the anxiety of encounter. Gradually the talk shifts to the girls in residence and one of the staff comments that relationships are different with the long-term girls who are admitted for residential treatment and the shorter stay pregnant girls. The impact of a continuing relationship vs. that with a built-in time limit becomes the focus of the discussion. Someone asks whether it is really useful for the long-stay youngsters who have known so much loss and separation to live alongside a population of girls to whom they become attached, but who they also know must soon leave them. The consultant responds by saying that it is better to have loved and lost than never to have loved at all. Ultimately the girls cannot be protected; girls will come and go, staff will come and go. The youngsters must surely be given such stability as the staff can offer, but there is no way to keep them from the experience of loss and separation. What can be done, both in therapy and in the life-space work, is to prepare them for the losses and teach them how to cope with them; indeed, teach them how to mourn.

With this the topic seems to come to an end and another issue is raised. Fran and Gypsy are asking to room together. Several staff members react sharply to this—Fran is really a mess and Gypsy is neat as a pin. What in the world would a match like that mean? Why would they even consider it? It turns out that an odd sort of attachment has developed between these two; Fran is certainly a slovenly housekeeper, but recently Gypsy has been pitching in a good bit and helping Fran clean up.

The consultant notes that the appearance of one's room is a good index to a person's self-concept. Getting a girl to change the way she manages her quarters can be more of a problem than it may seem; ultimately it involves getting her to change her inner image of herself, and that sort of thing takes time. The nurse observes that, in any case, at the moment Fran is dirty. Her chief rewards seem to lie in a wolfish kind of orality. Whenever she can she gluts herself. As a result she's a huge, solitary, friendless slob. For the most part other girls ignore or tease her; she's the butt of much hectoring and humiliation. Fran and Gypsy are great contrasts—the one so dirty, the other so clean. A child-care worker chimes in with an account of a child in her neighborhood who is dirty and treated badly by everybody. The nurse continues; Fran doesn't seem to know the most elementary things about personal hygiene. The child-care worker responds that she has taught many girls how to wash out their own clothes and she will take Fran in hand. She'd helped that neighbor child, and she knows how to reach Fran.

With this the consultant observes that the kind of teaching Fran needs is not so much the kind that provides instruction as the kind that makes for identification. We don't teach her to wash clothes so much as we teach her to like us, value us, and want to be like us, and to wash and keep clean because we wash and keep clean. We value these things, and if she wants to be like us, that's the kind of things she'll have to do and value.

The child-care coordinatory brings up a problem that has been troubling her: What is one to do with Riba? She lies all the time. How is one to respond? The consultant rejoins that these are not really lies, at least not in the usual sense of the term. Riba suffers from a sense of painful, inner emptiness, a condition she finds almost intolerable. She is constantly at work trying to fill this aching void or escape it, and she does this by a kind of verbal clinging. She says things that strike people as odd or dramatic or interesting. This has very little to do with the truth or falsity, it's a way of hooking on, of drawing people to her. Her lies are a means of gaining attention, but not the attention sought by the show-off; it is the attention needed by the child who is always collapsing inward unless she can grab ahold of someone.

The social worker observes that Cindy, one of the other girls, complains about this a lot and accuses Riba of lying. This is a baffling business; what do you tell Cindy? The consultant ponders this a bit and observes that the only thing the social worker can tell her is that this is Riba's problem. Riba hurts inside, feels lonely and tries to draw people to her with her stories. The worker says that Riba's stories tend to make it seem as though she has everything she wants. For example, when she talks about her wonderful family, she incites Cindy, whose family is so unhappy. The consultant repeats that it is going to be very important for Cindy to have some of this discussed. This should be said during her daily activities as well as in her individual session, that's where an awful lot of the therapeutic work for her will be carried on. For Riba, too, frank talk is recommended, direct response to her behavior by teachers, by child-care staff and by others as she engages in this pattern. He says this will provide the necessary input to help her change and grow.

A staff member asks about something else. It seems that current policy dictates that once a girl is taken to the hospital for her delivery, she spends three days there and then goes directly to her own home, a foster home or wherever she's headed, and doesn't return to the agency. This means the abrupt breaking off of what are sometimes intense relationships with other adolescent residents. And this happens rather suddenly at times. A girl may disappear in the middle of a school day or during the night. Yet when the staff tries to talk to the youngsters about their feelings and about separation, they just scout the whole idea and refuse to discuss it. "Is there any way we can get them to face their feelings?" the staff members ask.

To this the consultant rejoins that perhaps these girls have had too much separation in their lives, to the point that they don't want to know any more about it. Perhaps the best way to handle this, he says, would be to institutional-ize the response, to have a sort of routine. Whoever leaves would get a card that everyone signs, or perhaps everyone could write a note and the notes could be bound together to make a little book that would then be sent to her. Or per-haps a pillow could be provided, and those who wished could sew their names on it so that it then could be forwarded to the new mother. The social worker agreed; noting that some of the girls organize that sort of thing among them-selves and that it might be useful to do something like that for everyone who leaves. The consultant remarked that the idea was to give them something active to do in the face of separation so they don't feel like passive victims but rather can respond with at least a measure of mastery.

We can interrupt the account of this portion of the day's consultation to look at some of these exchanges in order to better understand the nature of some of the issues and the way a consultant works with them. Some aspects of care have the quality of endemic problems: they recur, are always troublesome, and never cured. The issues posed by the simultaneous management of pregnant and nonpregnant girls, the inevitable tensions that arise between short-term and long-term treatment cases, the group stress that are implicit in this kind of mixture need continuous address. The psychologic overtones are endless.

The long-term client sees someone not unlike herself who, by dint of her pregnancy, is favored with a shorter stay in residence and with a baby to take with her when she leaves. The staff members, on the other hand, see a tragic

destiny—already burdened with fourteen or fifteen years of mistreatment, rebellion, and developmental failure—now curving even further downward under
the load of a responsibility which cannot possibly be well-discharged. Ready
or not, the pregnant client makes major life-decisions almost weekly about her
relationships with the alleged father, with his family and with her own family,
her post-hospital dwelling pattern, the management of the baby, her current and
future educational course, her financial plans, her acceptance or rejection of
therapy, and so forth.

This extraordinary three-cornered structure is of course profoundly influenced by a host of external factors such as community funding patterns, availability of community agency workers, the girls' families (or foster families)
and their attitudes, boyfriends, girlfriends, and the people who live as neighbors
to the program. With the complexities implicit in all this, no single, straightforward solution is likely to emerge unless one group or the other is discharged,
producing a less complex patient population. Since that was not likely to happen, the consultant decided to treat such issues in a partial way as they arose,
looking at the specific behavior presented each time and trying to help the staff
to accommodate as best it could.

In the discussion of separation feelings during the consultation just described, the larger issues of pregnancy vs. nonpregnancy were underplayed
because no ready solution to the conflict was available. The consultant spoke to
the inevitability of this sense of loss and to the possibility that a group form of
response could conceivably be introduced, one which, if it caught on, would in
time become a ritual. Tucked away in the back of the staff member's question
was the difficult matter of dealing with the staff's sense of loss as well as the
girl's. Staff members had often put in months of work with particular youngsters. They too needed the ritual.

The case of Fran and Gypsy illustrates a common path that consultative
discussions tend to take. A question is raised at the outset—what to make of the
wish of two youngsters to room together—and rapidly evolves into an issue
about management of the one who is considered specially problematic. Indeed,
so absorbing is this latter problem that the original question never gets addressed. Nor is this a great loss; it is a commonplace of consultative work that
the initial question posed is often only tangential to the main issue and that it
takes the work of the group process to reveal the issue really needing consideration.

The consultant tries to use the material as it comes along to translate the
everyday clinical events into a recognizable formulation in dynamic theory. It
is a form of teaching dynamics that will, in time, train certain staff to think and
talk in those terms so that a common vocabulary emerges and a girl's messiness
becomes a problem involving body image and self-concept. This is not a form
of teaching that all staff will accept. For those who do, it often stimulates

reading about the topics raised and pursuing their grasp on this form of conceptualization. The others may prefer to confine their attention to the empirical problem at hand.

It should be noted, too, that the consultant offered no solution to this
problem. One of the frequent aspects of consultative experience is to be faced
with issues for which there are no answers or at least no answers the consultant
knows. What he does know something about, however, is how to help a staff
look for answers and how to recognize a good answer when it's available. One of
his mainstays in a residential setting is the reality that when a lot of staff members encounter a problem, their very heterogeneity will lead them to seek solutions in a wide variety of forms. Hence, one can pretty well depend on the fact
that by the time a given question comes to consultation, a great many different
efforts have been made in the quest for a solution. This leads to one of the most
common and useful inquiries he can make: What have you tried so far, and what
has and hasn't shown any possibility of working? This question has been the
take-off point for a great many positive and instructive discussions about patient
management.

On this occasion, however, he didn't have a chance to ask this because one
of the more enterprising and experienced child-care workers had offered to
teach the girl the rudiments of hygiene and personal care. With this, the consultant's task changed. Now he had to take the course that was agreed on and
try to make it into the most dynamically useful approach possible. By stressing
the essential role of identification in teaching he was both continuing his efforts
to inculcate dynamics and thus make the staff more sophisticated, and encouraging the child-care worker to add that extra fillip of warmth and interest to
her teaching that could encourage the girl to incorporate her teacher along with
what she was being taught. This would work toward structural change.

In the case of Riba, the difficult issue was what to do about the com-
pensatory acting out of the depressed youngster and, particularly, about other
kids' reactions. Again, there was no magic button to push. As with so many
management issues, one can only work bit-by-bit and the consultant spoke to
such a gradual educational, supportive approach. But he used the occasion to
underline once again the enormous importance of working on these issues in
the life-space, with child-care worker, nurse, teacher, therapist, everyone giving
a comparable message. Certainly the therapist will ultimately do more with the
data, give the patient more encouragement to explore its every dimension, and
link it up with other aspects of the teenager's life. But the basic stance is still
the same: Riba behaves as she does because of her problems, Riba has to explore
her problems and find a better way, and Cindy has to consider why she is so
vulnerable to Riba's behavior. This is the kind of effort that needs to be made
constantly.

It is a difficult lesson for staff in a residential setting to learn, how to form a wavefront, a communal approach to the difficulty the individual teenager presents. But this is the essence of milieu therapy. It is precisely to the extent that a setting learns to take a consensual approach to particular problems, putting together the different stances of a disparate staff so they address central behavioral issues in a coordinated way, it is to this extent that it is not merely housing a youngster or containing her, but treating her. To get all of this integrated is a difficult task, and it is here that the consultant has so much work to do: to help formulate the dynamics at the outset, then to translate them into practical things to say or do when one is in the life-space coping with the child and, finally, to help identify and work with the group resistances to doing these things.

In any case, that brought us to the end of the first consultation hour. The next was spent in a small group. Three caseworkers and the consultant met for the supervision of individual psychotherapy. The custom was for one of the caseworkers to present her interviews in a particular case for several consecutive weeks, preferably in a process fashion. The group would then react to her material in the traditional fashion of such supervisory efforts. On this occasion, the youngster was an infantile, eruptive fourteen-year-old who had been in many foster homes and had been thrown out of or had run away from all of them. Such a history makes for a dim prognosis. In spite of this, she had formed a meaningful relationship with her therapist and the discussion turned on the question of how to handle a forthcoming vacation the therapist was planning. The youngster had missed her hour, then burst in on the therapist unannounced later while the therapist was on the phone making travel arrangements.

This sort of contretemps is rather typical of residential work, where a special intensity colors the nature of all interactions. This arises out of the fact of living together so that the personal details of many lives mingle to a remarkable degree. There is no evading this and the burden on the consultant is to help the therapists cope with the special circumstances in which they work. This is compounded by the singular character of adolescent problems. The drugs, sex, and running away that form the core of so many adolescent difficulties are here compounded by the intellectual advances of the time, the physical size of the clients, and their transitional developmental status which makes for shifting and uncertain attachments. Therapy is at best hazardous under these circumstances, and much clarification of the developmental implications and complications is constantly in the forefront of the supervision.

One cannot leave this area without remarking on the extraordinary vulnerability of supervisory exchange. It is a delicate interaction, all too easily overwhelmed by the realistic pressures that thrust themselves into residential life. Thus when someone high on the administrative ladder announces that he's leaving, when a site visit has challenged some element in the program, when a reorganization is announced, when a rumor spreads that staff will be cut down, this material is brought up during the supervisory hour and tends to fill the space set aside for work on psychotherapy. The consultant has to be flexible in his management of such issues. He is all the more valuable to the staff, and ultimately to the patients, if he helps staff members maintain their equipoise and objectivity in the face of the sometimes harrowing stresses that troubled times can bring to a social agency. At the same time, the work of therapy supervision can be crowded out by the insistent yammering of external difficulties that can beset even the most dedicated professionals in a residential setting. Some fine judgments need to be made from time to time about when to go along with the abreaction of current stresses and when to urge a return to the supervisory context.

In any case, this hour completed, the consultant moved down to the administrative area to meet with the executive director and the coordinator. Here the discussion tends to be around financial issues. The agency is facing difficult times; it depends on community referrals and the communities are short of funds; referrals are down; inflation is making it necessary to raise fees and complex negotiations ensue. All this surfaces before the internal difficulties of reorganization are addressed. Here the consultant is less likely to offer advice and serves instead as a sounding board for problems as they arise. Occasionally he is asked to recommend one alternative or another among several courses of action. Sometimes he performs a technical function such as meeting and interviewing a candidate for an important post, but chief among his responsibilities is to hear the clinicians' concerns and to represent them to the administrator at an appropriate moment and in an optimal fashion.

In this role as spokesman and advisor, he must be ready for some experiences of frustration and disappointment. He is in the midst of what can at times be a most intense and trying kind of interchange. Often he is at his best as a facilitator of communication. On one occasion it appeared that the State of Maryland was not going to continue its support for a number of the girls in residence. The director felt that there was literally nothing to do but terminate their treatment. The consultant probed gently to learn if there were any degrees of freedom. Could they be kept longer pending further negotiation? Were there alternative funding sources? Was there any other resource? The director explained that the facility served a three-state area, and that if he established a contract with one jurisdiction he could not charge less to the others, at least not without inviting an administrative storm. His hands were tied. The consultant pushed a little saying the staff was deeply involved with these girls, that most of them had been here a year or more, that several difficult cases had come around well, and that for most of the youngsters this was as close to home as they had. They needed more help and were now eager to get it; a lot of time and effort had been invested in them, and it would be tragic to have them suddenly uprooted and dismissed in spite of the clinical indications.

The director responded that things were awfully tight. If the staff were willing to do without a couple of people and cover for them, then maybe something could be done.

"In that case," the consultant rejoined, "I think it would be most helpful if you could meet with them soon, spell out the problem, and give them a sense of what we are all up against. This does mean a lot to them and they need the chance to discuss it with you and to hear from you just how things stand." This was satisfactory and the two made their way to the next meeting, the full clinical case conference where the director took a few minutes to set up a time with the caseworkers to discuss the plight of the Maryland girls.

The case conference itself involved a late-adolescent girl whose father had a lifelong history of mental illness and whose mother was retarded. Because of the family's instability the girl had been placed in foster care at age three, and had a number of different placements in her adolescence. She began hallucinating and was admitted for a time to St. Elizabeth's Hospital which, in turn, arranged for her transfer here. She did well in this setting, finished her high school credits, made arrangements to take her college entrance tests, and regressed. She had never allowed herself to participate in therapy; she couldn't stand self-examination and was terrified of her inner life. The therapist had established a cautious relationship reflecting what the youngster said—and it had to be almost word-for-word—and discussing the immediacies of concrete everyday events. Now the patient was talking to herself in class, telling people in the milieu that she was hearing voices, and acting bizarrely on her job. This was occasional and sporadic, but when the therapist tried to broach the idea to her that approaching college might be stressful, the youngster exploded and almost physically forced the therapist to leave the room. Subsequent attempts to deal with this met with less ferocity, but no more success. What was the therapist to do?

The consultant urged a course of initiating antipsychotic medication and managing the patient by teaching her to rebuild defenses. If she began to get upset or act strangely, the therapist was to tell her to put the disturbing thought out of her mind. He should get her to talk about a neutral subject, something concrete and immediate, and change the subject from whatever was upsetting her. In brief, he was to be active, help her avoid and repress, help her contain the intrusive ideas. Above all, he was to avoid interpreting or confronting her with the underlying dynamics of her situation. The surge forward that comes with graduation and the separation that comes with discharge together comprised a goal at once sought and feared, inspiring and terrifying. It meant independence, with its awesome promise of aloneness; it meant greater maturity, with its inevitable consequence of greater responsibility. Above all (and most meaningful from the standpoint of the mental health professional) it meant the abandonment of one's identity as a child, and therein lay the danger. For this renunciation at the close of adolescence meant that all debts were cancelled, all claims relinquished. Regardless of how much one failed to get during infancy, regardless of how much unsatisfied, childish need persisted, regardless of all the many hoped for reunions and gratifications one has fantasized about and yearned to receive, it was now the moment when it must all be given up. The gratifications one has been calling for but never gotten are now perceived as never to be gained; the parental giving one has been denied but always expected would someday arrive is recognized at last as something one will have to do without. This is hard, very hard. And many a youngster cannot make this step, face this deprivation, give up on these secret but urgent wishes. So he clings to the methods of childhood, fails the test, drops out of school, runs away, or otherwise declares his refusal to grow up.

In particular, it is a hard time for the youth with a psychotic nucleus in his or her makeup. For this intensifies one's sense of vulnerability and sharply accentuates the state of neediness. To interpret these things, then, is to confront the youth with this painful quality that approaches bereavement; and the response is to wince, to fly from the interpretation, and to avoid the therapist. All one can do is stay with the youngster and, through one's consistent and even presence, offer at least a little of the need gratification that is so desperately yearned for and yet denied. One can offer a restructuring of defenses, a support of the fragmented efforts to control the chaos within. By shifting away from overwhelming topics one teaches avoidance and displacement; by focusing on concrete immediacies one directs the youngster toward realistic coping and reality involvement; by occasionally giving instructions to "put this out of your mind," "don't think of that now," and "try to forget about it and concentrate on activities," one strives to reinforce repression. The combination of adolescent process and psychotic potentials is a perilous one and the therapist has a lot of hard work to do if the patient is to get through.

Thus, the consultative work carries forward a great many kinds of effort over a wide range of interactions.

In summary then, the need for consultative work with adolescents arises out of the special character of adolescent adaptive style and the complexities of adolescent life relationships. This is compounded by the multiple, changing demands, on expectations, and social roles extended to these young people as they go through their transitions. Set within the framework of larger cultural shifts, the interplay of multilevel processes can easily prove overwhelming for the individual youth and profoundly stressful for the social agency attempting to help the boy or girl. Since the adaptive style of these youngsters includes such elements as combativeness, flight, seductiveness, sexual harrassment, and negativism, the problems are inherently difficult.

It falls to the consultant to such an agency to help the staff meet the stress of cultural transition. This means helping the administrators understand the vicissitudes the staff members experience and the clinicians the burdens the administrators bear; it means teaching the principles of development to everyone concerned with the youngsters and helping translate the developmental schemata into applied and practical tactics for case management. Finally, it means instructing and informing staff about therapeutic methodology, whether in individual or milieu approaches. Often this comes down to finding a way to aid staff in selecting the right question to ask so that a useful answer can be forthcoming.

The Consultant
in the Clinical Setting

6

Child Psychiatry Consultation in a Pediatric Ward

William H. Sack and Herbert M. Woodcock

This chapter provides a practical description of the process of child psychiatric consultation on a pediatric hospital ward. The need for such a guide has come to us from our experiences as teachers in the child psychiatry–pediatric liaison service at the Oregon Health Sciences University over the past decade. The new child psychiatry fellow, despite previous consultation experience with adults, often approaches this activity with uncertainty about both concept and procedure. We have noted some of this same confusion while serving as examiners for the child psychiatry boards. Therefore, we will attempt to spell out as clearly as we can the elements of pediatric consultation, in a stepwise fashion using case examples.

Traditional hospital consultation by our colleagues in the medical and surgical specialties focuses primarily on the clinical problem *in* the patient. The process of the consultation is given less emphasis. Not so with the psychiatric consultation, where the process and procedures involved in seeing the patient are as crucial as the clinical problem itself. Furthermore, child psychiatry consultation requires not only a broad understanding of diagnosis and treatment, but a pervasive understanding of child development, family dynamics, stress, the meaning of illness, and the hospital ward as a social system.

We hope such a description will be useful not only to professionals with a variety of backgrounds who are new to this work, but also to the practicing child psychiatrist who does only occasional pediatric consultation and wishes to refresh his memory. Many child psychiatry services now emphasize pediatric liaison rather than consultation as the conceptual foundation for these activities (Naylor and Mattson, 1973). While we also have moved in such a direction, we believe that knowledge of how to do a competent consultation still remains a core skill for the child psychiatrist, despite the variety of other activities in which he partakes. Before we describe the procedural steps in child psychiatry consultation, we will first review basic information about the child (reactions to illness and hospitalization) and the hospital (social and system aspects).

THE CHILD IN THE HOSPITAL

It is the rare child who grows to maturity without having gone through some physical illness. Some of these illnesses require hospitalization, which then brings the child into a new and often frightening environment. About three to four million children younger than 15 are hospitalized each year (Prugh et al., 1975). About one-third of young people will have been hospitalized once by the time they reach adulthood (Ibid., 1975). Each child will react to the hospital both in an age-specific fashion and in a highly individual fashion. Both child and family will bestow their own meanings on this experience. Many years ago, William Langford (1948) pointed out that children are prone to see the hospital as punishment, are prone to aggressive and dependency reactions (not to mention rebellious and provocative reactions), but also have the capacity to grow and mature by coping successfully with this stress experience. They may leave the hospital emotionally stronger and more mature than when they entered.

We wish to remind the reader of how varied children's reactions are to hospitalization at various stages of development. Examples we give should not be understood to cover the extent of such possibilities, but only to illustrate the essence of this phenomenon. The emotional risks of hospitalization of the neonate and the premature infant led to the pioneering work by pediatricians Klaus and Kennell (1976) on maternal–infant attachment. The child psychiatric consultant also has seen the psychological dangers to infants of prolonged hospitalization in terms of this same issue.

A psychiatric consultation request was made because of the increasing infrequent visits of parents of an 8-month-old infant who had remained in the hospital with a trachestomy since birth for a congenital laryngeal malformation that precluded home care. When the mother was interviewed, she complained that her child seemed like a stranger to her, "I don't feel like he belongs to me anymore." The nurses felt guilty for the strong attachments they had to the child, and their hostility toward the mother compounded the problem.

Spitz (1945) developed some of his ideas on maternal deprivation from hospital observations in the 1930s and 1940s. At that time marasmus was a frequent clinical problem and its psychological etiology unknown.

The classic work of Bowlby (1961) on parent–child separation began by observations of preschool children in the hospital. His well-known stages of a child's reaction to separation–protest, despair, and detachment, can unfortunately still be found on current pediatric wards. Most hospitalized children do not now suffer prolonged separations from their parents by reason of hospital policy. Yet parents may live far away from the pediatric hospital, and children at the toddler stages are still vulnerable to the trauma of separation. The long-term emotional effects of such an experience can be significant.

An able and conscientious junior medical student caused concern to her preceptor because she was showing increasing withdrawal and poor performance on her pediatric inpatient rotation. As he sensitively explored the reasons for the student's difficulties, he learned that the student had herself been hospitalized as a preschool child on the very ward where she was now a clerk. A transfer to a new ward immediately improved her performance.

One developmentally specific reaction of the Oedipal child (i.e., aged three to seven years) may be particular fears of bodily mutilation (Blom, 1958). Surgical reactions to hospitalization, he may, at times, feel that his illness is a punishment for past thoughts or misdeeds. He may further confirm his fears by receiving punishment on the hospital ward because of provocative acts or reckless behavior. Such provocation usually engenders a hostile response in the hospital staff and often elicits a request for psychiatric consultation.

The child in the developmental stage of preadolescence or early adolescence has been shown frequently to have fearful fantasies around "losing control" (Blom, 1958). When facing major surgery, it may be the anesthesia and not the surgery the child fears most. Fears of regression or loss of sphincter or impulse control may create an emotional crisis in a seemingly well-adjusted child.

Schowalter (1977) has elegantly highlighted the age-specific concerns around body image during adolescence. When physical illness threatens this new awareness of the body, self-esteem precipitously drops and emotional and psychological symptoms frequently result. The fear that "I'm different" is almost ubiquitous in adolescence, and if illness amplifies such self-perceptions, it may be helpful to link such adolescents to older persons with similar problems who can serve as effective models for identification.

Angie, a fifteen-year-old girl with newly diagnosed ulcerative colitis, was facing the prospect of a colectomy with subsequent colostomy. A week before the surgery she was withdrawn, uncommunicative, and depressed. At a staff meeting, one of the young nurses, who had the same illness, suggested we introduce Angie to an eighteen-year-old girl who was returning to the outpatient clinic soon, a year after her similar surgery. After three discussions that included the patient, the nurse, and the older teenager, Angie's mood was much improved and her postoperative course was remarkably smooth.

Rollins (1979), in her followup of a group of previously hospitalized girls with anorexia nervosa found that their most frequent positive comment about the former hospital experience was the friendship they had made with another anorectic patient. (Psychotherapy and weight gain were rarely mentioned.)

These descriptions of how children may react to hospitalization do not exhaust the possibilities. It is the nature of children to regress when facing stressful experiences; that is, they fall back on earlier modes of functioning and relating. Hospital caregivers may be baffled by such behavior and find themselves reacting impatiently and irritably to such babyish tactics of the child. Likewise, the child with a chronic illness may fear that his own place in his family will be lost (i.e., he will not be contributing as a family member) (Geist, 1979). Children may then revert to regressively sacrificing their autonomy in an effort to hang-on overcompliantly to the parents.

For the consultant working in this setting, it is hazardous to concoct generalizations from one clinical situation to others. Too many variables and too few empirical data hamper our efforts (Jellineck, 1978). This is why every pediatric hospital consultation brings with it a creative challenge.

THE PEDIATRIC WARD AS A SOCIAL SYSTEM

Not only must the consultant appreciate the nuances of childhood development and psychopathology, but he also must appreciate that the hospital is a complicated psychosocial system. The system will determine how the consultant is received and also how and where he may intervene. But before we describe the position of the consultant in this system, we must remind ourselves that the child temporarily lives in this system while in the hospital. For instance, in an informal head-count, one of our hospital nurse clinicians counted *40 people* (hospital staff) who interacted with one child on an average day. This kaleidoscope of strange faces ranging from janitors to medical students, nurses, and laboratory technicians must in itself have a significant impact on the child's sense of security and continuity. In years past a number of child psychiatrists joined with influential pediatricians to "humanize" the children's wards (Powers, 1948). Yet, a recent review of pediatric hospital practices by Prugh and Jordan (1975) indicated that many hospitals give psychological issues only lip service.

Every hospital that admits children should now have the following basic services:

1. Unlimited visiting hours and opportunities for parents to "live in" when appropriate.
2. Well-organized recreational and play programs.
3. Educational facilities and programs.
4. In-service training programs for staff that emphasize special emotional needs of children, such as their different sense of time and their ways of expressing fear and anxiety (Prugh, 1975).

Once the consultant steps into a pediatric ward, he should keep in mind a number of principles that have been described as the consultation set. Here the consultant enters into a relationship with the treating physician, patient, and hospital staff, yet remains outside of the system to study the patterns of these relationships. Miller (1975) outlined a number of system principles of hospital consultation that are applicable, as well, to situations involving children. We will list each principle and give a relevant example from our own experience to illustrate the issue involved.

(1. The consultant is working with a multiperson system that interacts in complicated ways with the individual hospitalized child.)

The consultant was asked to see a six-year-old child to consider the diagnosis of hyperkinesis. When he arrived on the ward, he quickly learned that the real problem was the child's boisterous behavior on the ward in the evenings. This behavior was particularly upsetting to a certain nurse. By arranging evening activities for the child through a volunteer assistant, the immediate ward problem was solved. The question of hyperactivity was also investigated.

(2. The consultant is an outsider to the system and may need to learn special meanings, customs, and even languages that are a part of that system before he can begin to understand it.)

One new child psychiatry consultant arrived on the pediatric ward to see a cardiology patient while cardiology rounds were in progress. In talking with the referring resident, he was summarily quizzed on the anatomy of the child's heart defect. Answering the cardiology questions correctly as his rite of passage, he received a friendly smile from the staff cardiologist and proceeded to do the consultation. As time went on, he was particularly esteemed and respected by his pediatric colleagues. He had become a "real" doctor.

(3. Responsibility for members of the system lies primarily within the system. Although a consultant must at times accept major responsibilities for a member in the system, and at other times may have to help a poorly functioning member to move out of the system, an ever-present and major purpose of his actions is to help the system cope with its problems.)

The psychiatric consultant was called by a pediatric resident who had just come from an interview with a young mother, one of whose twin infants was about to be discharged from the hospital. The mother broke down in tears, claiming she could not take the child home, because the father openly rejected this smaller twin with a congenital defect. The mother's emotional state so moved the pediatric resident that he was close to tears as well, and wanted the psychiatrist to take over the subsequent interviews. The psychiatrist resisted this suggestion, helped the pediatrician deal with his own feelings, suggested an approach to the next interview, encouraged the pediatrician to continue to be the active case manager and to motivate the social service worker, and remained only indirectly involved. The case moved to a successful resolution, and the psychiatrist praised the pediatrician for his persistence and sensitive intervention.

(4. While keeping his position as an outsider and observer of the system, the consultant may simultaneously become a temporary partial member of the system to facilitate its functioning, that is, attend a staff meeting, make disposition suggestions.)

The psychiatric consultant was presented a case of a very damaged infant with multiple congenital anomalies, including a severe meningiomyocele. The parents were told the prognosis was hopeless and that prolonging the child's life was futile. The nurses were told by the medical staff not to intervene actively in caring for the child. The nurses appealed to the consultant with their distress and frustration, feeling they could not carry out this plan. The consultant arranged a staff meeting with all of the involved parties. The various viewpoints on the case were aired. The consultant's ability to accept a variety of emotional appeals with openness and without judgment or rebuttal seemed to create a model for acceptance by nurses and house staff of each other. The volatile nurse–physician tension was defused during the meeting and a new, more flexible care plan was established. The physicians relented and allowed the child the care that made the nurses more comfortable.

(5. The consultant's most important input to the system often is as much the gathering and synthesis of information, the contribution of concepts, knowledge, and techniques, and the provision of modeling as it is decision making about the patient or therapy. Naylor and Mattsson (1973) and Sack et al. (1977) in surveys of consultation work have found that one-third to one-half of the time of a pediatric consultation may be spent in this aspect of work.)

A teenaged girl was seen several months after a bone marrow transplant for leukemia. The immediate problem was the girl's reluctance to be discharged. She was markedly cushingoid from steroid treatment and, on being interviewed, was clearly anxious and depressed. The consultant found the family to have considerable anxiety about the possibility of relapse. There were also issues of adolescent freedom and control. The psychiatrist spent time explaining the issues to the pediatric staff, helped to effect a compromise on the time of discharge, called a local mental health clinic, explained the problems, and arranged for immediate followup. This indirect effort took between two and three hours of additional time.

(6. An appreciative empathy for the affects of all hospital caregivers working in a stressful system is crucial to making appropriate responses.)

A two-year-old child was hospitalized repeatedly with exacerbations of leukemia. Each time the child was hospitalized, the mother would become severely critical of the nursing staff. She was predictably antagonistic and often sarcastic. The consultant interviewed her and found her to have a rather primitive personality, but also found her to be in chronic anxiety and fear over the child's impending death. Her anger covered a great amount of guilt and fear. When the consultant interpreted the mother's anger as not personal but a part of the grief process, the nurses began to have more tolerance and empathy. Two months after the child's death, the mother returned to the hospital ward and spent the day individually thanking each of the nurses for their splendid care of her child.

(7. Affect can be intriguingly transmitted through the hospital system in almost a hierarchical fashion. Whenever a patient stressfully experiences a particular emotion strongly, those around him often experience it as well. This can move along the system until it reaches the consultant [often in a surprising and "jarring fashion] before its source is recognized [Powers, 1948].)

A pediatric resident requested a psychiatric consultation, through the usual channels, on a fourteen-year-old girl who had been brought in because of an overdose the evening before. An hour later, when the psychiatrist had not

*yet arrived on the ward, the pediatrician paged him and critically berated him
for not responding immediately. The consultant refrained from retaliating but
did come to the ward and, in discussing the case, quickly recognized that the
resident was acutely anxious that the girl might repeat her suicidal attempt. The
pediatrician felt helpless about knowing how to manage this problem. With a
structured management plan worked out, and close availability of the psychiatrist, the pediatrician relaxed and became much more amiable.*

The sensitive consultant can detect a certain emotional climate on a particular ward the moment he embarks on his task. Geist (1977) described well
the elusive, subjective ward atmosphere that has so much potential for enhancing or undermining the consultant's efforts. This "ambience" remains
hidden behind ward traditions, activities, and the mechanics of everyday hospital
life. It can be sensed better than described. An unfortunate yet familiar fact is
that a large group of children with chronic and life-threatening illnesses now
occupy most university pediatric beds. The deterioration or death of a particular
child can affect the mood of the entire ward. It is well for the consultant to
know the general tenor of the ward as he sets about his individual tasks. He must
be familiar with the defensive ways staff can handle feelings of guilt, depression,
or helplessness. In the resident staff it may occur in the form of a flurry of
extraheroic, life-saving but futile activity, or in turning the very ill child back
into a case. For the nursing staff, it may be an inordinate amount of anger about
a particular issue that protects them from the pain of depression (1978). The
consultant must plan his intervention with a grasp of these "milieu" issues
in mind.

THE STEPWISE PROCEDURE OF THE
HOSPITAL CONSULTANT

The Request for Consultation

The hospital consultation begins when the child psychiatrist receives a
formal request for consultation from another physician. The consultant obtains
important initial information about age, location, medical or surgical status, and
duration of hospitalization.

The wording of the request may contain important information about the
attitude of the referring physician toward the patient and the consultant. The
psychiatrist begins to listen with his "third ear" for clues to not only the overt
reason for the request but a "hidden" problem as well (Schwab, 1979). For in
the mundane wording of the request, one may detect the kind of role the psychiatrist is expected to play. For example, "Please see this suicidal adolescent for

psychiatric care" might suggest that the pediatrician wishes her transferred to another service. Or "This child is a behavior problem" suggests a ward management problem in which the nursing staff is sure to have strong feelings. "Patient has persistent pain, please evaluate" suggests that the problem will be to differentiate "organic" and "functional" conditions.

The amount of detail and focus of the request, or the lack of them, may indicate the level of involvement of the physician in the problem. On the other hand, vaguely worded requests may indicate a basic confusion about the situation and a genuinely receptive plea for help. The urgency of the request may be not only a measure of the problem itself but a statement about the anxiety level of the referring physician and his staff. It is our policy to respond by telephone to all requests for consultation within a matter of hours, and immediately for urgent requests. Telephone contact alone usually allays the anxiety component of the request and ensures the interest and responsiveness of the consultant. Since consultation can occur only when a certain level of trust exists between physicians, it is crucial to build this alliance as early in the process as possible. Nothing confirms the stereotype of the passive, unresponsible psychiatrist "working behind closed doors" as much as his delay in responding to the request for help. The consultant is particularly alert to the "Friday afternoon" phenomenon in which he may be asked to see a child several hours before discharge and is expected to arrange for disposition. A prompt response is crucial, but *how* and *when* the rest of the consultation is done often can be gently and skillfully negotiated by an experienced clinician.

Discussion with the Consultee

It is wise, whenever possible, to talk with the referring physician in person before seeing the patient, family, or both. This allows for a deeper understanding of the overt and covert reasons for the request (Hackett, 1978). It allows the consultant to begin to grasp the referring physician's relationship to the child and family and gives the consultant a brief overview of the case history. Verbalizing his views allows the consultee to clarify his own attitudes, expectations, and involvement. It is also important to clarify how the child/family have been prepared for the consultation. The psychiatric consultant may be called to see particular children as a "retaliatory" threat for bad ward behavior or as a thinly disguised disciplinarian. Or, the total lack of preparation may result in the family's angry surprise and refusal to cooperate. It is our policy to be sure the child's family is informed of the request and the reasons for it *before* any intervention occurs, unless a psychiatric emergency is present.

A ten-year-old diabetic boy was causing ward problems, and the nursing staff was angry with the parents' overprotective and overly involved handling of

*the child. The psychiatric consultation request was made without the family's
knowledge. The consultant did not check on the preparation and so surprised
the parents that they threatened to remove the child from the hospital prematurely. They became more distrustful of hospital personnel during the remainder of the child's stay.*

Discussion with the Head Nurse

It is our policy always to meet with the head nurse. Much practical and
useful information can be obtained about the child's social skills, mood, play
interests, or parent-child interactions that are not the usual province of the
physician but may have important bearings on the consultant's evaluation.

Since every consultation request implies that the child in some way is dis-
rupting the smooth flow of a complex system, it is well to "tap" the system at
more than one level. Nurses are often (as every child psychiatry consultant
knows) the covert instigators of the psychiatric consultation request, and some
appreciation of their role and recognition of their opinion pays later dividends
when laying out specific treatment recommendations that involve nursing
management. Ward schoolteachers and recreational staff should also be contacted.

*The pediatrician sought psychiatric consultation for a 7-month-old failure-
to-thrive child. The medical staff felt the mother's parenting abilities were
marginal and wanted the child moved to a foster home. They had, however,
little direct evidence of the mother's parenting failure. Two of the nurses who
observed the mother feeding the child noted her generally tense handling and her
overstimulation of the baby with the nipple, so that after a few minutes the
child gagged and vomited. Two sessions with the psychiatrist allowed the mother
to ventilate her anxieties, and gentle correction of the mother's feeding style by
the nurses allowed the baby to eat, gain weight, and go home with its mother.*

Reviewing the Medical Record

A brief review of the record is essential and supplies important time-
saving information from a variety of sources.

1. A review of the medical history may reveal the evolution of the need for a
    psychiatrist's help. It may be fragmentary or cohesive. It may, for instance,
    reveal disputes by other consultants about the etiology of the symptoms.
    Sometimes physician attitudes toward the patient can be "read between the
    lines."

2. Laboratory findings may be helpful in interpreting strange ward behavior. Electrolyte imbalance, a high BUN, or blood glucose levels, or other hormonal deviations may be contributing to a behavior problem.

3. A careful review of the medications may also illuminate the situation. Phenobarbital, antihistamine, and other medications can cause unusual behavioral side effects. Sometimes stimulant drugs for hyperactivity only exacerbate the behavior or, rarely, can cause a toxic psychosis. Cortisone is a well-known behavioral-change agent in children as well as adults. The dates of any recent medication change should always be noted.

4. Nursing notes can be a rich source of behavioral data about the child over a 24-hour period, but may also contribute directly to the differential diagnosis.

The psychiatric consultant was asked to see a 12-year-old girl for "psychotic behavior." A perusal of the nursing notes showed that the child's worst behavior was always recorded in the early morning hours. When he brought this to the pediatrician's attention and further evaluated the child, diagnosis of psychomotor seizures was eventually made.

Approaching the Child and Family

The authors prefer to see the child's family first whenever possible. Gaining their alliance may result in making it easier later to gain the child's trust.

This not only allows one to gather the usual psychiatric developmental data on the child and to inquire about family perceptions and stresses, but also permits tapping the hospital system at another level. Frequent parental behavior, as manifested on the pediatric ward, may be the generating force behind the referral. It occurred in 20% of psychiatric consultations during our year's survey (Sack et al., 1977). With unlimited visiting privileges and overnight stays on wards, parents now bring onto the ward their own coping styles and defensive structures, which may add stress to the system. "Managing the parent" can become a heated ward issue, particularly when parents project or externalize their mood onto the staff and so generate further conflict.

The consultant was asked to see a child who was in the hospital for undiagnosed symptoms of fever and abdominal pain. However, the "real" reason for the consultation was not long in coming. The nursing and house staff were increasingly irritated by the patient's mother, who was coercively "sidetracking" a variety of caretakers into extended discussions about laboratory findings,

*X rays, films, diagnosis, and prognosis. "We can't get our work done," they
complained. The consultant, after interviewing the mother and allaying some of
her anxiety, suggested that one nurse each shift, and one house staff member
each day, set aside 15 minutes* at a specified time *to discuss the day's events
and progress. This gave the mother "something to hold onto" and gave the staff
control over a troublesome situation. Things quickly quieted down.*

In approaching the child, the psychiatric consultant always clearly states
his identity and the reasons for his visit, adding that he works with the child's
physician in trying to make things go better for children on the ward. Since
hospitals are busy and often crowded, it is frequently difficult to find a suitable
place to conduct the interview. The consultant has to be flexible in dealing with
the unpredictability of ward life. To obtain the necessary privacy, the consultant may need to arrange ahead of time the kind of quiet place he needs.
An interested nurse is usually the best ally in such a situation.

"How did you happen to come to the hospital?" linked with a question
about the child's understanding of his medical problem or illness often yields
important misperceptions from children about what is wrong with them. More
than 20 years ago Gofman and associates (1957) surveyed a pediatric ward time
(100 admissions) and found 75 percent of children had little understanding of
the reasons for their hospitalization or what might be causing their illness.
Unfortunately, the same problem is encountered far too frequently by psychiatric consultants today. Complicating the situation even more is the fact that
the child may prefer to give his own "secret" meaning to the events, despite
accurate explanations from adults. Pursuing this discovery task may also be
fruitful to the consultant in uncovering such themes as punishment or loss of
love in the child's explanation.

Occasionally the consultant finds the child acquiring a piece of misinformation from cavalier bedside discussions by physicians, as if the child were
not present. Although it has been many years since Powers called this practice
(1948) "a hoary rite" that should be abandoned, hospital routines and rituals
change slowly.

*A ten-year-old boy told the psychiatric consultant he thought he was going
to die because his physician said the drug he was taking "wasn't working anymore" (information overheard from ward rounds about antibiotics). He became withdrawn, irritable, and weepy, until this misinformation was corrected
by an explanation of the change in antibiotics and reassurance that he was
getting better.*

Particular children may remain mute or angry during the initial interview,
yet also give more subtle "reaching-out signals" that keep the psychiatrist at

the bedside. Remaining *with* the child who by his silence may be communicating much about his anger and frustration often pays later dividends in establishing a relationship that reveals the child's underlying fears and feelings. It may be appropriate for the consultant to begin early to put the predominant mood into words to help the child gain a sense of relatedness and mastery.

A psychiatric consultant spent three consecutive interviews unsuccessfully trying to get a mute 11-year-old girl to discuss her illness. She had ulcerative colitis and was not only sick but depressed and frightened, awaiting surgery. When the psychiatrist didn't visit her on the fourth day, the child angrily asked where she was. When the consultant did come, the child was ready to talk about her fears of possible abandonment by her family and anxieties about the upcoming surgery.

The flow and direction of the interview follow no set format. The consultant always conducts a mental status examination of the child and spends sufficient time with the child to reach a reasonable formulation of the problem. At times, a family diagnostic interview is appropriate. At other times, a series of interviews may be necessary (or interviews at different times of the day). The consultant occasionally is confronted by an older child or teenage patient with requests for confidentiality. Patient and consultant need to clarify at the beginning which parts of the interview data are to be kept private and which are to be shared with the staff, so the patient does not feel betrayed. The consultant always gives the child the opportunity to ask "that last question" that so often yields significant insight near the end of the interview. Asking the child to compare the actual experience of the interview with his former fantasies of what he "thought it was going to be like" is another way to bring out hidden perceptions and preoccupations.

The Consultant's Reply

The consultant must now transmit his knowledge to the hospital caretakers in a useful way. For unless the hospital staff finds in the consultant's report diagnostic clarification or practical suggestions for ward management, the consultation will be considered a failure despite the consultant's intellectual prowess or lofty insights. Here, the temptation of the consultant may be to display his psychiatric sophistication among "lessers"; that is, to gain a sense of superiority over his professional colleagues by throwing in psychological jargon and speculation. But the pediatric ward is not a psychiatric ward, and such displays of brilliance will not be well received. As one pediatrician said after hearing a lengthy formulation by a very bright consultant, "He's brilliant. I never could do that.   What do I do with this patient?"

It is our feeling that the report in the chart is not a substitute for a face-to-face sharing of findings with the consultee. Explanations should be clear, relevant, and geared to the immediate situation. This is actually harder to do than giving a lengthy written summary. The psychiatrist, without being condescending, should give the consultee some understanding of how the problem originated. This stimulates both curiosity and empathy in the consultee and staff (Nadelson, 1978). Practical recommendations should flow naturally from such an explanation and be geared to the hospital environment. The consultant may suggest that a staff meeting be arranged to discuss his findings. Including the staff in this way often "closes the loop" of communication with those who sought such a consultation in the first place.

Throughout the report the good consultant integrates knowledge of the child's early development, medical condition, family dynamics, and social and cultural meaning, and gears all of this to the personalities and style of the consultee and hospital staff on a particular ward at a particular time.

A twelve-year-old boy was neglecting his diabetic management and increasingly getting into fights with his mother, who had raised him by herself. In consultation, the psychiatrist learned that the pediatrician recently cut his clinic visits with the boy because of improvement. The boy expressed dismay and disappointment that he was not seeing his pediatrician as often. He obviously held the pediatrician up as an ego ideal and was depressed by what he felt as abandonment. Helping the pediatrician to use the power of his already good relationship quickly solved the diabetic management problem.

If the consultant cannot come up with a clear formulation, he should share his ignorance with the consultee in a straightforward fashion and express willingness to stay involved in any further way that the consultee requests.

Sometimes arranging a disposition for continued post hospital care, if not clarified, can become a problem between consultant and consultee. Each may expect the other to carry through, and so nothing happens. The step from hospital to community is a big one, and major gaps in the continuity of care occur at this point. To facilitate this process, the consultant may wish to help the consultee clarify "who is to do what." Particularly in chronic illness, with the anticipation of repeated hospitalizations, it is important for the consultant to take a longitudinal perspective on this issue and help to build relationships that bridge the gap of hospital and clinic.

The chart write-up should be brief and legible. The following outline is suggested (Schwab, 1977):

1. The reasons for the request should be stated.
2. The basic problem is outlined.

3. The medical history is interpreted in relation to the problem.
4. The developmental and family history is briefly summarized, when relevant.
5. The psychiatric interviews are summarized.
6. A brief, cogent formulation is outlined.
7. Clinical impressions are stated.
8. Recommendations are given and appreciation expressed.

Empathy for the Consultee

It is important for the consultant to recognize that certain dichotomies in patient care exist on hospital wards (Geist, 1977). Physicians and surgeons maintain a somewhat detached and objective relationship with their patients for good reason: they may be called on to inflict pain or invade another's body in the service of healing. The authors notice a certain impatience and irritation that new psychiatric consultants show toward their medical and surgical colleagues for not caring or for being unfeeling or aloof. The implicit assumption is that the surgeon should be able to conduct a therapeutic interview the way we do. While it is true that physicians can improve their bedside manner and their sensitivity toward patients, it is also true that physicians need to maintain certain defenses so that they can best carry out their primary functions. An intuitive sensing of how much emotional care the consultee can handle is important for the consultant to judge as he plans his recommendations. At times it may be important that the physician not change his role in patient care, and the consultant may need to use himself or someone else than the physician to deal with the ongoing emotional problems in hospital care. After all, the physician does not ask the psychiatric consultant to assist him in the operation room.

One of the authors recalled an early consultation experience in which he was asked to see a six-year-old child who suffered from extensive burns over 60 percent of her body. She was not eating and seemed depressed to the surgical resident, who asked for a child psychiatric consult. The child was indeed depressed and withdrawn because of pain and loneliness. The author indicated this and agreed to see her on a daily basis. He read stories, played games, and functioned in a generally supportive way, wondering whether or not such activity was really useful. While it did seem useful to the child, the author was surprised to realize how extremely valuable the surgical team considered this psychiatric intervention. It was only later he realized that by assuming the emotional care of the child, he was relieving the surgical resident from providing this kind of care for which the resident felt neither qualified nor capable of giving.

Care of the Dying Child

Care for a dying child has been reported in surveys to be the most stressful part of a physician's practice (Paykell et al., 1976). Nonpsychiatric physicians and medical students, in a recent study, rated as core psychiatric skill the ability to understand the emotional aspects of the chronically ill and dying patient (Johnson and Warner, 1977). This seems strange, since psychiatrists usually do not have direct caretaking responsibilities in this area. Courses in death education in American medical schools are taught most frequently by psychiatrists (Smith et al., 1970). These statements are intended to introduce the fact that the psychiatric consultant is highly valued by his medical colleagues in rendering service in this painful area of medical practice.

For the physician, death is always felt as a professional failure. Physicians, like everyone else, use ego defenses to protect themselves from the reality of death. These defenses can take various forms, such as the following:

1. Withdrawal (subtle or not subtle) is the most common way of sparing oneself pain, and the most difficult for the dying child and family to comprehend.

2. Depression over the relentless course of the illness can be translated into anger at other physicians and nurses.

3. False, deceptive hope can spare the physician but usually fools no one, and may have later repercussions.

The death of a child may awaken in the physician one of our own deepest fears: death before fulfillment. The consultant can help the care-giving physician deal with a dying child in the following ways:

1. He stresses the importance of clear, open communication among physician, patient, and family. Anticipating the next step and helping the family cope with what lies in the immediate future are paramount.

2. Steering a course between reality and hope is vital. Parents want the truth, yet they must maintain some hope, even in the face of relentless illness. If the physician errs on the side of too much hope, the family may later feel they were deceived. If too much reality removes hope, the family may prematurely disengage from the child and begin their mourning process too soon, thereby emotionally abandoning their child.

3. Psychological coping takes time. Studies have shown (Stillion et al., 1970) that it takes parents a minimum of four months to work through feelings of acceptance about the possibility of their child's death, once the fatal illness is announced.

4. Careful judgment is needed about how frank to be in discussing death with a particular child. Most children understand more about their own serious condition than they are willing to put into words. Morris Green (1966) stated that most all latency age children who are dying have three questions of their physician: (1) am I safe. (2) will a trusted person keep me from being alone, helpless, or in too much pain, and (3) will you make me feel all right? Coping with these questions honestly in talks with the physician may be sufficient for the dying child to be at ease. Creating a climate of psychological safety is important in the terminal phase.

The Generation and Disposition of the Child Psychiatric Referral

Our pediatric–child psychiatry liaison staff are often surprised by the unpredictability of requests for consultation. Why is this child referred and not another (who seems to have greater emotional problems)? Stocking and colleagues (1972), in a carefully constructed survey, found two-thirds to three-quarters of children on a hospital ward laboring with significant emotional problems, yet rarely more than five percent to ten percent were referred for psychiatric consultation.

This question motivated our liaison team at The Oregon Health Sciences University to gather data on the little-understood issue by reviewing the kinds and frequency of consultations done over a several-year period in which new liaison support personnel in the form of child life therapists were being added to the pediatric wards, and in which more liaison activities were being started (such as conferences, attendance at work, and ward rounds). We found that total formal consultation requests declined for the handling of ward behavior problems (with new help of the child life therapists) but that consultation requests for problems in differential diagnosis remained the same over this period. That is, the child psychiatrist as consultant was needed for better understanding of the obscure symptom. We thought this represented a "core" function of psychiatric consultation (Sack and Blocker, 1978–79). Bolian (1971) has pointed out that the child psychiatrist can gauge the amount of consultation work he stimulates by his visibility, interest, and involvement. The particularities of any hospital situation and the relationships between particular services will also determine who is referred.

Yet, overall, it has seemed to us that it is not the mere presence of emotional problems in hospitalized children that generates the psychiatric consultation. Rather, it is whether those emotional problems directly interfere with the smooth diagnosis and treatment of children in a medical setting. If it does not so interfere, the child's emotional problems will likely go undetected. Pozanski and associates (1979) recently reported the failure of hospital nurses to recognize depression in about 50 percent of overtly depressed ward children.

As for the posthospital disposition of children who received a psychiatric consultation, little information exists. Sack et al. (1977) tried to contact all child patients who had been seen for hospital consultation one to two years before, and reached about two-thirds of them. Many described the hospital consultation as a crucial experience that made things better. Patients from the middle classes followed through on recommendations for continued mental health therapy, whereas patients from the lower socioeconomic classes found more value in immediate environmental manipulations and often did not follow through on such recommendations. In the opinion of the authors, the hospital experience for many of the families had served as a form of "disguised crisis intervention." The consultation had a strong therapeutic aspect in helping to bring about solutions to problems mounting in intensity during the year preceding the hospitalization.

Types of Consultation on a Pediatric Ward

In a recent national survey of child psychiatry training programs, Anders (1977) reported that while 80 percent provide consultation services to pediatric inpatient units, fewer than half engage in other forms of pediatric teaching and service activity, such as ward rounds. The authors have found that regular rounds on the pediatric wards have been both fruitful and well received and cut down the need for that urgent Friday afternoon consultation one hour before the patient is to be discharged. We will list some of these ongoing activities that provide liaison continuity with the pediatric staff, but that also require every consultative skill that a child psychiatrist can muster.

1. *Behavior rounds.* Twice a week, a child psychiatrist hears a case from the pediatric wards in which emotional or psychosocial issues are discussed with the pediatric house staff. At times the child is interviewed in the presence of house officers, and at times the case is presented without the patient. Mattsson (1976) has well described the benefits and hazards of this approach.

2. *Consultations to specific groups.* Our child psychiatric staff has found it advantageous to meet with groups within the pediatric wards on a regular basis. Nurses in the intensive care unit and on the renal dialysis transplant team work in high-pressure environments with children who are often terminally ill. Both groups benefit from airing their frustrations and stresses. Bioethical questions often loom large. Another popular theme is how to deal with parents' reactions to their very ill children. Regular psychiatric conferences have been useful vehicles for getting busy professionals together to plan psychological treatment approaches and to share their feelings of hope and despair in a supportive fashion.

3. *Growth and development rounds.* The authors have recently initiated on the pediatric wards a weekly growth and developmental conference in which a child's case is presented so as to teach approaches to evaluating childhood development. This serves as a useful vehicle to underscore issues of regression as they relate to hospitalization of children. Making pediatric house officers more sensitive to the general field of growth and development has been useful in introducing psychological issues in a palatable and relevant fashion, rather than as something foreign to their pediatric work. It is conducted jointly by a pediatrician and a child psychiatrist.

4. Finally, the child psychiatrists in our liaison service have responded to short-term requests for support groups among the pediatric house officers. There is nothing more stressful to a physician than to attend a dying child. The pediatric house officers formed a group that met weekly for three months in 1980 and in which the residents shared their handling of their own grief when one of their child patients began to deteriorate or had died. The child psychiatrist who convened the group did no probing and made no personal interpretations. Rather, he encouraged the common sharing of experience, which legitimized the actions of the pediatricians as common and natural.

From Consultation to Liaison to Collaboration: Is It Possible?

With the move from consultation to "liaison" (Naylor and Mattson, 1973) (a term that can be defined as a close bond or connection in order to foster communication for establishing a mutual understanding), child psychiatrists and their mental health colleagues have become more visible on pediatric wards. Liaison work can be described as a form of pediatric live-in. The services must be readily available, predictable, and reliable in order to be seen as useful by pediatric colleagues. Unfortunately, however, the psychiatrist is still the provider and teacher, while the pediatrician is the recipient and student. Such an unequal relationship develops its own strains over time. The authors have found that liaison work must eventually move toward a more equal collaboration with pediatricians in order to feel comfortable and to endure.

Over the past ten years our liaison team has always received crucial support from the chairmen of pediatrics. But more recently several pediatricians have begun to work closely with us while maintaining their pediatric identity. This has enhanced our relevancy and acceptance among the pediatric house staff as no amount of psychiatric expertise could have done. The pediatricians present their points of view and develop their expertise among us, so that the child psychiatrist is again the recipient and the student. Thus, to be a good consultant, the authors have found, one must not only be a good teacher to pediatricians, but a conscientious learner from pediatricians. Collaboration with interested pediatricians who feel "equal" to us in the broad arena of psychosocial pediatrics may be one solution to the professional tensions that have so long plagued these two specialities (Eisenberg, 1967; Richmond, 1975).

BIBLIOGRAPHY

Anders TF: Child psychiatry and pediatrics: The state of the relationship. *Pediatr* 60(4):616–620, 1977.

Blom GE: The reactions of hospitalized children to illness. *Pediatr* 22:590–599, 1958.

Blotchy MJ and Grossman I: Psychological complications of childhood genito urinary surgery. *J Am Acad Child Psych* 17(3):488–497, 1978.

Bolian GC: Psychiatric consultation within a community of sick children. *J Am Acad Child Psych* 10:293–307, 1971.

Bowlby J: Childhood mourning and its implications for psychiatry. *Am J Psych* 118:481–498, 1961.

Eisenberg L: The relationship between psychiatry and pediatrics: A disputations view. *Pediatr* 39(5):645–657, 1967.

Geist RA: Consultation on a pediatric surgical ward: Creating an empathic climate. *Am J Orthopsych* 47(3):432–444, 1977.

Geist RA: Onset of chronic illness in children and adolescents. *Am J Orthopsych* 49(1):4–23., 1979.

Gofman H, Buckman W, and Schade G: The child's emotional response to hospitalization. *AMAJ Dis Child* 93:157–164, 1957.

Green M: Care of the dying child. *Care of the Child with Cancer*, Proceedings of a conference conducted by the Association for Ambulatory Pediatric Services in conjunction with the Children's Cancer Study Group A, on November 17, 1966, Bergman AB and Schulte CJA (eds.) 1966, pp 492–497.

Hackett TP: Beginnings: Liaison psychiatry in a general hospital. *MGH Handbook of General Hospital Psychiatry*, Hackett TP and Cassem N (eds) (CV Mosby: St. Louis) 1978.

Jellinek M: The hospitalized child: General considerations. *MGH Handbooks of General Hospital Psychiatry*, Hackett TP and Cassem N (eds.) (CV Mosby Co: St. Louis) 1978.

Johnson J and Warner R: Focused psychiatric curriculum selection: Student, psychiatrist, and nonpsychiatrist physician expectations. *Am J Psych* 134:1126–1130, 1977.

Klaus MH and Kennell JH: *Maternal-infant Bonding* (CV Mosby Co: St. Louis) 1976.

Langford WS: Physical illness and convalescence: Their meaning to the child. *J Pediatr* 33:242–250, 1948.

Mattsson A: Child psychiatric ward rounds on pediatrics. *J Am Acad Child Psych* 15(2):357–365, 1976.

Miller WB: Psychiatric consultation in the general hospital. *Psychiatric Treatment: Crises, Clinic, Consultation*, Rosenbaum CB and Beebe JE (eds.) (McGraw-Hill: New York) 1975, pp 472–495.

Miller WB: Special issues on consultation: The psychosocial interface. *Psychiatric Treatment: Crises, Clinic, Consultation*, Rosenbaum CB and Beebe JE (eds.) (McGraw-Hill: New York) 1975, pp 496–504.

Nadelson T: Psychiatric consultation in the hospital. *Psychiatric Annals* 8(4): 184–188, 1978.

Naylor KA and Mattsson A: For the sake of the children. *Psychiat Med* 4: 389–402, 1973.

Paykel ES, McGuiness B, and Gomez J: An anglo-American comparison of the scaling of life events. *Brit J Med Psychol* 49:237–247, 1976.

Powers GF: Humanizing hospital experiences: Presidential address. *Am J Dis Child* 76:365–379, 1948.

Poznanski ED, Cook SC, and Carroll BJ: A depression rating scale for children. *Pediatr* 64(4):442–450, 1979.

Prugh DG and Jordan K: Physical illness or injury: The hospital as a source of emotional disturbance in child and family. *Advocacy for Child Mental Health*, Berlin IN (ed.) (Brunner and Mazel: New York) 1975.

Richmond JB: An idea whose time has arrived. *Ped Clin NA* 22(3):517–523, 1975.

Rollins N: The treatment of anorexia nervosa. A paper presented to the 26th Annual Meeting of the American Academy of Child Psychiatry, Atlanta, GA, Oct 1979.

Sack W and Blocker DL: Who gets referred? Child psychiatry consultation in a pediatric hospital. *Int J Psych Med* 9(3–4):329–338, 1978–79.

Sack W, Cohen S, and Grout C: One year's survey of child psychiatry consultations in a pediatric hospital. *J Am Acad Child Psych* 16(4):716–727, 1977.

Schowalter J: On facing death: Perspectives of a child psychiatrist working in a medical school setting. Paper presented to the 25th Annual Meeting of the American Academy of Child Psychiatry, San Diego, CA, Oct 1978.

Schowalter J: Psychological reactions to physical illness and hospitalization in adolescence: A survey. *J Am Acad Child Psych* 16(3):500–516, 1977.

Schwab JJ: The psychiatric consultation: Part IJCE. *Psychiatry* 40(2):17–27, 1979.

Smith MD, McSweeney M, and Katz BM: Characteristics of death education curricula in American medical schools. *J Med Educ* 55:844–850, 1980.

Spitz RA: Hospitalism. *The Psychoanalytic Study of the Child I*, 1945, pp 53–74.

Stocking M, Rothney W, Grosser A, and Goodwin R: Psychopathology in the pediatric hospital. *Amer J Pub Health* 62:551–556, 1972.

Stillion J and Wass H: Children and death. *Death, Current Perspectives*, 2nd ed., Shneidman ES (ed.) (Mayfield Publishing Co: Palo Alto, CA) 1980.

7

Consultation with Highly Stressed Mental Health Professionals— The "Anchor Worker"

Susan M. Fisher and Irving Hurwitz

The discussion of supervision of highly stressed community workers is based on the effective prevention and treatment program for severely acting-out children established by the Child Psychiatry Department of the New England Medical Center in Boston. The primary therapeutic agent in the program, known as the Juvenile Delinquency Prevention Program, is the anchor worker, an individual whose role is to meet the multiple needs of children living in an economically deprived and socially unstable environment. The conceptual framework of this program regards most delinquency as a distinct clinical phenomenon, having significant intrapsychic pathology at its core originating in severe life-stress, and complicated by and interacting with deficits in the current social and educational systems in the child's life. The problem is viewed as one of ego failure at multiple levels, and as such, requires a comprehensive, creative approach that takes into account the deficits existing in both the defensive and adaptive aspects of the ego. To deal with these needs, the anchor worker is involved in virtually all aspects of the child's life including family, school, and community. He or she operates as a stabilizing force, promoting the development of

---

controls, the establishment of secondary-process functioning, and providing a sound identification model, anchoring or stabilizing, to whatever extent possible, the often chaotic, fluctuating, and erratically inconsistent conditions of life under which these children exist. Furthermore, the task implies coordinating and integrating the activities of the many agencies and institutions whose influences impinge on the lives of the children, beginning with the school and extending to social service resources, courts, the police, community, recreational agencies, and so forth. The project relies on independently formulated, self-generated strategies of intervention on the part of the anchor workers, each attempting to create as individualized a program for his or her case as possible.

THE REFERRED CHILD

The typical referred case was between the ages of 9 and 11, sent by the school for severe aggressive behavior involving peers and often teachers as well. Educational performance was generally two to three years below grade expectancy despite the fact of at least average intelligence. Many of the children had had previous psychiatric referrals, and diagnoses ranged from neurotic problems to severe ego fragmentation and borderline psychosis. The typical child was described as demonstrating perceptual motor problems, dyslexia, deficiency in basic skills, and showed low motivation for school work. Hyperactivity, distractability, and fighting were frequent complaints with impulsivity, provocation, and defiant behavior toward teachers occurring as repetitive themes. In peer relationships, the children vacillated between friendlessness and isolation, being teased and scapegoated, and relating by aggressiveness, picking fights, and assuming the facade of the unchallengeable tough guy.

The modal referral came from a chaotic home situation in which parental discord, abuse, fighting, alcoholism, unemployment and severe psychopathology were the rule. The families were multi-sibling with a loosely organized structure of caretaking, wherein household responsibilities were assigned among the children as frequently as among the adults. Personal hygiene was poor and the children were constantly described as unkempt, disheveled, dirty, or characterized in even stronger terms of personal distate by the teachers or other adults with whom they came into contact.

The children in this population suffered a wide range of physical illness including chronic upper respiratory infections, dental caries, gastrointestinal disturbances, enuresis, and other somatic disorders. Delinquent behavior covered a wide gamut of acting out including automobile theft, shoplifting, larceny, assault, and various drug related offenses.

There was an overwhelming characterization of the affective life of these children as depressed. In fact, of 53 baseline data reports in which affect is described, 44 of the children were identified in those terms. The remainder were described as fearful, withdrawn, or inhibited, terms which themselves may be substitutes for depression.

In the families, the children were subjected to harsh discipline often to the extent where not only was physical beating involved, but at times the parents expressed a wish and/or fear that they might kill the child. The parents' image of the child is constantly negative: he is seen as "bad," "evil," "crazy," "sexually abnormal," "stubborn," "a liar," etc. All of these comments conveyed the massive sense of rejection, alienation, and outright condemnation of these children as the embodiment of all that is unacceptable and intolerable in themselves and which served as the rallying point for their own frustrations and inadequacies. By the same token, the child's self-image is equally dysphoric and negative. They identify themselves as "a nothing," "helpless," "bad," "an idiot," "a clown," "an ugly buck-toothed freak."

The parents were also depressed, angry, often helpless people in their own self-characterization and felt incapable of managing the pressures of their own chaotic lives, their economic and social failure, and their feelings of rejection at the hands of social agencies and other institutions to whom they turned for help. Many of the parents were themselves physically ill, some quite seriously, so that available energy, even under positive conditions of motivation and desire to look after their children, was limited and even depleted.

In recognizing the importance of dealing with the stressful "here and now" in the lives of these children, the anchor worker begins with the fundamental issue, by active outreach and energetic engagement.

Clearly it can be seen that this is no small task. To provide these seriously damaged boys and girls with the opportunity, through the efforts of the anchor worker, to develop new psychological, social, educational, and community activity skills, involves a major investment of time, energy, and personal commitment.

IMPACT OF THE DELINQUENCY PREVENTION PROGRAM

In discussing the impact of the program, we shall first review the interaction between child and anchor worker, the influence of the program on the family and finally on institutions and agencies in the community. These comments are based on an analysis of the qualitative summaries maintained by the anchor workers in their week-to-week contacts with the children.

One of the significant variables to consider in an attempt to evaluate the impact of the program, is to describe the evolving nature of the relationship between the child and the anchor worker. The interaction was at the outset a highly positive one. The anchor worker was initially perceived as a potential and, indeed, actual gratifier (i.e., a "fun" person). However, as the relationship progressed, it passed through various stages of development in which the definition of the interaction underwent a number of significant alterations. The anchor worker was progressively identified as a counselor, a social worker, or a "shrink," without the necessity of any perjorative implication in the latter term. On the contrary, as a confidante and as someone possessing genuine empathy and understanding of the child, a feeling of support and protection began to crystallize in the child's attitude toward and perception of the worker. At the same time the limit-setting and controlling capacity of the anchor worker further refined the definition of his or her role, extending its positive significance to the child. This limit-setting process led to the emergence of notable ambivalence in the child, a process which could be considered as inevitable and posed significant possibilities for crisis in placing a strain on the anchor worker/ child relationship. However, this very tension or strain forged a more realistic understanding on the part of the child of the complex significance of the experience of being in the program. The shift that occurred was away from the more primitive or infantile good times or gratification-orientation toward the definition of the anchor worker's role and identity as more articulated and differentiated in terms of multiple therapeutic functions. The range of roles of the worker encompassed, in the later stages, that of a tension releaser, an external source of motivation for more positive and constructive attitudes and behaviors toward school, family and community, the source of a change in self-image and an accompanying rise in self-esteem. Eventually, a stabilization of the relationship took place with more reality oriented patterns of consistency in the underlying attachment despite surface variability. Positive effective involvement on both sides established a systematic therapeutic pattern.

From the standpoint of the families, the "positive outcome" cases in the group remaining in the program for two to four years, showed the parents becoming more responsive to the children's physical and emotional needs, achieving greater independence in the management of family issues, decline in such pathological behavior as drinking and sexual acting out, and a willingness to enter into collaborative interactions with the anchor worker in attempting to formulate strategies for dealing with their own and their children's problems. Parents were described as "having more insight into the nature of the child's problem," "a new ability to give active as well as emotional support to the child's expectations of a positive outcome to his life," "greater willingness by the parent to take the initiative in helping the child with school and social problems." The last observation is an especially important one since it emphasizes that the goal of the program is to shift the focus of initiative for change from the anchor worker to the parents and to the family itself. It seemed to represent a process of disengagement from dependency on the anchor worker to one of increased autonomy and self-direction.

Improvement in the children enrolled over a long period was described in terms of the emergence of greater self-assurance, confidence and self-esteem, a recognition of the "value of talking out problems rather than acting," and the ability to accept and internalize more secure limits and restraints. At the social level, there was observed a notable increase in the child's participation in community recreational resources such as boys clubs, summer camps, and the general willingness to participate in social activities within the neighborhood in groups not oriented toward antisocial goals or behaviors.

ANCHOR WORKER SELECTION AND ANCHOR WORKER TECHNIQUES

The methods of approach adopted by the anchor workers were variable and at times highly individualistic depending upon the philosophy and viewpoint of the anchor worker as to primary strategies and resources which could be utilized to formulate methods in the treatment approach. Such variability was to a significant extent supported by the very nature of the procedure by which anchor workers were selected and incorporated into the program. Few formal criteria existed or even now exist by which anchor workers were hired. Major factors included the age of the worker inasmuch as they had to be young and vigorous people with a strong sense of commitment to and an involvement in the process of working with difficult children. The mean age of anchor workers entering the program was 24. All were college graduates and the majority of the fourteen who have participated in the project in the initial six years of operation have had graduate work in a variety of fields including psychology, special education, social work, and sociology. Three had had experience as teachers in both conventional and special needs classes and the remainder had had extensive contacts with children in settings for the care of delinquent, retarded, or other special populations. The candidates were interviewed by the program director and one of the psychiatric consultants. The major criterion employed for selection was that the anchor worker be able to work independently and be capable of self-determined decision making in arriving at a plan of action either for an individual child or for the group of children assigned. This independence was organized around the supportive processes of supervision and consultation so that it existed within a framework of ongoing in-service training activities which provided the anchor worker with guidelines for his or her functioning in his or her therapeutic role. The approaches adopted by individual anchor workers were shaped by supervisory contacts, consultation, and case conferences, where a consistent conceptual framework was articulated. Within this context the anchor workers evolved their individual style and practical approach. This emphasis on independence and autonomy was extremely important since the anchor workers had the responsibility of dealing with a number of different community agencies which varied in their own attitudes and viewpoints toward the management of acting out children. Related to independence was the factor of diplomacy on the part of the anchor worker. They frequently found themselves operating in settings where there was distrust, suspicion, and even open hostility toward their goals and functions, and where the attitudes toward mental health efforts were openly challenging and antagonistic. The anchor worker had to be able to reconcile prejudices on the part of different community agencies and schools toward the families of the children in such a fashion as to enhance the degree of the institutions' sympathy, empathy, and understanding. A nonevaluative, nonjudgmental point of view was an essential attitude of the anchor worker role so that, despite the personal opinions and attitudes they might have toward specific practices and viewpoints that prevailed in these agencies, they often had to be adept in their ability not to take sides, a step which might compromise the best interests of their clients. An additional practical criterion for selection was the worker's willingness to commit long hours and severely taxing personal schedules to the implementation of their work. They were on "beeper" call 24 hours a day and had to have the requisite strength and patience to confront the multiple crises and problems that constantly arose. The choice of anchor workers was influenced by the sensitivity they conveyed to the ethnocultural issues of the community. Initially, the project involved primarily children of Irish–American Catholic background, living within a closely knit community with considerable internal cohesiveness and solidarity. Family, social, and neighborhood attitudes were rigidly defined and were characterized by a kind of insularity and provincialism. This placed a heavy burden on the tact and sensitivity of any new person entering this area, in order to insure maximal acceptance.

The worker frequently combined efforts with social workers in welfare and foster care agencies, representatives of the housing agencies and employment services to seek more adequate life conditions for the families involved. Often this entailed protracted and demanding efforts by the worker to arrange job interviews for parents, searching for apartments or obtaining repairs on housing in which the families currently lived. Once the step was taken to encompass the total family milieu in an environment so characterized by deprivation and stress, it was inevitable that multiple agency negotiations followed.

CONSULTATION AND SUPERVISION PROGRAM
FOR ANCHOR WORKERS

Anchor workers felt alone in their work. They functioned best using their own individual style and gifts in their interaction with the assortment of people and agencies in the child's life. The permission to be themselves, the lack of authoritarian expectations as to specific ways to perform, often combined with the solitariness of the enterprise to produce in the new worker feelings of floundering and a wish for a clear set of expectations, externally presented. In an ongoing, weekly, hour-and-a-half didactic group, the major initial task of the group leader was to confront and share the isolation that underlies complaints and demands for hard knowledge.

Consultation and supervision followed three major approaches.

1. Weekly conferences occurred, at which time the program director, psychiatric consultant and anchor worker staff met to review the intake or "baseline" material on new cases in order to pass on the appropriateness of referrals and to assign those cases that were accepted. These conferences also were the forum for discussion of the progress of cases that were already a part of the program, with emphasis on planning specific strategies, program revisions, formulation of diagnoses and psychological and psychosocial issues pertinent to the understanding of events in the lives of the children, and to assess the impact or effect of specific intervention procedures that were underway. The material discussed in these conferences was entered into the child's record in order that a continuous source of data would be available to monitor the planning and activities and to provide the basis for eventual review of the project for research purposes.

2. The second focus of training for the anchor worker in the delinquency prevention project was small discussion group conferences (2 to 3 workers) provided by senior staff from the department of child psychiatry.

3. The clinical issues brought to the third group which was ostensibly didactic in format, often, interestingly enough, repeated the exact clinical material brought up at the regular weekly case conferences where it *seemed* that they had been dealt with satisfactorily. In these sessions however, repetition brought with it the worker's statements of personal anxieties, doubts about his competence, and the questions he felt he had dared not ask earlier because of fear of compromising his own image or of challenging the authority

of the supervisory staff. This then frequently became a group issue and it was often possible to demonstrate parallels between the worker's feelings of rage, low status, competitiveness, helplessness before authorities in the program (usually unrealistic), and the feelings of their clients, the socially marginal population they serviced. The wish for an outer set of concrete rules and practical guidelines diminished and the workers were able to evolve a genuine sense of empathic awareness of those issues that were central to the needs and experiences of their clients.

This capacity to experience and yet objectify parallels, formed the basis for the specific steps articulated by the workers themselves in therapeutic interventions. For example, an anchor worker becomes deeply sensitized to the feelings of devaluation and lowered self-esteem experienced by a child in the classroom when the worker's own feelings of professional vulnerability are discussed in the group. The worker then can explain the meaning of the child's feelings to him or her and clarify their source and the possible management in more constructive alternatives in behavior. It is in a sense, bringing issues not unlike those involved in countertransference in traditional therapy to light in supervision, clarifying these and turning them back to the worker and client. Supervision makes it possible and is essential in order for the anchor worker to serve as a therapeutic agent who utilizes more than what can be accomplished on the basis of a relationship alone. It is clear that while the positive interaction between the child and the anchor worker is critical and necessary, it is not the sufficient condition to bring about the changes necessary to alter the behavior of the children. The consultation work bridges the areas of intrapsychic conflict, ego impairment, and the impact of the practices in the community institutions both on a theoretical and practical level for the anchor worker staff. The entire consultative process occurred against the backdrop of the relationship between the community based, less prestigious anchor worker program (Juvenile Delinquency Prevention Project) and the established, hospital-based child psychiatry department. Anchor workers frequently felt slighted and "low on the totem pole" within the establishment, while at the same time, they felt they did most of the hard work. The consultants were psychiatrists, frequently psychoanalysts, who, in several instances worked with anchor workers *rather than* with child psychiatry residents in their individual one-to-one encounters. Consultants, therefore, while they represented the ambivalently viewed establishment, also belonged to the anchor workers and had earned their trust. This complex mixture of roles, transference phenomenon (momentary displacements onto consultant) and realities made it possible in the group setting to sort out many feelings the anchor workers had. Just as important, however, the workers were able to see how their own feelings of being disregarded and disdained mirrored and echoed what their impoverished or helpless clients felt in the face of a complex welfare and mental health bureaucracy.

The consultants functioned for different workers in different ways. For some workers, they ultimately represented the ego ideal of the highest ambition and standards, and for some of this group, it reinforced their enthusiasm for further education (law school, medical school, social work school, and so forth); for others it elicited rivalrous feelings that were expressed and used didactically in the group to emphasize how their own clients may feel about the discrepancies between their social and educational level and that of the worker. For most workers, the consultant was a highly supportive, back-up person who would be available for crises with their clients and occasionally in their own personal lives. Because the anchor workers did not take responsibility for conventional psychotherapy, the consultant frequently acted as the bridge person to help the worker determine when the child was ready for (i.e., would profit from) the addition of regular, time-limited sessions with a child therapist in the usual outpatient treatment model, and serve to integrate this procedure with the specialized task of the anchor worker.

A CATALYST FOR INTEGRATION

The relationship with the consultant provided the literal and psychological space in which the various areas the anchor worker functioned in, areas that were so disparate, could come together and be reviewed, considered, and conceptualized in both theoretical and practical terms. It cannot be emphasized enough how alone the workers are, and how utterly dependent they are on their own resources—they have no offices, no professional spaces—it is this very flexibility that contributes to their fine results. In some way the consultant anchors *them* and promotes the integration of their complicated world of courts, welfare offices, schools, prisons, psychiatrist appointments, ego-alien and ego syntonic mechanisms, defenses, depression—areas of life and language they move in and out of—from the most concrete to the highest abstraction and metaphor.

BIBLIOGRAPHY

Aichorn A: *Wayward Youth* (Vanguard Press: New York) 1956.
Bandura A: *Aggression: A Social Learning Analysis* (Prentice Hall: Englewood Cliffs) 1973.
Berman AE: *Delinquency and Learning: A Neuropsychological Approach* (Unpublished Manuscript from Bradley Howe) 1976.

Eissler K (ed.): *Searchlights on Delinquency* (International Universities Press: New York) 1955.

Fisher S and Hurwitz I: Juvenile delinquency in girls. *The Woman Patient*, vol 3:Aggressions, Adaptations and Psychotherapy, Notman M and Nadelson C (eds.) (Plenum: New York), 1982.

Glueck S and Glueck E: *Physique and Delinquency* (Harper and Row: New York) 1956.

Hurwitz I, Makkay E, Monahan W, Fisher S, et al.: *Juvenile Delinquency: A Model for Prevention and Treatment of Acting Out Youth*, in press.

Kaufman I, Makkay ES, and Zilbach J: The impact of adolescense on girls with delinquent character formation. *Am J Anthrop* 29:1, 1959.

Kety S: Neurochemical aspects of emotional behavior. *Physiological Correlates of Emotion*, Black P (ed.) (Academic Press: New York) 1970.

Lewis DO: Diagnostic evaluation of the juvenile offender. *Child Psychiat Hum Devt* 6:198–213, 1976.

Masterson JF: *Treatment of the Borderline Adolescent: A Developmental Approach* (Wiley: New York) 1972.

Miller NE and Dollard R: *Frustration and Aggression* (Yale University Press: New Haven) 1948.

Redl F: *Children Who Hate* (The Free Press: Glencoe, IL), 1951.

Rutter M, Tizard J, and Whitman K: *Education, Health, and Behavior* (Longmans: London) 1972.

Warren MQ: The community treatment projects. *The Sociology of Punishment and Correction*, Johnson N, Savitz L, and Wolfgang ME (eds.) (Wiley and Sons: New York) 1970.

8

Consulting to a Rural Guidance Clinic

Joseph M. Green

Two maiden ladies, who had to some degree outlived their times, had a tomcat whom they loved and whose main joy in life seemed to be roaming the neighborhood at night. He would return in the morning, usually mangled, torn, and bloody from a fight. Their concern increased as the cat grew older, and they finally consulted their veterinarian as to whether there wasn't something the vet could do to stop these dangerous and violent tendencies. The vet said he could perform an operation which should take care of the problem and it was agreed. The tomcat returned home after a short period of convalescence, but the ladies were chagrined to discover that he continued to roam the neighborhood at night. However, he no longer returned bloody and bruised. They consulted the vet and reminded him of his failed prognosis. His response: "The only explanation I can offer is that he must be acting as a consultant." Such is the responsibility and authority of a consultant. He advises but often avoids the heat of battle. He has little actual authority, and as is often true of the parents of adolescent children, his influence is dependent on his moral suasion and the consultee's acceptance of his sagacity.

In practice, a child psychiatrist working in a rural mental health center generally alternates his role between that of consultant and that of medical director for children's services.

CONSULTANT

Let's speak first of the consultant's hat. If the consultant is to be effective, he must identify with the agency and get to know the community through the eyes of the agency. Rural clinics function within a tight system. The agency staff must identify with the community in order to be effective, and the consultant identifies with the community through staff members. The importance of maintaining the relationship to the agency over a long period of time cannot be overestimated.

It takes a while before the consultant is accepted into the system in a small town. As the consultant becomes known, his or her usefulness to the clinic increases and the experience becomes more gratifying as interpersonal relationships develop. Too often, however, consultation is merely an income supplement for the child psychiatrist to buy groceries while he is building a private practice. As his private practice grows, the consultation to the agency, which usually is less financially lucrative and may require commuting to an urban center, is passed on to the next newcomer. I would suggest that the private practitioner hold tenaciously to at least one day each week out of his office, out of town, and away from his practice. Private practice becomes very lonely and as his practice grows, the practitioner will welcome the change of pace provided by out-of-town consultation. The couple of hours of pastoral scenery without demands that the commute affords becomes one of those all-too-few times in a week which can be devoted to one's own thoughts about patients and to self. The private practitioner rarely has an opportunity to talk to anyone professionally. Listening and talking to consultees about their patients becomes a very educational experience. (Continuing Medical Education credits should be allowed.)

In developing a rural consultation at which child psychiatry trainees would spend one day each week for a year and then be succeeded by the next fellow, we felt it important to provide a long-term, consistent consultant figure as well, with whom the staff of the clinic could identify as the fellows came and went. It was decided that a University of Wisconsin faculty member would go to the clinics with the fellow one day each month as a permanent assignment. The fellow provides a valuable consultant service and much enthusiasm to the clinic staff, but the faculty member has become the consultant known in the larger community and through whom the community agencies relate to the fellow.

In one such small clinic, there had been considerable competitiveness and lack of cooperation between the county social service department and the clinic staff. Their responsibilities overlapped but their services were not integrated. When this consultant began his visits, the county social service department occasionally referred a patient for evaluation. The purpose of the evaluation was usually unclear, the problems were extremely difficult, and it almost looked as though the consultant was being "set up" to provide service of little value.

In an early consultation, arrangements had been made for him to meet with a child living in a foster home, his mother and his stepfather. He was asked to determine in an hour whether these parents were capable of good parenting and should have their child returned to them. The social service worker picked up the child in his foster home and delivered him to the clinic, where his mother and stepfather were sitting in the waiting room. It turned out that because of suspicion of child abuse, the child had been suddenly removed from the family six weeks earlier by being picked up at school and delivered to a temporary foster home. The child had not seen his mother since, and as might be imagined, there was quite an emotional scene in the waiting room. The mother was eager to cooperate because she wanted her child back home; she was also obviously joyous to see her child again after six weeks. The child, a boy of nine, had so much to tell his mother that he could not possibly respond to questions from an examiner. When the examiner suggested that the parents might go to another office and talk with a social worker, he became even more upset. The child perceived this as another separation from his mother, and the evaluation was limited to confirming a high degree of separation anxiety, which was hardly news to anyone.

It became a useful consultation, however, because the county social worker was invited and willing to become involved in direct cotherapy rather than referral and report. The consultannt became respectful of the social service worker's devotion to protecting the child and her ability to conciliate and negotiate with a hostile and threatening stepfather. The social service worker became respectful of the consultant's ability to help set goals and contracts to expedite the reunification of the family and the consultant's genuine wish to include the social service worker as a cotherapist, along with a clinic social worker, in exploring the family's problems.

As a result of several such cases, the social service worker began bringing patients and families to the consultant for mutual evaluative sessions and discussions, rather than sending them to the clinic on a referral. The worker now felt that she was getting meaningful help from the clinic. The clinic was delighted with its improved relationship with the county social service department and continuously tried to involve both the social service worker and the social worker/therapist of the mental health center in families in whom they had a common interest.

An important function of the child psychiatry consultant is to evaluate patients for a staff member. This is a different function than evaluating for the court or other agencies because the staff member remains the primary therapist. It is extremely important that the consultant does not usurp the primary therapist's relationship with his or her patient and maintains the role of consultant to the therapist, as well as to the patient. Most consultants would agree there is too little time to become directly involved in psychotherapy with patients and that his time is much more usefully spread out among several consultees. The consultant has both a clinical and an educative role. In his educative function, he offers to the consultee a different perspective with new ideas and options about treatment, rather than the final perspective. The latter seems to stifle creative therapeutic endeavor and is condescending to the consultee.

Time may be well spent consulting to the general psychiatrist, who may assume the responsibility for all clinic patients including children, even though he does not feel quite competent in treating children and wishes to talk over cases. The educative function may be further elaborated by assisting as a cotherapist, while other staff members observe through a one-way mirror. The following week the consultant may join those observing and discuss the conduct of the interview held with the patient.

In one small town clinic known to this consultant, there was a once-a-month community meeting (rural "grand rounds") to which all of the people involved in human services in the small community were invited. The policemen, a couple of teachers, the juvenile court probation officer, two ministers of different faiths, child-care workers from a local group home, an older retired gentleman with a Ph.D. (can't remember in what), and the clinic staff members gathered and discussed a general mental health problem with the consultant. The consultant became known to the community, who then availed themselves of his services, through the clinic. The clinic became the local center for mental health educational activities and the exchange of psychiatric ideas, in addition to its clinical functions.

Administrative consultant roles can be usefully filled by the child psychiatrist. Frequently, the director of a small town clinic is the person who was the best therapist on the staff but had had little administrative experience. The consultant can usefully advise from his experiences with the larger health delivery system. He may provide an objective view of the problems faced by an administrator in this small town setting that have to do with ethnic differences, cultural biases, and the larger integration of socioeconomic classes that takes place in a rural clinic.

In small towns, confidentiality becomes an even more important issue than in a large city clinic. The general conception of small town life is correct; people do know much more about each other's business. There is no private-practicing child psychiatrist available to families in most of these areas, so the more prominent, middle-class families, who in a larger city would go to a private practicing child psychiatrist, become clients of the clinic. They may expect special treatment. A parent may be a member of the board of the clinic or a supervisor on the county board which allocates funds to the clinic. In such a case, the clinical staff is understandably reluctant to become involved with the family on an intimate basis, and the family receives special treatment by default—no one other than the consultant is willing to treat them. The consultant becomes the VIP who treats the VIPs. In this capacity, he ceases to be a consultant and becomes a staff member.

The medical establishment is a necessary and useful adjunct to rural clinics and the consultant often bridges the interdisciplinary gap between the social workers in the clinical and the primary-care physicians in the community. The child psychiatrist-consultant adds respectability to the clinic and the primary-care physicians have more confidence in the clinic when they know the psychiatrist is involved in the treatment process there. It is a useful technique to involve the local physicians in any prescription of medications to patients from the clinic. Rather than to himself give the family a prescription for stimultants, this consultant prefers to call the local doctor and suggest that he place the child on medication. The physician thus becomes involved with the clinic and with the primary therapist at the clinic. The local physician is also involved and available if there is a reaction to the medication. This procedure is also in keeping with the role of consultant to advise, rather than assume the role of medical director to treat and to assume patient responsibility.

As is true in any consultation, the contract needs to be clear. What does the agency want of the consultant? What do they ask? What do they need? Is the consultant hired to fill a need of the staff or is he hired to meet certain bureaucratic regulations imposed by the board or, more likely, by the state government? His presence may raise the credibility of the clinic to those who appreciate quality of services but will his services, in fact, raise the overall quality of services and not merely the image of the clinic?

Since resources in a rural setting are much more limited than in a center of population, a much more creative use of those resources which are offered by the school and the court and the social agencies becomes a challenge to the consultant. Because he has a more objective view of and distance from the community than its staff members, he can more easily avoid embroilment in the interagency competition and channel those resources in an imaginative way. The competition between agencies in a rural community is much more personal than in the city and the complaining about colleagues is also much more personal. The gripes are about an individual rather than a system or a professional group. In the city they talk about the school nurse. In the country they talk about Wilma Clark.

MEDICAL DIRECTOR FOR CHILDRENS' SERVICES

As was suggested by the tomcat story, the consultant has little actual authority. The consultees are free to accept or reject his advice, although if they consistently reject, the consultant had best look for a different agency on which to bestow his wisdom. If the consultant accepts responsibility for the patient, is he still a consultant or has he become medical director? A small town clinic cannot usually afford to hire both a consultant and a staff child psychiatrist. Therefore, in addition to the above-mentioned duties of a consultant, one must also sometimes assume the role of medical director for childrens' services.

This will require expert diagnostic evaluations for other agencies, usually the court or the schools. The child psychiatrist likely is the most expert professional available to these agencies and his evaluations will build confidence in the clinic. Unless he wants to do all of the work himself, the medical director will avoid giving the implication that only the doctor is entitled to an expert opinion. Rather, he will involve a primary mental health clinician in the evaluation process whenever possible. He will strengthen his efforts to involve the primary clinician, as well as save himself many long-distance phone calls, if he avoids seeing any patient before that patient has seen a regular staff member of the clinic. In other words, he will not do any "intake interviews" and each patient will have a case manager who has already completed an initial interview before the patient sees the consultant.

Custody disputes will frequently be passed along to the consultant-medical director. In the cities, these will more likely involve visitation rights and custody after divorce. In the country, they will more often involve removal of the child from his or her family and temporary placement in a foster home. Juvenile and family court judges, even in the more sophisticated large city court systems, frequently have little training to help them to make these judgments. In a rural district, where the judge is handling cases of all kinds, he has even less expertise on which to make such a judgment. Most consultant child psychiatrists will only become involved in custody disputes if they are appointed by the judge as a "friend of the court." Particularly, when they represent a mental health center, they will avoid being engaged by one or the other parent's lawyer in the dispute. This becomes particularly difficult if one parent is or has been a patient of the clinic. Then the strong possibility of bias exists, but there may be no other expert for the court to engage. The psychiatrist representing the agency will certainly take pains to avoid letting the clinic become known as an agency which removes children from their parents, or future requests for services from parents will drastically diminish.

Evaluation for medication becomes an important part of the medical director's role in a rural clinic. Not only will he determine whether a child requires medication, but he also must play an educative role with the staff as to the appropriate role medication plays and the side effects about which one must be concerned. As mentioned above, there are decided advantages in involving the local physicians in this process.

Essentially the consultant is the expert and since he comes from out of town, he will occasionally be called upon to evaluate and treat a member of the staff who is having problems. One would probably not choose to do this in a city clinic where outside referrals are more easily achieved. In the rural clinic it can be done with tact and compassion and need not necessarily compromise one's effectiveness as consultant to other staff members. It does require, of course, a careful and continuing distinction between consultation and therapy.

ARE THE CLIENTELE DIFFERENT IN A RURAL CLINIC FROM OTHER CLINICS?

Middle-class therapists are often as out of touch with local socioeconomic and ethnic cultural factors in a small town as they are with those in an inner-city ghetto. The differences however, while psychologically as great, are much more subtle and less easily differentiated in the rural setting. Many of us enjoy fantasies about the bucolic life; few enjoy fantasies about ghetto life. The differences in life-style for children on a farm, as opposed to children in a city, is enormous. The child on the farm comes home from school and has several hours of chores to accomplish. These chores may allow the child to feel for himself an important role in his family; they may bring him closer to an appreciation of animal life. But they hamper his socializing with peers and put him at a social disadvantage with the town kids with whom he attends a consolidated high school. After the farm child has finished his chores, he goes in the house and joins his family more often than he goes out to join friends. Concepts of life and death are different (and more meaningful, probably) to the farm child because of his exposure to birth and death among the animals. One therapist spoke of the experience of an adopted boy among her clients who told of watching the birth of a calf. He had seen this process before; usually the mother cow licks off the calf, nudges it, encourages it to feed, and is protective. On this one occasion, he observed the mother cow walking away from her calf and the farmer having to find another cow to "adopt" the calf and raise it. Contemplate the fertile therapeutic field this discussion opened.

The consultant, in discussing family therapy and roles of family members with the staff in a rural clinic, will find their perceptions are somewhat different than those of the urban families around which he was trained. There is a great lack of anonymity among families in rural areas. The need for confidentiality was mentioned earlier. The limitations of social life in a rural community must be borne in mind in treating and understanding rural families. The differences between the life-styles of farm children and city children must be kept in mind in advising parents, especially as they are different from child rearing patterns in the consultant's own experience. There is a much more spontaneous follow-up and follow-along of families by the staff of rural clinics. People are less transient in the country. Perhaps this is why visitation and custody battles between divorced parents are less common. This also becomes apparent in school consultations. The teacher in a rural school knows the family history and knows the strengths of the various family members. When a staff member from the clinic goes to school to talk about a child, several members of the school team are likely to know that child and family. Families are frequently known to the staff of the clinic, including the secretaries, which complicates problems of confidentiality.

In some ways people in rural areas appear sicker. Their pathology is more grossly portrayed because of the lack of anonymity. A farmer beats a cow to death. An adolescent boy has sexual relations with an animal. These may be secret confessions to a therapist in a rural clinic by clients who are concerned about their impulses or lack of control. In the city, these persons would be observed and picked up by authorities, and might secondarily get to a therapist.

There are frequently pockets of pathology or systems of pathology with which the consultant has contact in a rural clinic, but with which he would not become involved if he worked at a mental health service in an urban area. This consultant recalls one "community of craziness" which existed in a trailer camp and was well known to the neighborhood surrounding the trailer camp. The first requests for service came from the neighbors and efforts were ineffective and not very enthusiastic. Later, when a grassroots demand for services came from members of the trailer camp, a useful mental health intervention resulted.

Churches are much more visible in small towns and they are more competitive with each other. The ministers are very much involved in mental health counseling. One clinic area, for example, included a town of 5,000 people with 22 churches. The larger county area served by this clinic and 100 clergymen and only 17 social workers available to the population. Ministers frequently mistrust the mental health agency because they feel they have not been included in the agency's evaluation and therapeutic intervention. Mental health workers often mistrust clergy and do not consider them colleagues in counseling. Referrals will be much more carefully made if the clinic attempts to educate the local clergy on the services the clinic can and cannot offer to the members of their congregations. They may well subsequently be able to offer some case supervision to the clergymen, who are usually not well trained for their counseling duties. This consultant found an annual ten-hour seminar series with clergymen to provide a valuable tool by which the clinic improved the quality of its referrals, the acceptance of its services, and the follow-up of its results.

Travel distances to avail oneself of services become a more important factor in rural clinics. There is no public transportation, and patients often have to drive long distances to the clinic building. Transportation availability and costs become a valid problem and not just a resistance to therapy.

ARE THE STAFF DIFFERENT IN A RURAL CLINIC FROM OTHER CLINICS?

Some staff members seek out small town or rural clinics because they prefer the professional isolation that such working sites provide. They will generally not welcome expert consultants. Other staff members choose the employment in a rural setting because they prefer the life-style affordable by open spaces and small town culture. They will initially keep some distance from the consultant and require the consultant to prove himself. When they are satisfied the consultant is not contemptuous of the rural scene, they will welcome the professional stimulation. There are others who much prefer city life and have accepted the small town working scene because only there can they find employment. These staff members will generally welcome and embrace the consultant from the city because they feel professionally isolated and embarrassed about their work place. They are usually less valuable workers in the community than those who have chosen it as a place to live, and they see their jobs as temporary. This is particularly true if they live in the city and commute to the rural setting. It takes time to become credible in any professional setting. It is particularly difficult to become credible if one lives in the city and descends on the clinic periodically rather than live in the town which the clinic serves.

Sometimes the professional behavior of the displaced worker, while appropriate in his or her desired working place, is inappropriate in the rural setting. An example comes to mind in which a bright and bouncy young lady, who had just received her master's degree in guidance and counseling, had taken a position in a rural clinic 100 miles from the city and the university. She continued to live in the city, spending only three nights each week in the clinic community. When the local high school asked the clinic if it could provide a speaker on the drug problem to the student body, the clinic director chose this new member of the staff, feeling that she was most knowledgeable about drugs, having just come from the university, and that it would be a good way for her to be introduced to the community. The new staff member, wanting to be accepted by the high school students, arrived at the high school for her seminar wearing sandals, a halter without a bra, and with a bandana on her head. She would not have been noticed at the university; the same could not be said at the high school. She gave a realistic talk about the dangers and nondangers of drug use, seeking to get people to explore and set priorities on their options. She was reasonably credible to the students, which made her presentation much more valuable than would have been an exposé of the evils of marijuana, but she so offended the teachers and administration of the high school by her appearance and manner, that for a time they were unwilling to have any dealings with the clinic. The damage had to be repaired by other staff members. The consultant, had he been asked, could have predicted the setback. The community is less tolerant of "strange lookers" and "loose livers" than are people in the city, and it does not serve the interests of clients if the staff insist on offering such models to the community. The role expectation of the doctor is much more clear in rural settings than in urban settings.

In rural clinics, as in ghetto clinics, there are more likely to be staff members performing functions for which they have not completed formal training than is true in clinics serving urban, middle-class populations. It generally seems to be true that the less training the staff members have had, the less use they will make of a child psychiatry consultant, and the more defensive they will be about the usefulness of formal training or their lack of same. They may be very respectful but do not feel very needful.

A teacher who was a referral source to a rural clinic, in commenting about the clinic, noted that she "appreciated the consideration we are given when referring a child. When I refer someone, I want to be able to suggest a therapist by name based on my knowledge of her expertise and the fact that the therapist will take the case." This will give the therapeutic endeavor a great initial boost, but the personalized referral is not often possible in an urban clinic. It may more than make up for the lack of specialized therapists in the rural clinics, where more likely all clinicians see all kinds of clients.

CONCLUSION

Everybody wants to see the doctor, and the doctor must always keep the primary therapist in touch with the patient. His role as consultant is as an expediter of therapy, a clarifier of dynamics, a voice of authority on the clinic opinions to other agencies and referral sources, a mediator of interdisciplinary disputes, a contact to centers of professional creativity and inventiveness, and a model to consultees.

A few suggestions are offered here for the prospective consultant to a rural clinic:

1. Don't come on as the expert to the staff; save that for the public who appreciates it.

2. Don't be too particular about the kinds of problems you are willing to see; there's probably no one else around who is better qualified than you to see them.
3. Attempt to make personal contact with each member of the extended family to whom the clinic offers consultation and evaluation services. Not only will your service be more useful, but your personal gratification in your work will be increased through the relationships.
4. Be aware that you are always setting a model as to how to relate to troubled people.
5. Play to stay awhile.

BIBLIOGRAPHY

Caplan G: *The Theory and Practice of Mental Health Consultation* (Basic Books: New York) 1970.
Caplan G: *Principles of Preventive Psychiatry* (Basic Books: New York) 1964.
Faguet R, Fawzy F, Wellisch D, and Pasnau R (eds.): *Contemporary Models in Liaison Psychiatry* (Spectrum: New York) 1978.
Pasnau R: *Consultation-Liaison Psychiatry* (Grune and Stratton: New York) 1975.

9

Consultation in Outpatient Settings

Norbert B. Enzer

In his survey of pediatric training programs, Anders (1977) found that services provided by child psychiatrists in these programs were significantly greater in the inpatient setting than in ambulatory settings. While this would seem in keeping with the history of consultative liaison psychiatry, it does seem contrary to a sense of the general need. In contrast, Lewis (1978) reported that of 128 child psychiatric consultations during a three-month period, the largest number of requests emanated from a primary care center.

Whatever the pattern, the ambulatory setting can be a fruitful area of consultation and collaboration between pediatrics, family practice, and child psychiatry. It is interesting and perhaps somewhat puzzling that until quite recently so little emphasis has been placed on this area of interaction within training programs, both in pediatrics, and in child psychiatry. Though one cannot minimize the concerns about the psychological issues in the hospitalized child, almost irrespective of the reasons for hospitalization, neither should the needs of the child or adolescent outpatient be ignored, nor should the educational opportunities.

Throughout medical education, the value of experiences in outpatient or ambulatory settings has been more apparent in recent years. The emphasis on inpatient work and on complex biomedical problems was a long standing tradition in American medical education. Large university medical centers which focused on tertiary care have provded settings in which students and residents could work alongside highly trained specialists and subspecialists. For some time following the end of World War II, these physicians, their clinical activities, their investigative work, and the problems presented by their patients captured the imagination of residents and students alike. However, in the last few decades, technological advances as well as some apparent changes in values have altered both the training and practice of medicine considerably. Whether in response to the pressures of public policy, particularly at the federal level, or to changes in less defined sociocultural values and attitudes, there has been an apparent growing interest in primary care practice, and in care settings other than the large general hospital. Clearly, there has been a growth in primary care training programs and greater emphasis on training in ambulatory care.

In the area of child health care, antibiotics, immunization, and other advances, along with shifting patterns of illness, have altered the indications for hospitalization dramatically. Concurrently, there has been a growing awareness of and interest in ambulatory care and chronic illness and a greater recognition of the potentially noxious influences of psychological and social factors on the growth and development of children and families. The report of the Task Force on Pediatric Education (1978) placed high priority on the importance of these factors in the spectrum of child health needs and strongly suggested increased training emphasis on knowledge and skill to address these needs. The President's Commission on Mental Health (1978), the Graduate Medical Education National Advisory Committee (1980) and the Select Panel for the Promotion of Child Health (1981) have all recognized the enormous unmet needs in the broad area of child mental health.

Over many decades, the decline of the extended family and geographic mobility of many families have created a situation in which primary care physicians are often seen as a resource regarding all aspects of infant and child care, even in matters in which they may have no unique knowledge or expertise. Books, newspaper columns, and television have expanded the potential influence of physicians beyond the consulting room and provide a means for physicians to offer advice, and in some cases, knowledge about child development, rearing, nutrition, preventive medicine, emergency care, and the treatment of illness. It is striking to note the prominence of psychosocial issues in so many of these presentations.

While there may be some general ambivalence regarding the medical profession, the public seems to view *their* pediatrician or family physician as an expert, and to seek advice about almost any matter which relates directly or indirectly to children.

Throughout this century, there has been a growing sensitivity to the needs of children and an expansion of the resources in the community. While even today, many needs remain unmet and some have pointed to trends in public policy and attitudes, growing resistance to taxation and dissatisfaction with government at all levels, including school boards, as indicating a lack of commitment to the needs of children, there are growing numbers of individuals, and both public and private agencies which do offer some assistance and profess some expertise regarding the development of children and their emotional and social needs. Nevertheless, physicians continue to have a prominent place in the minds of many, and for many are the first contact. Perhaps there is a greater sensitivity in parents to these issues and lacking a knowledge of other community resources, parents may turn to the physician. However, it may be equally likely that the physician is consulted because families do believe that there is a special expertise or comprehensiveness in the physician which they value. Furthermore, because so many children and parents have had contact with physicians through well-baby care and the treatment of the usual illnesses of young children, the physician may continue as the natural focus for questions and the concerns of families.

Just as there have been shifts in general health care of children and adolescents and in the training patterns, so too have there been changes in child psychiatry. In the recent past there has been a highly significant expansion of consultation–liaison training and a greater interest in the medical problems of children and adolescents. Where formerly much of child psychiatry training took place in child guidance clinics or rather strictly psychiatric settings, often rather isolated from general health care settings and training programs, currently there is a trend toward a greater involvement in general hospitals and clinics.

Historically, child psychiatry has had broad involvements with many social and community agencies, but the presence within the general health care system has been very limited in many areas. Even with the growth of interest in consultative-liaison child psychiatry, it would appear that most of the emphasis in consultation training has occurred in the inpatient setting and the focus has been upon the hospitalized child. Recently, there has been a growing interest in ambulatory settings and the nonhospitalized child. This development seems to parallel changes in pediatric training and the growth of family medicine.

In the practice settings, the relationships between pediatricians and family physicians on one hand and child psychiatrists on the other may vary greatly and depend on a wide variety of factors, including the quality of the personal relationships. Obviously, there are all too many circumstances in which no relationship exists and in which such an opportunity is very limited. In some communities, there are simply no child psychiatrists. In others, the child psychiatrist may be fully occupied in situations which decrease the likelihood of interactions with those physicians who provide primary health care to the children and to families. The child psychiatric director of an inpatient treatment center for children may be quite unavailable to the rest of the medical community.

Where there is some access to child psychiatrists, pediatricians and family physicians may have a variety of expectations and the professional services provided by the child psychiatrist may take several forms. Often these interactions are quite different from those experienced by both the primary care physician and the child psychiatrist during their years of training.

This chapter addresses the consultative work of the child psychiatrist within the health care system exclusive of the inpatient setting of the hospital. The principle focus will be on the consultative relationship with primary care physicians. For the purpose of this discussion all requests for professional assistance directed to child psychiatrists from individual physicians short of actual referral for care will be considered consultative. Many interactions with groups of physicians or others are best viewed as liaison activities or continuing medical education and will not be specifically addressed in this chapter. Certainly these activities have expanded considerably in recent years and though not within the scope of this discussion, they should be noted as an important part of professional life because of the potential for the communication of knowledge and skill, but also because they provide an arena in which professional relationships can be established which can influence the direct care provided to children and families, and an opportunity to influence professional behavior which can indirectly affect the care of children.

Possibly one of the more difficult roles for the child psychiatrist is that of consultant within the ambulatory health care system. Perhaps this is simply a reflection of the lack of emphasis in training. However, it may be that the very nature of child psychiatric training has created a tendency on the part of many child psychiatrists to suggest referral rather than to work with a consultee toward resolution of problems. It may be that it is often easier, more convenient or more rewarding to suggest referral than to devote the effort to consultation. But the patterns of professional life may also complicate and limit the interactions. For the most part, both in training and in practice, primary care physicians have very busy offices or clinics with large numbers of patients seen for a relatively short period of time. Visits are often very brief and even the moments between patient contacts are consumed with record keeping and telephone calls. Though contacts may be brief, they occur repeatedly and primary care physicians tend to accumulate a developmental perspective of the child and family over time. Decisions regarding both the nature of psychosocial problems and interventions frequently need to be made within the context of time pressures and the demands of more urgent medical problems.

Child psychiatrists, on the other hand, see fewer patients for longer periods of time and are accustomed to developing the history of both the child and the family in a highly comprehensive way at the time of referral for a specific problem. Interventions, particularly during training are often conceived in a more leisurely fashion and are less influenced by the pressures of time. Such differences in style may create a situation in which collaboration between child psychiatrists and primary care physicians is difficult. However, other factors may also interfere with the child psychiatrists' ability and willingness to remain in the role of consultant and work through others in the ambulatory health care setting. It may well be that consultation within that setting is viewed as different from consultation to schools or other agencies which may have been part of the training experience of the child psychiatrist. More often such activities, whether during the training years or after, are rather clearly defined in terms of specific hours, reimbursements, the focus and nature of the consultative activities and the individuals involved over time. Such may not be the case with other health professionals, particularly in the ambulatory setting. In hospitals where there are established child psychiatry consultation-liaison services, child psychiatrists participate in formal, direct case consultations in response to the requests of physicians and can be reimbursed directly for such services. In these settings liaison work with housestaffs, nurses, or other defined groups are also frequent. In such activities, the issues addressed may vary but they are usually limited by the setting and defined by the group of consultees and the consultant in a more or less formal and often predictable way. Such activities of a child psychiatrist are not directly supported by patient fees but rather by prior agreements with the institution. Child psychiatrists who function in these inpatient consultation-liaison roles develop relationships with the physicians and other hospital personnel which facilitate the consultative mode of functioning. Often there is a regularity and frequency which aids in understanding and some reasonable degree of consistency.

However, in many situations beyond the inpatient units of hospitals and their defined personnel, consultative activities may be more difficult to define and maintain. While the consultative problems of ambulatory patients may be no more or less complex, they may present uncertainties and complexities which are less apparent in the hospital. The familiarity with physicians, nurses, and other unit personnel and the regularity of contact which is so helpful to hospital-based consultation, may be lacking with outpatients. Clearly, this lack of regularity and familiarity can pose significant difficulties in the ambulatory area. The capacity to have a reasonable level of control over the immediate hospital environment may be a great asset in working with the hospitalized child. However, with the outpatient the capacity to control or influence the environment may be far more complex and limited.

There is a tenuous quality to consultative work outside of the hospital setting. While in any consultation activity there is no assurance that the perspectives or suggestions of a consultant will be accepted and implemented, at least within the hospital there is a ready opportunity for continuing interaction between consultant and the consultee and others involved. That continuity is often more difficult to maintain in the ambulatory setting. The level of confidence between the consultant and the consultee is especially critical.

Throughout the entire medical care system, physicians are accustomed to various levels of mutual assistance. It is a long standing tradition, and indeed a part of the ethical behavior of physicians, to ask for assistance and to provide it when asked. Interaction between child psychiatrists and primary care physicians occur at several levels and each has its own unique opportunities and limitations.

INFORMAL CONSULTATIONS

Informal consultations may be quite casual and may take place at times of chance contacts in common meeting places such as the halls or lounges of a hospital or over the telephone. Request for assistance may not even be identified as consultative by either party. Physicians may share their views with each other regarding various aspects of their knowledge, skill, and judgments. Exchange may involve experience with particular treatment approaches, the results of evaluation procedures, a particular pattern of symptoms, responses in a particular patient, or more general issues. Such informal consultation does not involve a direct contact between the consultant and the patient or other persons who may be the focus of the concern of the consultee. However, just as other physicians may be asked to review an X ray or the report of some other evaluation procedure, the child psychiatrist may be asked to comment upon or clarify a report of psychological studies or an intervention plan developed by a school. These "informal consultations" are often difficult to respond to. The consultee often presents such requests in a manner that implies that a brief answer is sufficient and that a full recitation of the situation is not necessary. Though the specific content may vary considerably, the consultee seems to be seeking some rather immediate reassurance or a quick answer to a brief question. Pediatricians may inquire about a child psychiatrist's experience with a new drug or an opinion about the effectiveness of a particular community intervention program. But complex situations may also be presented in an abbreviated way.

Informal consultations often arise out of prior relationships between primary care physicians and child psychiatrists. The assistance is provided without compensation and more often there is no written record of the exchange. At times, informal consultation may seem quite limited or even trivial.

In one informal consultation, a pediatrician sought the comments of a child psychiatrist regarding the very recent death of a two-year-old child. The exchange occurred in the hallway. The physicians were friends and had worked together with several patients and in planning a new clinical service. Though the contact was brief, the pediatrician indicated that a two-year-old child who lived in her neighborhood had died very suddenly two days before. The child had not been her patient but the pediatrician was aware that the cause of death appeared to be infectious and that there was no suspicion of child abuse. Many of her neighbors had approached the pediatrician seeking her advice about dealing with their own childrens' reactions to the tragedy.

The pediatrician indicated that she felt inclined to suggest that the parents deal with their children in an open and honest manner and that they encourage discussion and that they consider having the children attend funeral services. She felt that approaching this situation much as she had done with families in her own practice when there had been a death was most appropriate. She said a meeting of neighborhood parents at her home was already planned for that evening. Having observed a situation in which this pediatrician had dealt effectively with the death of one of her own patients, the child psychiatrist responded supportively and offered to be available if the pediatrician felt she needed further assistance.

Though, in this example, the child psychiatrist's role was very minimal, such situations do arise with some frequency. This pediatrician did not seem to need advice but the concurrence of the child psychiatrist and the offer of back-up were reassuring. The importance of such support should not be minimized. Aside from confirming that the pediatrician's views were appropriate and that she posed the necessary skills to manage the situation, the interaction may lead to further confidence in dealing with other situations and with the consultative process in the future.

In another situation, a pediatrician spoke to a child psychiatrist over the telephone regarding a six-year-old boy with frequent enuresis. The pediatrician indicated that several simple interventions, awakening the child to urinate, withholding fluids after supper, and the like had been tried with no success. The pediatrician felt that there was no need for an extensive urological evaluation but did report that the child's mother was greatly concerned about the possibility of a bladder problem. The specific reason for the call was to inquire about the advisability of using one of the electric alarm devices which are activated by urine. In discussing the situation even briefly, it became apparent that a conflict between the parents existed. The mother repeatedly asked about urological consultation, and the father felt the symptoms did not warrant such an approach and that the boy would grow out of it. Further, it emerged that the child was often very upset and fearful when the parents left him with a baby-sitter. Over the phone, the pediatrician and the child psychiatrist concluded that there was more to the problem and the psychiatric evaluation was appropriate. It was agreed that the pediatrician would meet with the parents and first, reassure them that he saw no need for urological evaluation; second, help the parents recognize that there were other symptoms which suggested internal psychological problems; and third, that their divergent views might be difficult for their son to understand. It was recognized that these goals might not be accomplished quickly but were essential prior to the suggestion for a child psychiatric evaluation. The pediatrician and child psychiatrist agreed to maintain telephone contact. This informal consultation did not result in a resolution of the child's problem but rather to a more reasonable approach to it.

There are times when informal consultation is clearly inappropriate.

A pediatrician asked a child psychiatrist how long it takes for a behavior modification approach to work in a patient with anorexia nervosa. The brief description of the situation indicated that the pediatrician had been treating a 14-year-old girl for about six months and that the girl had lost a few pounds during that time. The focus of the intervention had been on the girl's participation in regular family meals and the pediatrician said that he had repeatedly told her that her scrawny appearance made her look very unattractive. In keeping with prior family patterns, the rewards for eating with the family were to be money or new clothes. It seemed apparent that the pediatrician understood neither the complexities of the girl's difficulties nor the use of the therapeutic approach.

When the child psychiatrist attempted to explore the history of the problem and to request more detailed family information, the pediatrician responded with further questions about the effectiveness of behavior therapy. He reported that he had read reports of studies which established effectiveness and that he was sure that in time she would stop being so stubborn. The child psychiatrist's offer to see the girl and her family was met with the response that "if she isn't better in a couple of weeks, we'll talk to her parents about that."

In this situation, the brief, informal consultation was not appropriate or helpful. While it would appear that the request was for support of the therapeutic approach, when that was not forthcoming, the offer to explore the situation further was rebuffed.

Such a case illustrates a serious and real dilemma in regard to all informal consultations. In these situations, the consulting child psychiatrist is, in fact, not being asked to express a formal or official view of a clinical problem or the management of a patient. Nevertheless, even on the basis of limited information, at least there are questions regarding the basic understanding of the patient's problem and the adequacy and appropriateness of the treatment program. Despite the informal nature of the consultation, it is the responsibility of the consultant to convey to the primary care physician the issues and the questions clearly indicating that genuine concerns exist. How these concerns are conveyed may depend to a very large measure upon the quality of the prior relationship between the child psychiatrist and the primary care physician. The relationship may be one in which direct confrontation is possible but it is unlikely that in that case conflict would occur with any degree of frequency. More likely, the prior relationship would be more limited and characterized by less confidence. Under such circumstances, the consultants' views of the complexities and the potential for future difficulties should be conveyed directly and clearly and the expression of concern should be coupled with a standing offer to assist directly and *formally* or to aid in finding other appropriate consultation.

Some informal consultation may involve larger issues and may involve more time and interaction.

In one smaller community, a group of pediatricians was confronted with a significantly larger number of children for whom back braces were prescribed because of the diagnosis of scoliosis. In a joint effort between the school system and the health department in the community, a screening program for scoliosis had been established and a rather large number of children with this problem were identified. The group of pediatricians were concerned about the reaction of many of these children to the back bracing and consulted a child psychiatrist via telephone for advice in regards to their attempts to assist these children with psychological and social adaptation. As a result of these conversations, the pediatricians were able to help the children, most of them girls, and their families recognize the affective responses and assist in verbal expression of these affects. They were also able to assist parents and the children themselves in the selection of clothing which would minimize the unpleasant appearance of braces and aided in encouraging alternative forms of physical activity in which the children could productively engage. Furthermore, they were able to assist in the establishment of relationships between older children who had adapted reasonably well to the brace and to the treatment regimen with younger children for whom this was a new experience.

FORMAL CONSULTATION WITHOUT DIRECT
CONTACT WITH PATIENT

Formal consultations without direct contact with the patient, or others involved in the situation by the consultant, often involve a more lengthy and comprehensive discussion of a problem. Such requests for assistance may come to a child psychiatrist via the telephone, the mail or face-to-face contact, occasionally arranged in advance. The consultee more often does not expect an immediate response and indeed may explicitly request a more thoughtful and even on-going series of discussions. Reimbursement of the consultant by the consultee may occur in these situations and the maintenance of a written record may be appropriate. Again, the specific focus of the consultation may vary from specific cases to programmatic or more general issues.

A pediatrician, who was a former student of a child psychiatrist, called to ask his former teacher for some assistance with a child with several significant developmental problems. The pediatrician, who practiced in a rural area where there were limited services, said that an extensive series of evaluations had been obtained but that community resources were limited. He hoped he could get some help in developing interventions which could be implemented at home or in his office. He volunteered that he had discussed his call with the parents and offered to send all the records to the child psychiatrist. He further said that he hoped he could discuss the case over the phone as well as receive a written report. This case was not strikingly different from some others in his practice, and he felt his contact with the child psychiatrist could be useful to him generally. He said he intended to pay the child psychiatrist for the consultation and had indeed used the word "consultation" throughout his conversation. Records were sent and reviewed, and thereafter via telephone a series of intervention strategies which could be implemented were developed and later outlined in a letter to the pediatrician.

This example points to one of the major issues in consultative work in general, but specifically in the outpatient area. From the outset the pediatrician stated he was seeking formal consultation, and implied that he had the consent of the family to do so. He further indicated that he expected to reimburse the child psychiatrist. In a sense, a formal contract was established. However, it is important to note that the child psychiatrist in this example was operating on the basis of faith in his former student. Specifically, there was no documentation that the family had agreed that the pediatrician could share clinical information. Further, some of the clinical information was essentially hearsay or second-hand in that it was derived from reports of others. Again, a major concern is the quality of the prior relationship between the pediatrician and the child psychiatrist and the mutual level of confidence. While it is clear that such interactions can be useful, there are certain risks. Questions regarding the completeness and accuracy of clinical information which may be a problem in any case are compounded if the information is available only indirectly. These matters must be explored carefully and thoroughly.

Some primary care physicians are interested and willing to assist children and families with regular counseling and guidance. In such situations, the primary care physician may consult the child psychiatrist not only about the evaluation process and the treatment plan, but may indeed seek ongoing supervision regarding the treatment process itself. Where there is a reasonable level of familiarity with the work and the approaches of both the child psychiatrist and the primary care physician, such communication can often be very helpful. However, without such familiarity, consultation may be of more limited value and may even be inappropriate. Geographic proximity may be less of an issue than the familiarity between the primary physician and the child psychiatric consultant.

One successful example of such an interaction is the case which follows:

Susan, an only child, was almost fifteen when her mother consulted the pediatrician. Though this physician had cared for Susan throughout her entire life, it had been some time since he had seen her in his office. Her father had died about two years before (about three months after the diagnosis of a malignant disease was first made). The family had been a particularly close one. About six months after the death of her father, Susan's school work began to decline and progressively she withdrew from friends and from various activities. During the six months prior to her mother's consulting the physician, she complained frequently of vague physical symptoms and began to miss a great deal of school. Because of economic necessities, the mother had returned to work about a year after the father's death, and she acknowledged irritability and increasing tension with her daughter. Following a medical evaluation of Susan, the pediatrician spent some extra time individually with Susan and with her mother and had two interviews with them together. At this point, he consulted a child psychiatrist with whom he had been friends for many years. Though the pediatrician and Susan and her mother lived in a small community about a hundred miles away from the medical center where the child psychiatrist worked, this particular pediatrician and child psychiatrist had maintained a personal relationship and had often consulted one another by phone. The pediatrician indicated that his evaluation suggested that neither Susan nor her mother had actually adequately grieved the death of the father, and that, in fact, they had taken a mutually protective stance with one another, often deliberately avoiding comments about the father or expressions of their own grief in an attempt to avoid upsetting the other. He further indicated that because of his longstanding relationship with this family, he felt in a position to be of some assistance and spoke of his willingness to do so. Following further discussion, a treatment plan was developed in which the pediatrician would attempt to assist Susan and her mother in the expression of their individual grief as well as means of sharing that grief with each other. It was hoped that ultimately such expression would lead to an opportunity for the pediatrician to assist both mother and daughter in reestablishing a mutually supportive and gratifying relationship. It was agreed that there would be telephone consultation following each visit with Susan and her mother. Within a six-month period of time, the therapeutic goals had been achieved. Susan's school performance and peer interactions had improved, the tensions between mother and daughter had diminished, and the pediatrician, as well as Susan and her mother, felt that the regular ongoing counseling sessions could be discontinued.

Formal consultation requests may not involve specific patients. A family physician who had considerable interest in adolescence and who enjoyed working with adolescents, sought an ongoing consultation/supervisory relationship with a child psychiatrist. A contract was established for meetings every two weeks of one-and-a-half hour duration in which various patients and other issues could be discussed. Though, at the outset the focus was principally on patients, rather quickly the issues of the organization of the office, fees, appointment scheduling, and separate waiting area for teenagers were discussed.

FORMAL CONSULTATION WITH CONTACT WITH PATIENT

Formal consultation with a direct contact between the child and/or family and the child psychiatrist is necessary in some situations. Where there is a lack of familiarity between the child psychiatrist and the primary care physician this approach may be required.

In some situations the primary care physician may request a direct contact with either child or parents in order to have some assistance in determining whether or not there is a need for further intervention or evaluation.

In one such situation a pediatrician referred a ten-year-old boy and his parents for consultation. Approximately five months prior to the consultation the child had been injured in an automobile accident while riding with a neighbor. The child had suffered a concussion and a fractured femur and had required approximately three weeks of hospitalization. An older boy, the son of the neighbor, had been killed in the accident. During the child's hospitalization, supportive care had been provided by the hospital's department of social work. The pediatrician requested the consultation to determine whether further intervention at this point in time was appropriate or whether it was the opinion of the child psychiatrist that the child and his parents were coping adequately with the injury and with the death of the friend.

In other situations, it may be quite clear to the pediatrician or family physician that help is indeed needed, but it may be quite unclear what services are most appropriate and where they may be available. In such a situation, the request is often for a full evaluation and assistance in determining the specific needs and in arranging for appropriate care.

One such situation was that of an eight-year-old boy who was first seen by a pediatrician toward the end of his second year in elementary school. There was one other child in the family, a sixteen-year-old brother, whom the parents felt was doing well. The patient had considerable difficulty in school during his first two years. His academic work was below grade level, largely because assignments were not completed and often classroom tests were not accomplished at all. In addition, there were considerable behavioral difficulties at school with major conflicts between the boy and peers in which fights often occurred. There were episodes of considerable verbal abuse of teachers and other school personnel and although the school had attempted to provide special services to this youngster, he had shown little evidence of responding. At about age three, a significant problem in vision had been diagnosed and the boy had since worn rather heavy glasses. The parents described him as a youngster who was always in trouble at home and was very destructive of his personal property, including his favorite toys. The parents were poorly educated people who were clearly very angry with their son and frustrated by their inability to control his behavior. They seemed rigid and quite punitive in their report of their attempts to deal with the problem at home. Under pressure from the kindergarten teacher three years before, the family had sought help at a community mental health center, but had withdrawn suddenly and without warning after about three months of contact. The parents themselves had had considerable conflicts with school personnel and felt that their son had been singled out for unfair treatment. The parents' first contact with the pediatrician had been prompted by the parents' desire to have the child put on medication in an attempt to control his behavior. The pediatrician felt there was evidence of considerable difficulty within this child and family and requested a full evaluation in an attempt to determine the needs and the appropriate services for this child. At the time of the initial consultation, the pediatrician indicated his willingness to participate in coordinating the services, but also was quite clear in indicating his uncertainty regarding the nature of the problem and the appropriate approaches.

REFERRAL

Perhaps the final level of interaction around particular clinical situations is that of referral itself. In these situations, the primary care physician may refer an individual child or a family with the rather clear understanding and hope that the child psychiatrist will assume responsibility for the full evaluation and for whatever ongoing care is needed.

Most unfortunate, perhaps, are the situations in which a child who is under the care of a family physician or pediatrician has continued problems or symptoms which are addressed in superficial manner and in which consultation is not requested.

One such situation was that of a thirteen-year-old girl who was referred under considerable pressure from school personnel because of repeated and prolonged absences from school. There had been clear symptoms of a series of fears and anxieties dating back to approximately four years of age when severe nightmares and night terrors had occurred. These had been managed by the pediatrician with sedation. Upon entering the first grade, there was evidence of considerable school avoidance which had been approached as a disciplinary problem. Throughout the early years of elementary school, there were continuing episodes of absence from school and periods of emotional turmoil during the absence of parents from home. During the two years prior to the referral, the girl had complained frequently of a variety of physical symptoms, some of which had prompted hospitalization on three occasions. Interpersonal difficulties with parents and with peers had escalated. On several occasions the mother had reported to the pediatrician that she was "at her wits end," and foster placement had been discussed in the girl's presence. At the time of the referral, the pediatrician had indicated that it was his view that the parents should not hold out much hope for benefit from the referral and evaluation by a child psychiatrist.

One would hope that a referral might be suggested in a somewhat more optimistic manner. Had a telephone consultation with the child psychiatrist occurred prior to the pediatrician's discussion with the parents, the referral might have been suggested in a more positive manner. In this case, a good deal of the child psychiatrist's initial effort was devoted to dealing with the parent's attitude of "why bother?" Such a situation required considerable skill in dealing with the patient and family as well as with the family physician.

It is also appropriate for child psychiatrists to be mindful that the consultative process is not a one-way street. Children under the care of child psychiatrists often have needs for medical consultation or intervention. More often in cases where the medical problem is acute but not severe, parents or an older child or adolescent may seek medical attention spontaneously, and little if any action on the part of the child psychiatrist is required.

However, there are other situations in which medical evaluation or ongoing medical care is required. If there is a need for consultation or referral, the child psychiatrist does have the responsibility of discussing the concerns with the parents and the child and explaining both the reasons for the action and the need to share information with the medical consultant. Ethical considerations require that the concurrence of the family and the child patient be sought before information is shared with a consultant.

There are ambulatory settings in which child psychiatrists and pediatricians or family physicians work together on a regular collaborative basis. Some clinics which provide care for children with developmental disabilities or chronic illnesses have evaluation or treatment teams which involve not only physicians but other health workers as well. Such settings may offer very comprehensive care on a long-term basis in which the responsibilities for care are shared among the various professionals depending upon the specific needs of a child or family.

The focus of the consultation of a child psychiatrist with a primary care physician outside the hospital may involve at least the following categories:

1. Individual patients or families.
2. Groups of patients.
3. Systems in which the primary care physician operates.
4. Professional functioning of the primary care physician.

Examples have been provided which illustrate each of these foci of consultation.

Whatever the focus and irrespective of the setting, there are certain operational principles of consultation within the ambulatory health care setting which are important to the child psychiatric consultant. While these may not be unique to the ambulatory area, they are of central value.

1. The relationship between the child psychiatrist consultant and the primary care physician consultee is critical. If there is professional familiarity, trust and respect, a great deal more can be accomplished and more complex problems addressed.
2. The nature of the problem must be defined and understood by both the child psychiatrist and the primary care physician.
3. The nature of the consultation request must be understood by both and the type of recommendation expected must be clear. If the expectation is for greater appreciation of the complexities of a particular clinical problem, the response should be quite different than if the expectation is for a particular suggestion regarding some specific aspect of care.
4. The capacities and interests of the consultee should be clear to the consultant. The advice to the primary care physician who is interested in counseling and willing to engage in such work with families or children is very different from the advice offered to a pediatrician who may be overworked and perhaps not prepared either by training or inclination to devote himself to such work.

5. The consultative recommendations, advice or support must be phrased in terms which are meaningful to the consultee. Whether in written or verbal communication, jargon has little place. Verbal communication has the distinctive advantage of providing immediate determination of whether there is understanding.
6. Criteria, however informal, should be established so that the consultee and the consultant have some standard by which to assess progress or the lack of it.
7. Alternatives or contingencies need to be developed and discussed to provide some choice to the consultee. Such alternatives can often be invaluable should initial recommendation not have the desired results.
8. The availability of continuing consultative help should be defined and, where appropriate, referral possibilities should be described.

Child psychiatric consultation often raises a series of ethical considerations, the most frequent of which are issues of confidentiality. While each issue may need to be considered in its own right, there are certain general principles which are important. Honesty and openness are perhaps most critical. A primary care physician should explain the need for consultation and seek the agreement of patient and family. The consulting child psychiatrist should explain that information will be shared and obtain permission to do so. However, it is permissible to place some limits on what will be shared depending upon the particular situation and what is relevant to the continuing care of the patient and family.

While the establishment of formal consultative agreements or contracts may be very useful and appropriate, it is also clear that it is neither practical nor appropriate to expect or to seek such formal arrangements in all cases. Whether formal or informal, the consultative process does depend in large measure upon the willingness of the child psychiatrist consultant to provide perspectives or advice and yet not demand control and a similar willingness on the primary physician to consider the advice and to continue to accept the direct responsibility for the care of the child patient and family. Though the consultant may not have primary responsibility for the patient, there are indirect responsibilities to the patient and direct responsibilities to the consultee even though there may not be a formal agreement.

Pediatricians and family physicians are often confronted by a variety of questions and problems for which consultation with a child psychiatrist may be very helpful. The telephone and more direct personal contact between these primary care physicians and the child psychiatrists can in some cases provide assistance without the direct contact between the child psychiatrist and the child

or parents. On the other hand, there are situations in which the direct evaluation of the child and the family is appropriate. The nature of psychopathology
or of the interpersonal diffculties are not necessarily the determinants in regard
to the level of involvement between the child psychiatrist and the primary care
physician. There are situations in which rather significant and complex problems
can be dealt with by carefully planned advice and information sharing between a
child psychiatrist and a primary care physician who have a reasonable level of
familiarity with the work and attitudes of each other

Much emphasis has been placed upon the quality of the relationship between the child psychiatrist and the pediatrician or family physician. Very often
these relationships develop spontaneously and as the result of a variety of interactions which may involve mutual clinical activities such as referrals or participation in the evaluation of patients or participation in other professional
activities (e.g., continuing medical education, committee work). It is useful for
the child psychiatrist to be mindful that any of the contacts with primary care
physicians may result in consultation requests either formal or informal and to
attempt in any contact to learn about the practice patterns, attitudes and approaches of potential consultees. Developing a sense of understanding and
familiarity may encourage consultation but it may also lead to more effective
and useful assistance. The development of genuine confidence does depend upon
satisfactory experience.

The continuing collaboration between primary care physicians and child
psychiatrist clearly enhances the potential of both individuals. Earlier and more
appropriate intervention, whether on the part of the primary care physician or
the child psychiatrist may result from this growing familiarity. As such collaboration continues, the primary care physician may in addition be better prepared to deal with many of the problems with which he is confronted, either
through the direct involvement with the child or through referral. Furthermore,
ongoing consultation and supervision may result which will enhance the effectiveness of the primary care physician.

Outpatient collaboration and consultation in fact, can enhance the effectiveness of the physicians involved and of the family in coping with many of
the problems of childhood. It is essential that both pediatricians, family physicians, and child psychiatrists develop a level of mutual understanding and
familiarity, not only with issues of personal style and attitudes, but also with
the various pressures that confront the specialists. An understanding of the
nature of office practice in the health care of children is a critical piece of the
child psychiatrist's capacity to effectively become involved in collaborative consultative activities with these primary care physicians.

While ideally, increased emphasis should be placed upon these activities within the training period, it is possible for both child psychiatrists and pediatricians to advance their skills and understanding beyond the training period itself.

REFERENCES

Anders TF: Child psychiatry and pediatrics: The state of the relationship. *Pediatr* 60(4, pt 2):616–620, Oct 1977.

Lewis M: Child psychiatric consultation in pediatrics. *Pediatr* 62(3):359–364, Sept 1978.

The Task Force on Pediatric Education: The Future of Pediatric Education. A Report by the Task Force on Pediatric Education (American Academy of Pediatrics: Evanston, IL) 1978.

The President's Commission on Mental Health: Report to the President (Government Publication: Washington, DC) 1978.

Graduate Medical Education National Advisory Committee: Summary Report of the Graduate Medical Education National Advisory Committee to the Secretary. DHHS Publication No. (HRA)81-651 (US Department of Health and Human Services: Washington, DC) 1980.

The Select Panel for the Promotion of Child Health: Better health for our children: A national strategy. DHHS Publication No. 79-55071 (US Department of Health and Human Services: Washington, DC) 1981.

The Consultant
and the Educational System

10

Teachers and Classrooms

Philip DiMattia

OVERVIEW OF THE PROBLEM

Teachers and other educators rarely refer children to child psychiatrists because, among other things, referral requires a teacher to make a highly individual, perhaps unsupportable statement that a particular child's adjustment is significantly unusual. He must do it without definitions, without guidelines, without specific training, without standards of accepted practice, with potential risk to the child's future or to his own, and finally, without any assurance that it will bring full or effective service.

Yet, the teacher should be a good referrent. He sees the child in a variety of activities and social arrangements over a long period of time and, sometimes, throughout complete cycles of development.

Some issues that make it difficult to make referrals can be identified:

1. There is no universally accepted definition of emotional disturbance.
2. Etiology is still unknown, despite interesting conjecture.
3. Professionals have tended to be rivalrous rather than cooperative.
4. Well-intended normalization trends like "mainstreaming" and "de-institutionalization sometimes result in inadequate identification, therefore inadequate response to needs for services.
5. Family's rights to privacy and autonomy are sometimes in conflict with individual human rights.

---

6. The larger problems of maladaptation and its implications for the culture and the society is largely unhypothesized and unexplored.
7. Societal and government-funding commitment to prevention, intervention, and rehabilitation is limited.
8. The needs of care providers are generally unknown and unattended.

There are many other issues that lack statement and even form. Scrutiny of any one leads to the identification of many more. All conspire to deny the potency of the most likely observer.

Difficult though it may be to objectify criteria for evaluation, it is still well guided to continue discussion, experimentation, and compromise to make agreements as the foundation of a reference framework for teachers and others to use to help discover unusual needs. Clear and uniform social expectations and standards, even if marred by error, would be useful and supportive.

School districts differ widely in their organization, administration, and philosophy of service. The differences that reflect a healthy society's right to directly manage the course of education of its young can be mortally discriminatory, yet no responsible person would defend the denial of needed service to a child. The problem is one of perceived need.

It seems reasonable to expect that efforts at identifying deviations for making referrals would comprise a framework against which to examine conditions. The reader will find that the framework summary is very much in accord with Piaget's contention that the major task of childhood is to discover oneself as an entity among entities and to experience events among events.

It thus implies role parameters for both the child and those who assume the parenting role, whether the latter be the natural parent(s) or parent surrogates that include teachers, doctors, and a total spectrum of helping professionals. Upon reflection, it also calls to attention the spectrum of services required in order to accomplish the task.

Given the want of resources, the matter of a service spectrum gives rise to another question that clamors for resolution. Can we distinguish between optimal and adequate services and, if so, under what conditions?

BRIEF SUMMARY OF THE CHILD'S NEEDS*

What are children's needs? A detailed outline would include all of the content of developmental psychology. But fundamental to all of the specifics, about which there are large areas of debate and room for variability, is the need for

---

*Excerpt from published paper by Gair D, DiMattia P, "The end of the line, or a way back?" Fourth Annual Children's Advocacy Conference, 1978.

a stability and predictability, sufficient for the completion of the tasks of child-hood.

The task of childhood (here including adolescence) can be summarized as achieving an adequate internalization of the components of a secure relationship to parents and others sufficiently to allow the capacities of ego development (cognitive, emotional, physical mastery) to be matured. With this maturity the individual can become an adult capable of enjoying the struggles and oppor-tunities of adult relationships, work, play, and parenthood with the cultural limits acceptable to society and thus be part of the continuing stability of that society or have the unusual capacity to change or successfully leave that society.

Childhood thus can be defined as the time of life, beginning with birth, when the survival and optimum development of an individual in a society requires the authority, strength, and wisdom of adults at first totally and then by decreasing amounts until competence in self-preservation and internalization of society's values has been achieved sufficiently to allow the individual to be-come officially or de facto emancipated and accepted as a representative of the society.

Adolescence, the last phase of childhood, begins with the physical changes of sexual maturation and the coincident intellectual changes allowing the devel-opment of abstract thinking. Adolescence is characterized by confusion in both child and parents, and other caretaking adults, and frequently intense struggles between them about the degree of the continuing need for adult control and guidance as defined above.

The other sections of this chapter deal with degrees of significance of the child's problem, the leadership function, professional interactions, mispercep-tions, planning for change, emphasis upon service, and finally, several brief se-lected cases.

PROBLEM SIGNIFICANCE

Every child can be a candidate for referral to a child psychiatrist for study, evaluation, and treatment. The significant adults in the life of a child are likely sources of referrals by the very nature of their work and position of responsibil-ity for the child.

The highest priority that exists for helping children with emotional prob-lems is simply reaching the staggering number who are not receiving sufficient help. This priority includes children who experience severe emotional difficul-ties but never have been identified to be in need of service as well as those who have been identified but are not being served.

Several sources outline some of the components of this problem that may warrant review. The 1978 report to the president from the President's

Commission on Mental Health suggests that the overall prevalence of persistent, handicapping mental health problems among children age 3 to 15 ranges from 5 to 15%. By conservative estimates, at least two million American children have learning disabilities of varying sorts that could have profound consequences for both them and their families. There has been a dramatic increase in the use and misuse of psychoactive drugs, including alcohol, among young Americans and nearly a threefold increase in the suicide rate of adolescents. The September 1979, issue of *Kappon* reported that the overriding concern of the public about public schools has been the lack of discipline in the schools, followed closely by concern over use of drugs. In much the same vein, a survey of members of the New York State United Teachers revealed that dealing with disruptive students in the classroom is seen as the number one cause of stress for teachers.

The Bureau of Education for the Handicapped (BEH) estimated that two percent of children and youth require special education because of their emotional problems. The current estimate of school-age population in the country (ages five-seventeen is 51,317,000. A two-percent BEH estimate would identify 1,026,340 children in need of service. A review of Public Law 89-313 and state education plans indicate that there are 284,645 emotionally disturbed children receiving special education. This suggests that there are some 741,000 high-risk children not currently receiving any form of special education.

An analysis of 15 evaluation studies and two data bases conducted by the General Accounting Office, September 1981, to determine the extent to which P.L. 94-142 is being implemented, found evidence to indicate that preschool, secondary, and emotionally disturbed students are comparatively underserved groups. Of the nearly four million school children served (1980-1981), a "typical" child in special education programs is under twelve years of age, male, and mildly handicapped. The handicapping conditions of those served were learning disabled (36 percent), speech impaired (30 percent), and mentally retarded (19 percent). The next in frequency were the emotionally disturbed (eight percent), while other categories comprised low incidence conditions. This data represents only those served directly within public school programs.

In a recent report by the American Association of School Administrators, *Keeping Children in School*, it was reported that approximately 850 thousand students drop out of school annually and that the absentee rate nationally averages 5.5% on any given day. This latter figure represents only unexcused absences.

Granting the diversity of this data, it does appear reasonable to assume that the problem of emotional disturbance among school-age children is widespread in the United States. The child psychiatry resources available to respond to referrals from teachers are severely limited. The American Academy of Child Psychiatry (AACP) reports a membership of 1,900. This figure includes physicians who are in training as well as graduates of a child psychiatry residency.

The stated purpose of the academy is to stimulate and advance medical contributions to the knowledge and treatment of psychiatric problems of children. The shortage of qualified child psychiatrists has contributed to the omission of a viable role for them in recently passed national and state mandated special education legislation. When one considers not only the incidence factor, but also the severity factor, it is appalling that this is the case.

The natural consequence of this shortage is that an important resource for children is removed from first-person interaction to a consultation status and that this is an ineffective and unworkable role. Consultation within the medical discipline maintains repute and is of extreme importance in current practice. Within the educational community, however, consultive specialists are not well regarded, perhaps because they perceive failures of relevance resulting from the insensitive imposition of those consultants on classroom teachers by mandate or administrative arrangements outside of teachers' control.

It is reasonable to assume that the next decade will be a period of growth or decline for child psychiatry as a profession. It will also show changes in the nature and quality of service to the large numbers of severely handicapped children in our nation who have psychiatric needs. Clearly, if these needs are not met the resulting increased suffering will escalate and recycle the critical problems of society. The great threat is that many thousands of children will grow up without the experience of being cared for sufficiently for acculturation. The legacy they will leave will be dismal and stark. All mankind, for all time to come, will be affected.

LEADERSHIP FUNCTION

The diagnostic expertise and knowledge of child development that the child psychiatrist possesses may limit the usefulness of consultation upon referral as a primary interface with the teacher. The child psychiatrist contribution to clarifying the existence and extent of a problem suggest a more directed role. The psychiatrist should certainly set aside some time to gain an understanding of the implicit dynamics of the classroom and the teacher's response to it. A perfunctory examination of some of the factors of teaching will explain why this profession has the highest stress rate in the country, as evidenced by the number of hospitalizations, recently increased pressure for accountability, student competency, parent involvement, and the myriad of changing social factors within the classroom itself. The psychiatrist should recognize that these issues, summed up in teacher stress comprise perhaps the single most crucial problem that schools will be forced to deal with over the next decade. In a real sense it represents the teaching profession's challenge to growth or decline. The changing conditions that result from forces and social actions outside of the school community but have great impact upon it lead to much antagonism among various groups within that community and generate what may be characterized as a self-defense "me" mentality among teachers. What appears to others to be a lack of humanity may mask fear, self-questioning, and loss of self-confidence.

Then the psychiatrist must look at the students' backgrounds. If learning is an interaction among things that exist, and if personal confidence plays a crucial role in the influencing of interactions, then there simply can be no learning without confidence just as there can be no development of confidence without protective caring. If protective caring is in jeopardy, as evidenced by the predicament that so many of the nation's children are confronted with in their natural families, and if there is a heightening of tension and confusion within the classrooms around the country, then the learning that helps children to become adults able to contribute to new social stability will be jeopardized.

If child psychiatrists stay at remote distances by defining themselves only as consultants to the primary caretakers of the children, including teachers, in the near future it may be a long wait between phone calls from teachers and their colleagues. This will be a natural result of pressure upon the school community to provide in-system supports of varying degree which are more cost effective as the schools respond to current mandates. In the majority of referrals made directly by parents to child psychiatrists, the psychiatrist's work with the child and family—as fruitful as it might be—will not be likely to have great influence on any therapeutic maneuvering that may be required within the child's schooling. Often, the disposition resulting from an initial referral includes a recommendation for an alternative educational program which in many cases contains a live-in component. This sort of recommendation often results in conflict and requires resolution. In most cases either the parent or those delegated as advocates join with the child psychiatrist in seeking to force the school community to agree to provide certain services that are seen as needed, whether the school agrees or not. This unilateral process to secure services often results in lengthy bureaucratic procedures. Litigation follows conferences, meetings and correspondence. During these efforts the child and the classroom teacher are drifting further and further apart. The original referral, the study, evaluation and design of a treatment program were triggered by behaviors that were of concern to the meaningful adults in the child's life; whether in or out of school a less responsive environment results for the child because of the prospect of lengthy negotiations. Through the educational process the current placement of the child is considered appropriate until a determination of specific individual educational needs has been determined in accordance with local state and federal mandates as contained in the provision of P.L. 94-142 (Handicapped Education Law). The clinical process may become politicized and even higher barriers result between the teacher and the psychiatrist as the teacher's function is accorded little if any attention.

MISPERCEPTIONS

What emerges from a consideration of a referral is the awareness that, despite the desire to provide quality care for the child, the underpinnings of the structure through which members of the child's constituency operate are quite different. Originating in the dynamics of the change process, the key to the difference is anchored in the perception of the individual members of one another. Failure to deal with the individual professional helpers perspective generates fear and raises serious question regarding the effective collaboration needed to take care of the child sufficiently to allow and endure growth. Whenever members of the helping professions become aware of any negative perceptions and respond accordingly then what exists is the stuff of which conflicts are made. They are the types of conflicts from which referrals to the child psychiatrist will always be difficult.

Addressing the problem in a positive fashion, then, demands that the dynamics of the referral situation be attended in the early stages of planning. It requires that those enrolled (1) be aware of the possibility of distorted perceptions, (2) understand the sources of misperceptions, (3) deal with them at that level, and (4) avoid the possibility of reciprocal negative perceptions which are causal to conflict.

PLANNING FOR CHANGE

It is important for the child psychiatrist to realize that the potential source of teacher referral anxiety lies in the information or misinformation factor and to be effective must remain mindful that training is an extension as well as an interaction of personal relationships.

When teachers and other professional staff in the school community become concerned about certain behaviors in students, they are required to follow procedures which examine specific issues and problems. Schools and the teachers who staff them are rooted in a tradition that emphasizes content in academic areas and thus deals with curriculum accommodations and modifications as their major area of responsibility. In general, when teacher concerns about a student's inability to read are validated through formal evaluation procedures and are specified as an inability to make sound-symbol relationships, there is little problem developing corrective programs. When psychological problems appear, manifested in feelings and modes of expression that deviate from behavior to which teachers are accustomed, the inexperience and naivete of some teachers can be a serious limitation to obtaining evaluations. The current attempt to individualize education for all children falls far short of success. That schools must change from a total academic content orientation and become more expansive cannot be disputed. Some suggest that schools must also take responsibility for the physical and emotional well-being of the student, especially as they relate to his sense of personal worth and ability to contribute to his own destiny.

As school's attempt to realize the above goals through training, administrative decision making, planning, programming, and evaluation, they will require a substantial expansion of support. Child psychiatrists can best give this through planned, aggressively sought collaboration toward the goal of improving the quality of life not only of students but of their primary helping professional personnel as well.

Teachers who make referrals while identifying a wide variety of concerns about the individual child's ability to adapt and to meet adult expectations may also be reflecting their own feelings of isolation and uncertainty. They may question their own capacity to develop and sustain a learning atmosphere rooted in protective caring that is predictable and stable enough to reduce anxiety and induce growth. Their concerns are usually about panicky children, disorganized children, and those who throw tantrums. Above all, they are concerned for the child who is so explosive and unpredictable, so angry that the likelihood of his being managed and cared for within the school setting is in serious question. The most accurate word used by teachers to describe the children with exaggerated behavior patterns is "crazy." Hardly considered acceptable by the supporters of normalization principles, "crazy" might nonetheless be the most realistic of the popular terms in common use today.

If the teacher is to help the child by setting better and more consistent limits as the first task area, then he will need specific training and a practical framework from which to operate. This framework must differentiate between the limit-setting needs of young children and the needs of children who are entering adolescence. The central concern of the teacher is to eliminate and manage behavior difficulties that interfere with learning while continuing to teach.

Implicit is the assumption that limit setting and consistency are the underpinnings of a learning structure. The identification of supports outside of the classroom setting and the opportunity to participate with an active treatment team where the focus is less on why and more on how in an atmosphere of mutual trust and good will, can serve the child far better than perpetuating the myth of a simple prescriptive treatment which too often is the product of consultation. The treatment team concept and the problems associated with the teams' development have been given considerable attention; the need for such an entity is beyond dispute. The teams have been identified by many names as a by-product of national efforts in behalf of "mainstreaming" and "least restrictive" placements (e.g., individual educational planning teams, individual treatment teams, and individual rehabilitation teams).

Productive use of treatment team approaches warrants thought. The terms themselves are quite straightforward. Treatment, the less complicated of the two, simply connotes the application of remedies with the object of affecting a cure. Team, on the other hand, involves three social stages, (1) membership in a group (teachers identify with other teachers), (2) the extension of that membership (to include doctors, social workers, psychologists), and (3) the process of, or movement toward, absorption with peer status within the expanded group. A constant is the intent of the person or persons involved in the change process to become incorporated into a new group—a treatment team.

The intent must include a realization that the collaboration of the team will bring a more valuable collective response to problem solving than can any single member. It can also help to clarify the professional identity of the adult helpers to the child. The task of the team, the overriding motivation of all the efforts of its members, is to engage with one another to change something. Planning is done for this very reason. Team planning, therefore, becomes a function whose agenda can be stated in question form.

What is the child's capacity to understand the external boundaries of his own inner structure? For what degree of clarification of emotion responses does the child exhibit a need? Can the child take comfort from the adult who has temporary physical custody, such as the classroom teacher. What is the quality of his relationship to others? Does he see some others as allies.

Who are "they"—who are the enemy? Does the child give evidence of being developmentally closed? In what ways is encouragement being given to the intellectual, physical, social-emotional mastery that the child experiences? The answers to these and similar kinds of questions becomes the substance of the team's therapeutic intervention and maneuvers.

For the teacher, development of a mutual support system to help plan and implement becomes critical to his work with the student and the class. While remedying academic deficiency through corrective instructional activity, the teacher may grow in understading of the relationship between the child's achievement and the development of competence and self-confidence in the child, and its impact on social and emotional growth. Psychotherapy and other traditional clinical maneuvers can be viewed as additional strategies that help to support and enlarge the development of the child's positive self-image.

It is the integration of effective supportive services that results in quality care for children who demonstrate a marked inability to care for themselves. It is the collective helpfulness of the responsible caretakers that serves to unite team members with a common purpose. It is a thoughtful person's responsibility to recognize and correct, in a spirit of good will, any failures in service and to avoid blaming the victim, as sometimes occurs. What are viewed as children's failures are more appropriately service failures.

This paper has attempted to identify some problems teachers have in making referrals to child psychiatrists. It discusses the limitations of traditional consultative practice. It also has directed attention to the learning environment which will encourage growth when well prepared to do so. Unawareness of underestimation of the possibility of misperception between coworking professionals is a critical weakness of many team leaders.

Unless the teacher is an active partner and is able to exercise full membership in the treatment team, the expertise of the psychiatrist as it relates to the teacher function will be invalidated. Sometimes noncooperation will be obvious while in many other circumstances, though unapparent, resistance will be all the more powerful. For the child psychiatry profession to respond to teacher referrals it must assume some responsibility for an enabling leadership that assists the friends and helpers of children to cooperate with each other in working together toward a common purpose. This is a formidable challenge.

The remaining section of this paper presents three sketches. They are not intended as prescriptions. Rather, they are problems typical for referral in that they are complex and resistant to resolution. They are offered as dilemmas without answers, for the reader's thought and discussion. The more thought given, the more complicated they will seem to be—and the more demanding of a conscientiously managed array of resources and interventions.

Thus, the primary role for all professional helpers of children lies in developing effective models of collaboration and alliance that fosters a structured atmosphere of protective caring that is able to reduce anxiety sufficiently to indure the child growth. In the final analysis the quality of care of the children, whether it be in the school setting or any other, is dependent upon the professional's ability and motivation to creatively process their experiences and apply them in the design of treatment programs.

Eric is a five-year-old preschool boy who attends a full-day nursery program. He has been asked to leave three other schools in the past two years because his behavior was considered disruptive and unmanageable. Both of Eric's parents are practicing psychologists who have one other child, aged 18, who often baby sits with Eric. They were anxious to meet the teacher before school started to try to plan a program that would tolerate Eric's destructive behavior. They wanted some assurance that the teacher would be sympathetic and not frightened.

Eric is a curious, bright, motivated child. He wants to read and shows interest in daily conceptual lessons. He spends several thirty-minute time blocks each day building, gluing, painting, and putting together puzzles. Eric always prefers doing these activities alone. He usually refuses to answer questions or sit in a group for any activity. He leaves the room when the teacher gives a group lesson or reads a story and sits within hearing distance but away and alone. He can stand or sit next to another child to do an independent project, but he moves away if an adult speaks personally to him for longer than a few minutes or makes an attempt to cuddle or get close.

If an adult or child continuously demands a response, Eric will smash his own project and leave furious. It is likely that he will rudely tell the person to leave him alone, and he might even kick or hit. He often spends thirty to sixty minutes alone after being this upset, before he is willing to return to places where other people are. Eric seems a withdrawn, angry child. He is obviously torn between his interest in learning and his discomfort with other people in a school setting.

The closer the teacher or students approach to try to draw him out or include him, the more upset he is and he usually responds with behaviors that make a second approach unlikely. In a regular program, Eric would probably become increasingly isolated. If taken out of class and placed in a one-to-one or small-group setting, his emotional discomfort would probably increase because of added pressure.

While Eric is a curious, bright, motivated child who wants to read and does show interest in conceptual lessons, he also evidences severe discomfort with other people in the school setting. While much is not known of why he behaves as he does, the teacher's task is formidable in building an atmosphere of protective caring and trust sufficiently to reduce anxiety and allow growth for Eric as well as other children in the class.

A major goal of nursery school is the building of social and emotional experience. Eric's anger and withdrawal can be managed by modification of teacher behavior and expectation in the day-to-day ordering of the classroom and activities, assuring insulation from adverse stimulation that serves to trigger Eric's negative behavior and, indeed, may be a desirable initial phase for development. However, the need for an integrated treatment plan that addresses emotional feedback to Eric, to teacher, and to parents, as well as positive social interactions with peers becomes a major issue. The child psychiatrist can contribute to the emotional and social tasks by initial assistance in clarification of these as problem areas and in support to those elements of Eric's constituency to assure consistency of purpose and goals.

Thus, involvement would serve to establish an important link of helpers to Eric, as questions are generated around limit-setting issues and avoidance of fragmentation thereby, encouraging a more comprehensive planning that gives direction and integration. Support for the teacher-directed efforts becomes especially critical if the what, why, and how, are to be productive while at the same time realistic within the confines of a classroom setting. The involvement of the child psychiatrist becomes possible as "Team Evaluation" procedures outlined by federal and state mandates become implemented.

Jimmy is a large, somewhat overweight ten-year-old with blond hair, blue eyes, and a shy smile. He lives with his mother who went to work at a raquet club four years ago when she and Jimmy's father separated. She has worked her way up to a management position. Although his father often abused both him and his mother, Jimmy refused for several years to believe that the family no longer lived together, and even now expresses some confusion following his father's infrequent but tension-provoking visits. Besides making some planned day visits, the father has returned to the house unexpectedly, from time to time, late at night, drunk and threatening. The mother has difficulty limiting his access both because she is afraid of him and because she is ambivalent about denying him contact with his son.

Jimmy is assigned to grade five in a special class for children with severe emotional difficulties. He functions at a much lower level academically than his endowment would seem to warrant. He reads with primer level skill but is a little more competent in math. He can do three-digit addition and regroups in subtraction and is learning the multiplication tables. He frequently refuses work or demands one-to-one attention from a teacher. He often is overwhelmed before he begins if his assignment seems long, if he must work with another child or small group, or if the material is unfamiliar. He refuses defiantly. Shouting and threatening, he throws materials, desks and chairs and requires physical restraint by a very strong adult (or adults) to prevent him from harming the teacher or other students. He struggles violently, screams obscenities, and constantly threatens, "You die, Hennessy, you die," at his teacher. After about ten or fifteen minutes, exhausted, sweating, and crying, the tantrum having subsided, he returns to class as if nothing happened. He may have several of these episodes in a day or have none for several days.

Sometimes it seems as if he is out of control when this happens. At other times he seems to be able to use tantrums to coerce adults to comply with his demands: "I don't want to go in now. I want to go to the nature trail. If you don't let me you'll be sorry." If thwarted, a tantrum does follow. One time the scene at a school picnic was so dramatic and disruptive as to bring on the investigation of the local police. It is not really clear whether he is threatening or predicting.

Children are unwilling to risk his temper and tend to avoid interacting with him. His only outside school friendships have been very short-term and have usually resulted in some acting-out behaviors that have necessitated adult intervention. His mother has been threatened with eviction from her apartment because of his petty vandalism in public areas of the building. She reports that he is a model of good behavior when he is with her.

Jimmy is initially very seductive and ingratiating with adults. He seems defenseless and vulnerable, and although his body is over-large for his age, his features are immature and he seems young and little. Adults, sometimes even seasoned professionals have a tendency to overreact protectively toward him during the first few weeks of acquaintance. This has three important results:

1. *Staff are at odds and have difficulty finding common goals because Jimmy is perceived to be victimized by some and rescued by others.*
2. *Eventually, when Jimmy's tantrum behavior becomes familiar to those who had been rescuers, they sometimes react to their own feelings of humiliation and helplessness with a temporary anger equal in intensity to their earlier seduction.*
3. *As totally demanding, unremittingly violent behavior continues relatively unchanged (or worsen) over a long period, it exhausts the physical and emotional resources of adults who are trying to help.*

In this example it is easy for staff to become fragmented and lose sight of the students need for consistency in overall management. The contribution of the child psychiatrist to the teachers involved should include provisions for the development of a cohesive response to the protective needs of the student. Here consistency does not refer to responding to the child in the same way but rather to the central need of a cap on the narcissistic physical behavior needs of the student through an array of support services. Freedom for Jimmy must be defined by limits required.

Allan is a good-looking nine-year-old with dark hair, freckles, a quick smile, and twinkling eyes. He likes sports and is well coordinated. He is in a resource room in a public school and seems to be doing very well with this year's teacher who is fond of him and finds him rewarding to work with. He is academically capable in this arrangement (if not inspired), which is an improvement over the last two years in regular class when he was disruptive, mischievous, and unable to concentrate to the point of failing the grade and requiring a special program. His older brother and younger sister are seen as model students within the middle-class suburban school, but Allan is regarded as a bad boy.

Allan's chief difficulties this year seem to be that he fights constantly in the school bus and has, in fact, been twice suspended from school as a result. It is reported that he has been in trouble with the police for breaking windows in an empty factory building and has been caught stealing in a supermarket drug store. Although he was alone both times, he says that he was in the company of other youngsters who managed to avoid being seen. It is not known whether or not this is true.

Allan pilfers things he wants from school, from time to time, such as a pencil or eraser. He lies to avoid punishment but does not make up "tall tales" for the fun of the telling or to enhance his status. If reprimanded he cringes and sometimes even cries. The intensity of the reprimand has no relation to the intensity of his response; rather, his relationship to the adult determines how strongly he reacts. If the adult is a favored or important person to Allan, the mildest rebuke elicits as much emotion from the child as a strong rebuke from someone he cares less about. He has a good sense of humor and likes to laugh. He has many friends to play with who seem to enjoy him despite his fighting in the bus. Many find him appealing and readily able to make positive relationships.

The school's assistant principal, however, thinks of him as a troublesome child who is a disappointment and a trial to his family and who, on the evidence of his recent encounters with the police, is headed for more severe delinquent acting out. He states this openly to Allan.

Allan's father is usually unemployed. Though he has not sought steady work for several years, he thinks of himself as a painter. He is attractive and superficially well-socialized but is reported to have a drinking problem. His mother is also attractive and recently has been wearing fancy nightgowns all day while home from work pending surgery for a somewhat vague back ailment. The activities of the household center in the living room where she lies on the sofa with the television on throughout the day. The father seems to do all of the household work and caretaking, but the mother complains constantly that no one helps her and that she does it all.

Allan's brother and sister are in and out of the living room and are vocally approved of by mother and father. Allan, on the other hand, spends much of his time in his room (routine punishment for infractions of various kinds) and is not often seen as a participant in family life. At one time, in fact, Allan's paternal grandparents filed an abuse charge against his parents because Allan was locked in his room so much of the time. Now the room is unlocked, but he still spends most of his time there.

The mother and father vehemently disagree about the children's management. He thinks she is not firm enough. She thinks he in too harsh. Neither is firm or lenient in routine practice; both are whimsical and inconsistent.

There are peculiarities and discrepancies in the family's presentation of itself. The school thinks the parents are dedicated, heavily invested, average middle-class parents. The grandparents differ with this view. They also believe that Allan is treated like an outsider. Though Allan's mother awaits surgery on her back and cannot work, she taught an eight-session roller skating course at a local rink. Sometimes, when school personnel call home, she claims to be her own sister and takes a message for herself even though she knows that the caller recognizes her voice.

At the request of the Evaluation Team, a school social worker recently conducted a ten-week casework evaluation in the home of the family. She feels that the parents are unwilling to change that there would be little justification to suggest to try to intervene with a casework approach. They simply do not perceive the need for counseling, and except for Allan, their energy is invested in maintaining the status quo.

CONCLUSION

As a member of a resource classroom within the public school it appears that Allan is achieving a measure of success academically. Concerns center about his behavior on the school bus and an over identification with delinquent behaviors. The administrators attitude of Allan as a and disappointment, the view of siblings as model students and the reported apathy as well as inconsistency within the home become important issues for consideration. The child psychiatrist contribution in this circumstance on the surface is difficult at least. Perceptions and expectations of Allan are indicative of outcome. Those who prophesied good encourage positive behavior while those who prophesied bad appear to encourage negative response. Dealing effectively with the distortions of negative aspects of the environment in order for graceful integration to occur is part of a larger educational problem that has a place for the child psychiatrist among others to develop innovative in roads that may be accessible through staff development opportunities within the schools and broader community for those directly involved with children and youth.

BIBLIOGRAPHY

Bourne R and Newberger E (eds.): *Critical Perspectives on Child Abuse* (Lexington Books, DC Heath and Co: Lexington, MA) 1979.

Dupont H (ed.): *Educating Emotionally Disturbed Children* (Holt Rinehart & Winston: New York) 1975.

Eekelaar J and Katz S (eds.): *Family Violence* (Butterworth & Co: Toronto) 1978.

Fenichel C: Psycho-educational approaches for seriously disturbed children in the classroom. *Intervening Approaches in Educating Emotionally Disturbed Children*, Knoblock P (ed.) (Syracuse University: Syracuse, NY) 1965.

Long N, Morse W, and Newman X (eds.): *Conflict in the Classroom*, 3rd ed. (Wadsworth: Belmont, CA) 1976.

Maslow A: *Toward a Psychology of Being* (Van Nostrand: Princeton, NJ) 1962.

Redl F: The concept of a therapeutic milieu. *Am J Orthopsych* 29:721-734, 1959.

Rhodes W and Tracey M: *A Study in Child Variance* (Univ Michigan Press: Ann Arbor, MI) 1972.

11

Administration and the Therapist: Consultation Conflicts and Alliances in the College Community

Elizabeth Aub Reid

It is essential to consider both the nature of the college itself, and the structure of the consultation service, to understand its relationship to the larger institution. Colleges and universities come in many sizes and varieties. Every university consists of bricks and mortar—its buildings—but its essence consists of the unique college community—its people. This includes students and faculty, as well as administration and a whole variety of support people—from buildings-and-grounds to health service personnel.

A university is a defined community in which each member has a position in the hierarchy. Students are relatively transient members but at any one time, they too have a defined position vis-à-vis the rest of the community. People have relationships, loyalties, grudges: they form networks, some transient, many continuing over long periods. Most members of a mental health service are among those who are permanent members of the community. They form friendships and loyalties too, and so they must take these into account lest they cloud judgment in professional situations.

Within the university, individuals, departments, and special services acquire reputations, sometimes deserved, sometimes not. Either way, however, reputations once formed are hard to live down. It behooves a group that wishes to be used by the community to worry about its public image or reputation, and remember that individual acts contribute to that image. It is reassuring to notice, for example, that many people come to a good mental health service or specific person at the suggestion of an acquaintance who reported being helped.

A university is a remarkably small town. People talk to each other. Although one might expect people to be reticent about having gone to a mental health service, in fact many are not. At one extreme is the young woman who saw me across her college dining room and shrieked with enthusiasm, "There's my shrink!" as she rushed across the crowded room to say hello. Then there are those who never share with anyone the fact that they have seen a psychiatrist. Enough do share their experiences so that the reputation of the service and the individuals in it rest to a great extent on reports (some first hand, many at several removes) of people's actual contacts. Thus, in the small town sort of environment found at most universities, doing one's job well builds a reputation which leads to new opportunities to be of service. Undoubtedly, the opposite is also true.

A health service's prime responsibility is the care of its patients. The health service is usually responsible for the health of *all* of the members of the university community. Whatever other functions a particular service performs, these must be in addition to fulfilling that responsibility and must be done in such a way as not to jeopardize, in any way, the ethics or quality of patient care.

Universities are in the business of education, for the most part educating young adults. This education often includes providing a living environment for much of the year—and hopefully addressing growth and quality of life issues which go beyond the narrower sphere of academic education. In this era of severe financial constraints, these latter responsibilities tend to take second place to strict academics, and people whose concerns may be in these spheres must make special efforts to keep their importance in the awareness of those making financial and overall policy decisions for the institution.

The members of a mental health service are skilled and experienced in helping people—especially young people—with psychological problems involving both severe pathology and the usual problems of normal development. They know a great deal about the normal maturation of this age group, as well as about the distinct problems prevalent in their institution. Those skills and that information can be very useful to the institution and its members. The issue is how best to do this without jeopardizing patient care by acceding to administrative pressures, or by divulging details of treatment. In the current climate of fiscal tightness, it may be necessary to persuade financial managers that personnel designated as patient caretakers in fact will be appropriately earning their salaries if they spend some of their time not in direct patient care but in helping to train faculty and staff by consulting with them.

INDIVIDUAL CONSULTATION

The most frequent form of consultation in a college mental health service is helping with a crisis, usually involving a single person (sometimes an already identified mental health patient, sometimes not), or a specific problem. Someone in the university has a problem for which he or she wishes help and calls on the mental health service or an individual in that service who is known and trusted. This kind of consultation is usually fairly straightforward. The psychiatrist tries to define the problem and to help in any way that is appropriate. Good individual consultation based on psychodynamic understanding and interpersonal skills is not very different from that in any other clinical setting.

In colleges, certain basic principles having to do with keeping priorities clear should be kept in mind. In most consultations all parties—including student-patients, teachers, and advisors—are members of the university community and are, therefore, equally entitled to the services of the mental health worker. Balancing responsibilities to all individuals, without doing damage to anyone, and helping everyone as much as possible, is the challenge.

In situations where there is conflict, the *patient* must *always* take precedence. If this means avoiding or failing another member of the community in some way, explaining the reasons will usually suffice. In fact, most people won't mind. They can themselves envision using the mental health services for their own problems, and get to see an example of how they would also be protected in that situation.

It is around confidentiality that this kind of conflict most frequently arises. If a permanent member of the university community (perhaps a dean or faculty member who is a long-time colleague of the psychiatrist) calls, worried and seeking information about a student-patient, it takes a particular forbearance on the part of the psychiatrist to deny the request of a friend or colleague for the sake of a patient who will soon be gone from the school.

Suppose a senior dean, a colleague (perhaps friend), who is influential in the university and may even influence the psychiatrist's position, calls to learn if a student is disturbed enough to move students from one dormitory to another. The psychiatrist's natural response would be to be open with the dean. The natural reaction of anyone with special information is to feel powerful and to want to share it. Suggesting that the information is privileged sounds like rejection, and perhaps contains implications that the dean cannot be trusted with a secret. Refusing to discuss the matter with the dean because the student has not given permission to do so obviously is ethically the best thing to do, but it will go against the psychiatrist's natural inclinations. He must use conscious, careful forbearance, accompanied by a polite, clear explanation; a breach of this sort rarely remains secret. Once such incidents get into the gossip-rumor chain of the community, it is very hard if not impossible to persuade anyone to use the clinical service. No one wins in that situation.

Interestingly, since passage of the Buckley Amendment which defines student privacy and access to information contained in the academic record, (such as formerly privileged letters of recommendation), faculty and deans are concerned about such issues for themselves and are much less likely than they once were to ask inappropriately for information.

These are strategies to lessen the difficulties:

One weekend night around Thanksgiving, two juniors—roommates—presented themselves at the Health Service Emergency Ward asking to see the psychiatrist. They were worried about a third roommate who was not studying, was behaving oddly, and discussing suicide. Her aunt who lived nearby had a chronic illness and a large cache of medicines. The roommate planned to steal some, return to the dorm around Christmas vacation, when the chances of being found were small, and take an overdose.

Clearly, this was not a situation where the roommates should be left as the only responsible people. Every effort would be made to take over responsibility by turning the suicidal roommate into a patient. However, at this time confidentiality constraints did not apply. Thus, the first thing we did was to discuss the situation at length with the very worried roommates who were themselves, at that point, patients. They were commended for their concern, reassured that the responsibility would be shared immediately, and told what to do in the future if they needed help, either for the roommate, or for their own anxiety in the situation—which was acknowledged as appropriate. They felt enormously relieved and clearer about what to do, and felt better understood in their own rights. Both continued to turn to the service for their own anxieties around the situation as it evolved.

Before seeing the patient, the psychiatrist wanted to be sure that the authorities would be apprised of the situation, so the service would not need to carry the responsibility of a worrying suicidal patient alone. So, the roommates were asked to go directly to the responsible dean. Thus, all channels of communications were open *prior* to seeing the patient.

The dean called and the situation was discussed, including how he might persuade the patient to see the psychiatrist, future monitoring of the situation, and ways to stay in contact, whether or not the patient gave permission to the psychiatrist to communicate to the dean. The dean was free to call the psychiatrist on his own initiative. If the patient proved not to be a genuine suicidal risk, and refused permission to communicate with administration, the psychiatrist would be forced to withhold any further information from the dean. The dean would also understand silence to mean that the psychiatrist felt the situation safe enough not to be forced to break the usual confidentiality rules. In short, by communicating *before* there was a patient, a discussion and working alliance was established among all of the people involved.

The young woman proved indeed to be intent on killing herself. However, with intense psychiatric intervention and a lot of support from those around her in the dorm, who were themselves supported by the mental health service, she was able to remain in school and out of a hospital that year.

This is an extreme case, but it does illustrate how the mental health worker, with planning and tact, can serve both patient and the surrounding people who are not designated as such but are also clients, without breaking patient/doctor trust and doing anyone a disservice.

The mental health service can be useful in dealing with behavior problems or psychoses which may require dismissal from college or hospitalization. Both upset the college community. The mental health service may also be called upon to help where there is not a designated patient, but a crisis situation involving some specific group in the university. An example of this is when someone has left abruptly because of psychosis, death, or suicide. We may be asked to help many people in different relationships to the episode and each other. The following will serve as an example.

A young woman disappeared from a cabin in the mountains, leaving an ambiguous note which implied suicide. The mental health service's first knowledge of the situation came when a tutor discussed with one of the psychiatrists his own grief, and his worry about the roommates, other students who knew the girl, and the larger dormitory community. After this discussion, the psychiatrist asked the roommates, who felt somewhat responsible and also were very upset by the loss of their friend, to come in as a group and later as individuals to work on their own grief reaction and guilt feelings.

The more senior admistration in the living unit also called for help again because of the contact already started and perceived to be helpful. They too were dealing with their own grief and at the same time trying to decide how to handle a difficult situation among the students. Discussing their own feelings, as well as the pros and cons of how to handle the dorm community was very supportive to them. Our offer to talk to any students who wished to come was declined at that point though at other times such visits have helped students share, understand, and come to terms with their reactions better.

Later, somewhat to my surprise, we saw several students, either in the office or more informally, who were more peripherally involved with the suicide victim. For many, this was the first experience with the death of a peer;

*they needed help with their feelings and came after hearing we had helped some-
one else.*

*By using knowledge of the grief process and suicide, the psychiatrist was
in a position to be helpful. By remembering what the needs of each of these
people were, she could tailor her response—helping faculty, administrators, and
students not only to deal with their own feelings, but also with the needs of
others.*

Another form of consultation which centers around an individual consists
of the administration asking for and using psychological advice in making certain
administrative decisions, e.g., whether or not to postpone an academic requirement (paper or exam) or to allow either a nonroutine withdrawal or a readmission following a leave for emotional reasons. In all of these situations, the
institution needs an established policy which should be worked out between the
health service and the administration. It is preferable that any psychological
opinion offered be *advisory* only, for two reasons. First, sitting in judgment is
something at which mental health workers are not good. In readmissions, for
example, our track record as predictors of performance is no better than experienced administrators. Second, it is absolutely crucial that administrative functions, if they are undertaken at all by the mental health service, should not
interfere with the normal use of the service, either by the individual in question
or by the general population. Thus, it must be very clear to everyone that the
opinion is voluntarily requested and is advisory only. The student can either request or refuse it; for readmission, for example, the consultation must be at
most recommended, never obligitory.

When a patient comes for administrative relief there are two tasks, one
administrative, but the second and more important if indicated, to make therapeutic help available to the student. This can be difficult, and there will be situations where it is preferable to refuse the administrative function in order to
preserve the therapeutic one. In a small school the grapevine is more pervasive
and the choice of therapists smaller. Getting involved in difficult administrative
questions, such as readmission after a psychotic episode, may not be worth the
price of risking the image of the service as autonomous and separate from the
administration.

In a setting where the health service is routinely used to advise the administration in certain situations, the dual function should be carefully discussed
with the patient, and whatever communications is to be made to the administration should be reviewed in advance with the patient and *written* permission given
to send it. This aspect of the encounter is separated from discussion of whether
the person needs further help and offering that. Further visits to the health
service should be explicitly explained to be like other contacts—privileged, and
not shared with the administration.

Whenever there is a conflict, it is essential to preserve the interests of the individual patient. This is primarily for the sake of the patient, but will also serve to preserve the reputation of the service as reliably separate from the administration.

GENERAL CONSULTATION

Consultation within the university can take a more general form. It can directly serve to educate the staff following the liaison model. Courses in psychology or anthropology come under this heading. So would requests by a person or group for the purpose of learning or sharing, where the stimulus for the contact is not an immediate problem needing a solution. This can be either a one or two encounter sort of contact, or an ongoing consultation over time.

The single encounters are useful not only for disseminating information, but also for getting seen by a wider audience than one would by just waiting for people to come to the office. These encounters take many forms. Examples would be at meetings of advisors or house residents, and at orientations for freshmen or new employees. Members of the staff who are good at this become known and are asked back for similar occasions. It is interesting, however, to note that such occasions, usually consisting of lecturing, with relatively little comfortable discussion, do not become ongoing consulting situations. Lectures are useful but they rarely lead to further consultation requests.

For significant relationships to form, or for deeper learning to take place, a more extended period of time is necessary. Much more can be done in an ongoing consultative relationship: scheduled meetings with a person or group which meets either regularly for some purpose of its own or specifically with the psychiatrist.

In all these situations, consultation should be requested. A doctor can offer service, but until there is both trust and a felt need, the offer will be politely ignored. How a mental health service or person gets into the position of being used varies enormously, but there are two general routes. The obvious one is doing good clinical and consulting work. The grapevine in a university is amazing.

The other route which should not be ignored is through other contacts which are social or professional but not psychologically oriented. Contacts of these kinds make both for actual consulting relationships and for a reputation which can lead to requests for consultation.

I was asked to be one of a heterogenous group of professional women to serve as friends and role models for undergraduates. The venture was not a great success itself, but it led to several relationships which resulted in invitations to do specifically psychological consulting. For example, through that group I met the then-chairwoman of the admissions committee who invited me to observe and contribute to the admissions committee. Several of its members, whom I also met this way, have continued to call with various problems for which they seek psychological consultation.

I had a consulting relationship for many years with a dean in which we met regularly to discuss various problems from medical to psychological questions. It never would have begun if I had not been associated with her college and met her on many occasions, usually social, until we became comfortable enough with each other for her to ask me to do this.

This leads to varied patterns of consultation with ongoing groups. As with the admissions committee, the psychiatrist can sit with an ongoing group as a regular participant, contributing a psychological viewpoint to the proceedings. Experienced educators know their business. We do have something to offer, but less than one might think. This observation is worth remembering if one does not want to wear out one's welcome.

Other counseling services on the campus (such as career-planning services) turn rather naturally to the mental health service for consultation or supervision. Because their members are already trained in the use of such help, supervision usually proceeds much as it would with any other group of professionals. Working with groups who are not used to such supervision is much trickier.

Busy college counselors will not spend time doing something which is not clearly useful. A lecture format usually is not pertinent enough to current problems. People also feel, probably accurately, that they could get similar material more quickly by reading. General discussion, either with or without a prearranged agenda, in my experience usually falls flat as well. What seems to work best is discussing an actual current problem brought up by one of the group. An issue worrying one person will have aspects reminiscent of problems being carried by other group members and a general discussion ensues. Someone genuinely worried about something will, if the session goes well, leave with a greater understanding of the problem and perhaps some new ideas on how to handle it. Anxiety will be noticeably decreased and some learning will be perceived as having occurred. Those are the goals of this sort of work.

The discussion itself makes a difference. Experience would suggest that it helps very much to have a group which is homogeneous. Mixing people whose problems are very different makes it less likely for everyone to resonate to a problem one member brings up—and it becomes harder to keep everyone involved. If one or two members (deans or chairmen) are in positions of authority over the rest, then candor, admitting ignorance, and sharing doubts will probably not happen. Not much learning about psychological problems can occur that way, significant problems are not brought up for discussion, and no one feels satisfied.

How the discussion is led shapes the process. The cardinal rules are to diminish anxiety and to clearly teach something. The latter is the easiest. Acquiring and dispensing knowledge is what a university is all about. One should make a point of including some didactic time in every session. Depending on the problem presented—alcoholism, depression, suicide potential—time is spent on a minilecture usually late in the session. This is valuable by itself, and also lends credibility to the entire process.

Most of the time is spent helping members share problems, solutions, and puzzlements. They teach and learn from each other's successes and mistakes and also learn to feel more secure and free to share feelings and insecurities.

Most groups have their own issues and rhythms. For some years, we have run a seminar of deans, each of whom is responsible for a group of upperclassmen and staff in one housing unit. Most of the group are doing this for the first time, but they are all struggling with essentially the same issues. The first part of the year is spent getting acquainted as a group and establishing a sense of commonality. Red-tape issues and how to handle certain fairly common problems (rowdy parties, security breaks, no-show to summonses after poor grade reports) usually predominate at first. This is the way the group gets to know and feel comfortable with each other. How to refer students to the health services is the usual subject used to get to know the psychiatrists. We discuss methods, go over confidentiality rules, talk about what sorts of problems might be considered suitable to send and the like. The hidden agenda, however is, "Can we trust each other?"

As the year progresses, more personal problems of the people the deans are responsible for surface. Psychosis, depression and suicide, inability to study, and alcohol and drugs come up, usually early in the year. Parents, and how to handle them, are another problem for this group of people, who are themselves fairly young and often still working out problems with their own parents. For instance, how much responsibility, or quasi-parenting, should they take on vis-à-vis their students? Should they call parents if a student asks? What should they say to a parent who calls them to complain or interfere? Young themselves, they see the students' side most easily and are less likely to readily perceive the parents' worry or capacity to be helpful. They also can see quite easily their own conflicts between wanting to "help" by giving concrete advice and realizing the student might prefer to work something out himself. Through issues like this, which are relatively clear, they can begin to sort out their own wishes and needs from those of their students.

In a group that works well together many issues will be covered in the course of a year, but emphasis seems to fall more on those that are important to group members than the issues that concern their students. If one of the group has suffered a significant personal loss, then loss will be discussed more often than in other years.

An important goal is to help the members learn to trust themselves, which means noticing their own reactions to situations and making some sense of them. Getting into this with a lay group is a sensitive business. If psychiatrists move too fast, people get scared and don't return; too slowly, and sessions get dull. As the group gets comfortable with each other, it becomes more and more possible to persuade whoever brings up a problem to describe the person in considerable detail and include what sorts of reactions the person elicits. Helping the members notice and use their own feelings is one of the goals of such consultation. Professionals are used to such probing; lay people are not, and one must be careful to have the process allay, not increase, embarrassment or anxiety. However, the feelings are there; acknowledging them and showing how they can be helpful and instructive allays anxiety and makes the whole experience seem satisfying. With successful groups, some of the last sessions are often spent discussing their own personal issues: family, future job concerns, feelings about their current work, and the like.

If problems do not suggest themselves to group members, or they have trouble describing them vividly enough for the others to make sense of them, role playing can be used to liven up the proceedings. Many people use this very successfully. My own predilection is to use it more to get discussion going than as an ongoing teaching tool, but that is a matter of personal style.

This kind of group consultation can be done with many groups in a university: student peer counsellors, junior faculty, teachers or advisors, resident proctors in dormitories—the list is long. As mentioned before, however, mixing too disparate groups will not work well. Meeting frequently enough to maintain intensity and continuity is also important. Weekly or bi-weekly meetings work well. Monthly ones, however, get a good deal more attenuated.

The college consultant functions as a catalyst on two major fronts. The personal development of students through education and direct therapy is facilitated. And the staff and faculty can grow and develop their own skills through group consultation and teaching. In the care of individual students, the doctor is known in the college community as a *real person* with student and faculty friendships, and an assigned job which the college funds. This context of complex relations with administration and patient maintains conflicts which must be kept clearly in mind and firmly and diplomatically managed to function effectively in the long run.

In sum, I think there are two crucial factors which make for the success of ongoing group consultations. In the first place, the group should be homogeneous in the sense that everyone in it has the same or similar jobs. No one in the group should be seen as much more experienced or hold a position which puts him or her in a supervisory capacity over the others.

The second factor is keeping the agenda spontaneous, allowing discussion of problems brought up by members of the group. Thus, the discussion is always dealing with an immediate, pressing problem of at least one group member and others in the group will have similar situations with which they too are struggling. Much of the discussion consists of sharing and comparing among themselves problems and various means of coping. This becomes very supportive but will be inhibited if someone is present who is much more experienced, preventing that kind of mutual admission of uncertainty and doubt.

The purpose of such a seminar is not to make amateur counselors out of the participants, but rather to help them do better what they already do, with less wear and tear on themselves. The aim is to improve listening skills and help participants trust their own judgment at the same time that they learn to see more clearly their own limitations. They thereby will become better judges of what falls within their capacities, and what should prompt their seeking outside help.

BIBLIOGRAPHY

Farnsworth DL: *Psychiatry, Education, and the Young Adult* (Charles C Thomas: Springfield, IL) 1966.

Glasscote RM, Fishman ME, et al.; *Mental Health on the Campus: A Field Study* (American Psychiatric Association: Washington, DC) 1973.

Hanfmann E: *Effective Therapy for College Students: Alternatives to Traditional Counseling* (Jossey-Bass: San Francisco) 1978.

Reid EA: Consultation in the college setting. *Am J Psych* 134(5):568–570, 1977.

Reid EA: The college psychiatrist as a consultant. *Psychiatr An* 8(4):164–168, 1978.

12

Consulting at Boarding Schools

Richmond Holder

While Tom Brown would not, Oliver Twist certainly would have been surprised to learn he attended a type of boarding school; Holden Caulfield not only knew it but loathed it and ran away. All three fictional characters lived in the special subdivision of the educational system known as boarding school and by such less flattering epithets as "foster home for unwanted rich kids," "prison," and "glorious residential setting for the birth and growth of the ole boy network." Before discussing the process of psychiatric consultation in these institutions, we might briefly examine their history.

In one form or another, and usually under the auspices of the church, such schools have existed for many centuries. For practical purposes, though, in pursuing the American genus of the species, we find its precursors in England. There the landed gentry, frequently synonymous with the aristocracy, felt the education of heirs was best left to the professionals, away from home, and in an atmosphere that today ironically might well be called a therapeutic milieu. Though very private and still at least intellectually exclusive, these schools are called "public" and are very much alive and well—Eton, Harrow, and Rugby to name but a few. They provide homes for the boys (only many years later did girls enter the picture), fine teaching, and last, but not least, training in the manly art of competitive sports. In a country rapidly expanding its empire (with attendant battles and hardships), this was no small part of the total educative process. The Duke of Wellington, himself a product of the system, was not indulging in idle chatter when he stated, "The battle of Waterloo was won on the playing fields of Eton."

At least three schools comparable to the English ones previously mentioned were founded in the United States in the eighteenth century and still flourish to this day. These schools had an interesting and quite important difference, however, in that provisions were made from the beginning to see that boys of all socioeconomic backgrounds would be admitted and generous scholarships provided. A century later in England, in 1874, the United Services College was established by a group of army officers who wanted to provide their sons with an education suited to class and family but could not afford to send them to the more expensive schools. Out of this sprang one of the most delightful books ever written about adolescents and their lives at boarding school, Rudyard Kipling's *Stalky and Company* (1899). It rivals or surpasses the adventures of Holden Caulfield in *Catcher in the Rye* (Salinger, 1945). The development of American aristocracy was interwoven with the evolution of private schools, especially boarding ones, which helped prepare each new generation to assume its position and consolidate economic and sociological gains. Finally, in a kind of reverse snobbery, American schools in this century dubbed themselves "independent" instead of "private."

Social historians claim that the "robber barons" of this country were much impressed, during their tours abroad, with the great English public schools. Just as they fabricated coats-of-arms and built chateaux more suited to the forests of France than the beaches of Newport, R.I., so did they attempt to recreate the public schools on our shores. Doubtless if they had found one for sale, they would have bought it, carefully taken it apart, and reassembled it in an appropriate spot here! Failing that, they set about replicating the originals, brick for brick, tower for tower, and eventually masses of ivy to enshroud the hallowed halls with the mystique of age and exclusivity. Only one thing remained missing—some semblance of unifying dress for the students which would evoke the ancestral organizations and yet not be out of keeping with the customs of the new country. It was clear that top hats and similar adornments were *de trop*, but school ties, insignia on blazers, and occasionally even caps could and did pass muster. Some observers of the scene felt the unification of dress, especially in the girls' schools, was designed to prevent competition in displays of sartorial splendor. Perhaps a blend of both views approximates the truth.

The system saw perhaps its finest hour in the political scene when its adversaries referred derisively (derogatorily?) to the old school tie or, currently, "the old boy network." Whimsically or otherwise, the schools themselves are called in some quarters Saint Grottlessex, a witty synthesis of three of the older names, and a tribute to the fact that most of them, in keeping with their European ancestors, had a minister as leader and were closely allied to the church.

Writers from Thomas Hughes, author of *Tom Brown's School Days* (Hughes, 1849) about Rugby, through Horace Vachell's *The Hill*, a novel about Harrow, and perhaps the most noted of all to American tastes, Salinger's *Catcher in the Rye* (1945), have not let the boarding school phenomenon go unnoticed. Indeed the second half of this century has seen a proliferation of books about it. The *Rector of Justin* (1964) by Louis Auchincloss exhaustively analyzed life at Groton while *A Separate Peace* (1959) by John Knowles chronicled Phillips Exeter and *The World According to Garp* (1978) by John Irving also satirized Exeter. Two plays—*Tea and Sympathy* (1953) by another Exeter graduate, Robert Anderson, and Lillian Hellman's *The Children's Hour* (1934)—addressed themselves to some of the darker problems of school life. Even the periodicals have been producing articles, of which perhaps the best known is Nelson Aldrich's "Preppies" in the *Atlantic Monthly* (1981).

Most of the schools have slowly shifted from accepting only boys—a few took only girls—to accepting both sexes. Only one or two of the boys' establishments remain unconverted to coeducation. Their oft-repeated mission of preparing children for the business of living in the outside world goes on. This is amusingly and even chillingly dramatized in Irving's book about Garp. He names his fictional boarding school "Steering." From this precise appellation we are alerted to the fact that the founders and backers of these establishments wanted their children not just to be taught but to be *steered* in the right way to live life and become effective members of society.

Did they place them away from home for this purpose or, as some cynics would have us believe, to be unburdened by them in times of family strife or impending divorce? Whatever the reason, the outcome appeared successful and the organizations grew like Topsy. Success begat success, money poured into school coffers, and this small segment of the American educational scene produced significantly more than its share of magnates of industry, moguls of finance, and leaders of the ship of state, including not a few presidents. Senators, cabinet members, and lesser luminaries were turned out too, and often could be recognized around the world wearing the traditional tie while the network continued to function, much as Smiley's people did in John Le Carre's famous novels about the British secret service.

Partly because of the system's growth, partly because of the pressure of changing times, psychoneuroses were springing up in the boarding schools' garden of Eden. Actually, they probably were there all along, but the mechanisms for handling them were slow to develop. One must only recall that a department of child psychiatry did not begin at the Massachusetts General Hospital until 1948 and that, while various child guidance centers had been around much longer (such as the Judge Baker Guidance Center and the Thom Clinic, both in Boston), they had ready-made, long recognized as "troubled," inner-city populations to serve. By contrast, the schools, for the most part, were relatively isolated and probably suffered from the assumption that "It can't happen here."

Nevertheless, it *was* happening and the faculties, backed by their trustees, began to consider psychological help for their students. At first, one or more teachers were designated to provide it, as had been done for years by advisors, tutors, or others. When this proved too burdensome, or when some catastrophe like a suicide occurred, outside help was called in. Psychologists or psychiatrists, the latter having a possible added clout deriving from their medical title, would come to the schools more consistently, at first on a day basis and then in some cases overnight. This practice was pioneered by the Phillips Exeter Academy and a few others, which at first engaged one psychologist and one psychiatrist. These consultants achieved strong acceptance by faculties.

When the author arrived at Exeter in 1952 to replace the psychologist and spend two-and-a-half days a week there, the emotional climate was already friendly. A psychologist highly trained in group dynamics had worked with small groups of faculty members and had been quite successful in promoting their receptivity towards students' getting individual help. Being there overnight gave an entree into community life of both staff and students that could not otherwise easily have been achieved. The doctor could watch sporting events, occasionally play squash or tennis with friendly teachers, visit in their homes, and eat meals in the dining halls where much of the life is centered. Best of all, he was invited into the dormitories to discuss psychiatry and exchange views on life with the interested boarders.

Throughout these encounters, an informal gentlemen's agreement existed extending far beyond the ordinary demands of the Hippocratic oath, an agreement keeping medicine and social life separate. Occasionally this gave rise to what appeared to be a conflict of interest. On the one hand the faculty would see the consultant as a kind of rival "molly coddling" its charges, and on the other the students would see him as a member of management.

These views and others would dutifully be reported by the student press, the tone of which ranged from enthusiastic to negative. Not unnaturally, when a senior editor was in treatment (and going through a period of positive transference) the stature of shrinking gained in glory.

In other schools the consulting service, so-called, had many names and many locations. Perhaps the most satisfactory was to have it based alongside of or in the infirmary, as in Exeter, though even this had its drawbacks. Anonymity in the early days was one of the great needs of successful consulting. Achieving this was another thing. In one old-line school the author served in, the students, in conjunction with the librarian, worked out a system of sign-up by marking an X in a series of designated free times posted on a bulletin board. While this occasionally was riddled by pranks and no-shows, it worked about as well as the more formal system complete with form, name, and other data.

Fear of the system and what it meant to see a "shrink" was almost entirely based on public opinion, and that in turn rested on the adolescents' perceiving the doctor as a human being. Playing squash, attending games, eating in the dining halls, being ready to join in with a dormitory discussion, or submitting to a newspaper interview were all useful adjuncts to the job. Above all, those served wished to be assured of their privacy and freedom from exposure to management, especially in matters relating to alcohol, cigarettes, and more recently, drugs.

M. Jacobbi's article in *Boston Magazine* reveals the anguish of the student population at what they perceive as a double standard of the school regarding the smoking of marijuana. The penalty for this is expulsion at one school, an unusual way to handle a form of adolescent behavior which (while admittedly undesirable) is indulged in by a vast percentage of that age group in all kinds of schools, both public and independent. Such drastic punishment is highly dubious as a deterrent and even more questionable as a means of educating the young in the dangers of drug abuse. In a situation like this it is helpful when the consultant is seen as a real person in the real life of the school, but at the same time, he runs the risk of being identified as an enemy by both sides, especially the patients.

The use of the word patient raises another set of issues. From the start of boarding school consulting, the physician has been faced with a triple challenge: (1) selling the service to the students (2) selling it to the faculty, and (3) selling it to the families. The latter was and is perhaps the most difficult task of all. Due to the very nature of the population served, the families are often many miles away. Possibly because of the heavy percentage of scholarship students, some parents are unfamiliar with the concepts of psychiatry, and (were the truth to be known) even its existence. This means not only that the reality of a problem must be established, but also that the need for its remedy must be concurred in by both parent and child. All this requires backing by the administration (or "the Kremlin" as it was called in one school) and being fitted into a framework acceptable to one and all.

Much of the above may seem routine to any clinician experienced in the ways of a clinic or, indeed, private practice. However, in a boarding school milieu the difficulty of finding time for a therapeutic hour is at one and the same time both increased and diminished. It is decreased because numerous activities are provided for the young to enrich their lives, such as clubs, a variety of sports events, and a rigid framework of arising, meals, and going to bed. It is increased by the fact that they are on location, as it were, and readily accessible around the clock, including weekends should anyone wish to work then.

During my tenure at Exeter (1952–1962) for two-and-a-half days a week, about 12.5 percent of the population of 750 boys were seen for emotional problems each year. While this is a lower figure than the Manhattan Project came up with (25 percent) it parallels other schools and colleges and probably means about one-third of such a group or four percent were in therapy regularly. The difficulties presented ranged widely from ordinary adolescent concerns to severe academic failure and even suicide. In recent years it is understandable that the complaints have been greatly augmented by drug usage, ranging in severity from pot to heroin with a wide potpourri of mixtures in between including Quaaludes, Darvon, cocaine, and the ubiquitous Valium. Despite this, the overwhelming primary complaint of the referred adolescents in boarding schools has almost always been academic underachievement.

How did this group reach the psychiatrist at this particular school? Over a five-year period, referral of boys with emotional problems broke down as follows:

Self-referred	47 percent
Parent referred	13 percent
Faculty and dean referred	20 percent
Initiated at infirmary	19 percent
Student referred	1 percent

Year in and year out the percentage of self-referral stayed fairly constant at about 45 percent. It would have been interesting to correlate this with the number of young people whose parents had already been working with a professional in the mental health field, and who therefore had opportunities to see the usefulness (or lack of it) of consultation. Unfortunately this was not done.

Only one percent of students are referred by other students; but sometimes dramatically, as when two football players dragged a troubled student and threw him into the consulting room.

More often, notes from deans, other faculty members, or coaches after a marking period are a prelude to seeking help from the consultative service, or lengthy letters from family aware of pre-existing trouble in a boy, which was not mentioned to the admissions office at the time of application. Occasionally, too, an impending divorce or other family trauma precipitates a request for help at some distance from the school. The psychiatrist has to be flexible and functions somewhat as a family doctor at long range, a confidant(e) of a dedicated staff trying to help a group of adolescents away from home, and diagnostician and therapist. In the latter role, he has to be paid somehow. Let us now examine how the finances of consulting are handled.

Earlier on, it was considered that psychiatry could be thrown in as part of the medical package of schools, but when this proved to be too expensive, a sliding scale of fees was introduced with a two or three visit diagnostic procedure being paid for by the institution. On the whole, the fee for service worked better than other systems and in much the same way as it does in the outside world. Fee service was very often viewed with suspicion by this particular group of parents, as evidenced in one particular case where the father living in a big city far away indignantly refused services of the school psychiatrist. He insisted that his son see a renowned specialist whom he had heard about in Boston. As a consequence thereof, the consultant changed his hats and obligingly saw the boy in his private office in Boston, with considerably more difficulty and expense to the family than would have been incurred otherwise.

Fees, as might have been foreseen, were closely linked with maintainance of confidentiality. It had been hoped at Exeter that we could preserve the boy's visits in total confidentiality. A bill arriving at the family homestead, whether in prairie or metropolis, blew the whistle on that. By the same token, failing to inform parents that their child was being evaluated by a psychiatrist, much less treated, might well have produced some nasty legal situations. Hence, it was concluded that every effort had to be made to assure the patient that his secrets would be kept, but that we had to be in contact with his family.

Notification in the large majority of cases meant very carefully worded letters. One could not say "problems" even though young Aloysius Pumpernickle Throckmorton III was lighting fires and cheating. One had to fudge and say "potential difficulties in maintaining his academic career at St. Grottlessex." Therapy became "working with the school consultant" and so on, all equally palatable to parents, staff, and boy alike. After all, the elite population of such schools did not and could not have disturbed, sick, or anything less than all-American healthy boys!

Only when contact with the family had been established and a personal interview set up, if possible, did the complete question of money arise. Already paying hefty tuitions, the parents might well be outraged at having to pay out more money for something whose value they question. Once they had met with the doctor, however, things usually seemed to fall into place. All of this would seem to indicate that much of the project's success rested on the personality of the doctor and his relationship with the staff and the students. One of the biggest boosts to the psychiatric service was the social cachet of its acceptance by one or two key individuals such as newspaper editors or athletes who had worked with the doctor. This put the good housekeeping seal of approval on the process and from then on things would usually work well.

Like all good things, of course, the students' careers at the schools would eventually come to an end, and the astute clinician would learn to recognize hopefully before it arrived in spring term, the senior syndrome peculiar to the foster-home aspect of boarding school. It seemed to center around the approaching departure from what had been, for the most part, an excellent home away from home for these teenagers before transition into the outside world, usually college. Various forms of psychological mourning and acting out related to impending graduation could be spotted. Occasionally it would take the form of unconsciously attempting to do something to prevent graduation, such as one classical case of obviously plagiarizing his final paper. Other warning signs would be massive slipping in the marks before the college acceptances had come out and, rarely, more extreme forms of acting out to delay departure into the next life phase, including the ultimate penalty of getting bounced from school—an unwanted extension of the psychological self-destructive process.

Along these lines, the college admission applications almost invariably have carried some form of question relating to the presence of mental illness, most recently with assurances that responses will be used only after matriculation and by college health services. Probably many of these forms hark back to an earlier year when there was less preventive work done in psychiatry, and in many instances, they probably referred to actual psychotic breaks. However, one school in the forefront of the use of mental health facilities issued a blanket statement for every graduate that "Mr. X at some time in the course of his four years here may have used the infirmary mental health facilities, which in our opinion has no bearing on his college admission qualifications. Should there be anything that is pertinent medically, our school consultant will be glad to confer with the medical staff of the college of his choice." In one variation on this, some schools and individuals simply do not mention a psychiatric record on a student, but the trend nowdays is to make it part of a person's total medical and sociological history. Then even though further work is needed in later years, happily, it has appeared that seeing a consultant has not adversely affected the applicant's chances for getting into the college of his choice, and may even reassure a college that mental health awareness has been established in advance.

Perhaps now it is fair to say that most psychiatric work of the boarding schools is done by members of the staff trained in psychological counseling or by referral outside the school, since the availability of a specially trained person on the grounds for a period of time is becoming prohibitive in terms of logistics, time and money. However, it is also fair to state that the availability of someone of the counseling professions may make considerable difference to the population of a boarding school and help ease the transition into the life away from home. He occasionally can be helpful in preventing more serious mental difficulties, and often start a teenager into a therapeutic program at a time when it can be the most rewarding for him and, consequently, for the school he represents.

Thirty years ago, I started boarding school consultation by doing physicals to screen new students. One day I was hailed before the weekly faculty and staff meeting, all ninety seated two rows deep around a massive square table. The occasion for my presence, I discovered, was to know what I thought about the psychic state of a young freshman. It appeared he had been wetting his bed at age 14, was stealing in the dorm, and had been found setting a fire. After this case presentation the assembled multitude gazed somberly at me and asked through its spokesman if I thought this boy had a problem.

I was cautious. "It is possible," I said "that he may have a problem but, at the very least, I think the matter should be explored." No sooner had I spoken than the most senior master present pounded his fist on the table and roared, "He can't have a problem. I went to Harvard with his father." Happily, not everyone concurred with this early verdict, and later I was able to see, diagnose, and take into treatment the young fellow with quite happy results.

Not so happy was another case some months later where a lad who had been seen briefly by a psychiatrist the year before appeared at the infirmary quite depressed and seeking help. I saw him twice and left him on the second day to head back for Boston with his reassurance ringing in my ears that he would be all right until my next visit.

That night he came to the infirmary with a chipped tooth which he said had been injured in a fall in the dorm bathroom. It was duly noted, pills were prescribed for his pain, and he left. One hour later he hung himself with a window sash cord tied to the shower rod, in the same spot where he had earlier tried the act, falling and chipping his tooth.

These cases represent the extremes of diagnostic categories, obviously. Suicides in the independent schools is probably the most guarded statistic of all. As always in such tragic occurrences, both sides feel much guilt and it is considered that any publicity would only intensify an already bad situation. One can only guess at the incidence of suicide; an educated estimate of mine based on talks and experience in a number of settings would be possibly one case per average school of five hundred every seven or eight years. This is fairly low if one considers that self-destruction is the second leading cause of death among adolescents (automobile accidents being first). Whatever the statistics, in my opinion one must always take the threat of such an action most seriously. Notes, in particular, are an extra special cry for help. They should be dealt with promptly and openly. The very fact of discussing the proposed deed seems to bring considerable relief to the sick youngster.

In 1950, a boy left a note on his bureau with a Shakespearean phrase, "The only becoming note of his life was the leaving of it." By the time it had been discovered, the boy had run away. Happily he was found and returned to school to enter treatment with me for the next 18 months. Unhappily, five years later and with additional therapy elsewhere, he killed himself in a closed garage with a hose leading from the exhaust of his beloved sports car.

Turning into a cheerier aspect of the cases seen, one might consider those who act out as their primary symptomatology. This group of teenagers well may not fall in the category of psychiatric cases at all. Much depends on the wisdom and experience of the faculty handling the situation, and often the acting out points to pathology in the target of its shenanigans. One delightful episode illustrates the latter point.

A particular dorm master with a morbid propensity for spying upon boys after lights were to be out and catching them in some form of illicit activity earned the name of Slew Foot. His stealthy, carpet-slippered nocturnal raids were notorious and loathed by students and many faculty members alike. One evening well after curfew a nimble group of his charges took a sturdy sheet of canvas and glued it to the outside frame of the dorm apartment door from which he exited to conduct his raids. Quicksetting glue and a few thumb tacks almost instantly produced a trampolinelike vertical surface for our villain to encounter. Thus baited, the trap was sprung. Various scufflings and talking noises just loud enough to be heard in the teacher's domain resulted in his pulling his door inward and leaping forward to catch his prey.

Glue, tacks, and cloth held. Slew Foot bounced back like a ball from a bat and landed upon his derriere. Enraged, he charged again, not knowing what had hit him, with the same result (and with sounds of gratification heard without). Soon he was busy slicing his way out into a ghostly-quiet corridor with everyone tucked safely and legally in bed. Happily, after his initial fury subsided and the light of day dawned, he was able to profit by the experience.

Other examples of acting out are more complex as with trashing, a simple but tedious trick involving crumpling up numerous newspapers in large balls until the victim's room is filled to the ceiling and the door closed. Curiously enough, this sort of prank can be carried out against a boy who is disliked or in a benign manner against a member of the in-group. More extreme examples that have been tried include tying condoms over the outside door knobs of newly wed faculty members and killing pets by strangulation.

Most of this never gets to the consultant except indirectly. His job is to unscramble the normal behavior of bored teenagers away from home and separate it from occasionally serious psychopathology, sometimes quite a tough task. A close working relationship with the faculty and students, preserving the strictest confidentiality, was of enormous help. An especially wise dean can and did help the neophyte child practitioner sort out the subtypes of behavior. One has to be careful, however, about how one appears to be associated with the staff, administration, enemy, or whatever the adults in charge are called by their students.

As in the real world outside of school, fame, wealth, and power can pose problems for both sides. Though Hemingway, needling Fitzgerald, said the only difference between the rich and the rest of us is that they have more money, there are more subtle and significant issues. One of these arises when a potential patient is the son of a trustee or substantial benefactor of the school. Should the lad's marks be marginal he is described as "a late bloomer." His acts of vandalism can be attributed to "high spirits" and so forth. Of course, this is not always or even usually the case but the potential threat is still there, especially in the minds of those responsible for the overall administration of the organization. Happily, in thirty years only rarely did I see this affect the outcome of a case where the boy needed treatment.

Members of the power structure of the country pose a somewhat different challenge for the doctor. They are not accustomed to being hauled in, as they see it, to explain away their offspring's shortcomings. Some accept it thankfully and graciously, others not. Almost all appreciate frankness and a direct approach since so often in their businesses or professions (notably the entertainment industry) their understanding of what is really going on is cluttered by sycophants and "yes" men. Overall, if one sticks to the clinical facts and sympathizes with the true parental positive feelings (when present) one can do a good job professionally.

An odd but important aspect of VIP families is their way of dealing not only with their children, but also with what they see as extensions of their business, domestic, and in this case, medical staffs. This can be illustrated in the case of vacations, especially when exceptions to school procedures have to be made in the interest of the family empire and its travel arrangements, including meetings with the therapist. Letters will frequently come out of the corporate headquarters as if they were purchase orders or advertising campaigns for a new line of merchandise.

Typically, there will be a primary communique to the son and, on occasion, to the dean or headmaster. There will also be a carbon copy (*cc*) to the advisor including details of the travel plans such as who, what, when, and where even the trivia of baggage handling. Then there is the *cc* to the lowly consultant. Much of this might seem interesting or even funny, but to the patient it is often a cause of real humiliation. How often have I heard my patient say, "Gee, I wish Dad would write me himself, just once, in his own hand. Why does it always have to be his secretary?" Back of it all is the boy's feeling that he is a very small cog in a very large corporate empire.

Another important feature in the affluent offspring's life other than parents, although more and more replaced by maids, was the ubiquitous nanny. Either imported from Europe as useful status symbol or, if a native, treated as if she were an immigrant, she becomes in the young child's life not only a parent surrogate but often more important than the actual parent. This gives rise to competition with mother, and adds one more very poignant conflict to adolescent turmoil when the possibility arises of the nanny or governess being dismissed. The most likely time for this to happen is when her usefulness is diminished by the boy's departure for boarding school. As one client so poignantly put it to me in describing his new life at St. Grottlessex, "It's no girls, no food, and no home." Mercifully, the first matter has been largely eliminated by the almost universally coeducational population of the schools.

All these factors and many more must be appraised and handled by the skillful practitioner. In extreme cases he must even be prepared to hospitalize his charges and then fight for them to be readmitted to the school when appropriate. Tact, humor, attention to detail, letter writing, dealing with the faculty with warmth and understanding—besides safeguarding the clinical needs of his patients—are all part of the doctor's job. What makes it different from ordinary practice is the fact that he is on the spot figuratively and literally.

When I first started consulting and psychiatry was relatively new to the schools some thirty years ago, it was not always clear to the teachers that their young charges were suffering. They saw them variously as being stubborn, bad boys, lazy, spoiled, and even sometimes stupid. What adults often failed to see was the youngsters' pain. As in ordinary practice it was this pain which made them seek help and usually kept them in therapy. Happily, members of the school administration, often including sports coaches, would initiate requests for consultation which were almost invariably well founded as they became familiar with the psychiatric field.

Under special circumstances, I encouraged the advisor to handle the student himself. Three factors dictated this: Some referrals really centered around the normal patterns of adolescent adjustment reactions; second, as the load upon our services increased it was impossible to handle it all; third, in some instances, a good alliance between faculty member and student can place staff in the stronger position to lead a troubled youngster to safer ground, provided staff have good access to the consultant while this is done. Many teachers feared they would harm their students or get out of their depth in working psychologically with them. In point of fact, this is exactly what skilled educators have been doing for centuries and are trained to do. Also, the teenager is able to relate better and more quickly to someone he already knows. Obvious exceptions to this are when disciplinary issues are involved or when behavior has come to the attention of a dorm master or advisor the boy does not trust. Under those circumstances a diplomatic rerouting of the clinical care is needed. Occasionally a case may come first to the school doctor's attention, and he may wish to try his hand at the gentle art of psychotherapy (sometimes with disastrous results). Once again the role of diplomat must be called into play.

There are few meaningful statistics about the social class of my referrals or their diagnoses. I saw mainly well-to-do boys. Also, the cases from such a background (as in the recent film "Ordinary People") may have had greater exposure to the field of psychiatry. It may also have been that, unconsciously or otherwise, the faculty was paying particular attention to them. In a like vein, a disproportionately large number of medical offspring appeared and still appear in my office. Many years ago I was kindly and wisely advised by a senior colleague to set down my conditions of handling such cases from the start (i.e., they would be treated like any other families and the cases run by me, not the medical parents). I have found this especially useful in handling psychological colleagues' children, potentially one of the "stickiest wickets" in our work.

Perhaps my impression grows out of a screened memory, or even the changes in our society, but lawyers' offspring seemed to pose equal if not worse problems than those of their medical confreres. By contrast, the non-WASP, less sophisticated families fitted into the medical scheme of things as though born to it. This may well reflect the remnants of reverence for our profession still remaining some segments of society!

Just as impressions are hard to document, follow-up statistics are hard to ascertain. I read religiously the alumni bulletins of the half-dozen schools with whom I worked most, and I am gratified to get an occasional wedding announcement or even birth notice from former patients. Perhaps the most valuable form of follow-up is the check-in of students from bygone years seeking advice or mini-therapy sessions about current difficulties in their lives. This I find most gratifying. It shows that the attempts at therapy were not forgotten and were viewed as something helpful that could be incorporated into present-day life. Not all, of course, are success stories. Some merely hold onto the status quo, and one or two, as mentioned before, take their lives in later years. Hopefully the intervention of psychological assistance at a crucial time in their lives prevented deeper troubles in the future. One may well say, and the cocktail circuit does not hesitate to, that they would have improved anyhow. Time did the trick. I can readily believe this and have considerable faith in Father Time. Nevertheless, I also have faith in what a little short-term therapy can do for a young person with his whole life ahead of him and the vast powers of growth and adolescence going for him.

Perhaps in closing I should attempt to list some of the signs of potential trouble in the world of the teenager both in and out of boarding schools. Underachievement is the number-one symptom. A word of caution is in order here, however. If the youth is playing a varsity sport, acting in a play, and busy with friends, he is not underachieving. He is simply misalloting his time. He may also appear to be under-achieving when in realty he is suffering from dyslexia which afflicts as many as 20 percent of all teens. Only skillful psychological testing can ascertain this, and prompt remedial measures are then in order. It is vital to bear in mind, that the student may chronically feel inadequate due to years of suffering under the misapprehension that he was dumb. This in itself calls for help, sometimes of a substantial nature. It is all too easy to turn the case over to the remedial reading teacher and breathe a sigh of relief. Indeed children who have considered themselves stupid over any length of time sometimes require more therapy than those suffering from a simple maladjustment to adolescence.

Failing and falling grades across the board may be another sign of real trouble. In boarding schools there is usually plenty of information available from advisor or dorm master to understand what is going on. The positive family-like atmosphere of the living arrangement presents many of the same advantages of a milieu treatment center. On this account especially, a warm and trusting communication between teacher and consultant can work wonders in helping unravel potentially trouble-making factors, be they letters from home about an impending divorce or serious friction with a roommate.

Frequent class absences, sports excuses, avoidance of locker rooms, frequent visits to the infirmary, or isolation from his peers can all be seen as red flags of danger. One of the best methods of dealing with these situations, but needing the cooperation of a friendly English teacher, is use of the story told in a free unassigned subject theme. While many of these may be written only to jolt the adults, often they are real cries for help. Other such smoke signals are, of course, *consistent* flaunting of rules and authority. An important subsidiary area here is consistent failure to turn in written reports or complete lab work. The central theme of all this type of activity is consistency, since all of us do some of these things some of the time.

Just as in the regular clinical medicine, boarding school consultation requires a careful, detailed, and accurate history of the potential patient. One should know, for example, the reasons for the boy's being at the school. Was it because three generations had been there before, or because he himself wanted to be there? Was he pushed in obliquely by the possible family gift to the school of an indoor heated swimming pool, or did he make it on his own grades and wishes? No matter how skilled the admission officers of these ivyed halls, they can miss some of these points and more serious ones, such as an incipient or existing neurosis.

The world of Garp is a cruel and tough one. While not as savage as the world of Tom Brown or Oliver Twist, the boarding school presents the greatest psychic challenge a youngster has experienced up to that time in his life. The psychiatric consultant can treat students, educate their families about their children's real needs, and broaden the thinking of the faculty. If the consultant achieves this we can do much to minimize the casualties and ensure the survival of a new wave of young men and women to take hold of their futures.

REFERENCES

Aldrich NW Jr: Preppies. *The Atlantic Monthly*, Boston, 1981.
Amory C: *The Proper Bostonians* (EP Dutton and Co: New York) 1947.

Ashburn F: *Primer for Parents* (Coward–McCann: New York) 1945.

Auchincloss L: *The Reactor of Justin* (Houghton Mifflin: Boston) 1964.

Baser BH (ed.): *Psychotherapy of the Adolescent* (International University Press: New York) 1957.

Burnett FH: *A Little Princess* (JB Lippincott Co: New York) 1963.

Committee on Adolescence, Group for the Advancement of Psychiatry: *Normal Adolescence* (Chas Scribner's Sons: New York) 1968.

Gathorne–Hardy J: *The Unnatural History of the Nanny* (The Dial Press: New York) 1973.

Hughes T: *Tom Brown's School Days* (JM Dent & Sons, Ltd, EP Dutton & Co, Inc: New York) 1949.

Irving J: *The World According to Garp* (EP Dutton, Inc: New York) 1978.

Jacobbi, M: Private School Guide, *Boston Magazine*, 1981.

Kipling R: *Stalky and Company* (Collier Books: New York) 1899.

Knowles J: *A Separate Peace* (Macmillan Company: New York) 1959.

Krugman M (ed.): *Orthopsychiatry and the School* (American Orthopsychiatry Association, Inc: New York) 1958.

Marquand JP: *The Late George Apley* The Modern Library of the World's Best Books (Random House, Inc: New York) 1936.

Nesbitt E: *Treasure Seekers* (Ernest Benn, Ltd: London) 1962.

Salinger JD: *Catcher in the Rye* (Little, Brown & Co: Boston) 1945.

Sargent PE: *The Handbook of Private Schools* (Porter Sargent Publishers, Inc: Boston) 1978.

Wechsler J: *In A Darkness* (Boston) 1978.

13

Consultation: Two Worlds in a Factory Town

Robert S. Adams

CONSULTATION

The forms and course of consultation are determined by the needs, wishes, and goals of both consultant and consultee and by the constraints imposed upon them by their immediate environments and cultures. This interaction between personal needs and environment is a familiar paradigm. In this paper, I will describe two consultation experiences in related, but dissimilar settings. Common to both programs is the community in which they were set and the fact that they faced similar problems of limited community resources amid a growing sense of the need for more resources. Both are school programs, one public and one private. Both have perceived increasing needs for psychiatric and mental health services, and both are dependent on a community with relatively limited resources. There are significant differences, as well, both in the history of each program and in the demands made on the consultant. The focus of interest in this paper is an effort to understand the role of these differences and to derive from this some models of consultation in a particular kind of community and setting.

Both schools are located in communities surrounding a medium-sized industrial and commercial city. The city, with a population of two-hundred thousand, was created and grew as part of the expansion of industrial New England in the mid-nineteenth century. Recently it has been economically depressed because its principal product, brass, has been in less demand. The city has been geographically isolated from governmental, cultural, medical, and academic urban centers, although more recently the interstate highway system has increased traffic in and out of the city. The city is ethnically very diversified and traditionally very insular.

The population is largely blue collar, descendants of Eastern and Southern European workers brought in as cheap but skilled labor early in the century. There were, until recently, native-language Roman Catholic parishes and churches. Public schools were also identified with specific ethnic groups. There was a small managerial and professional class, but this group also lived in identifiable enclaves and, more recently, in the surrounding countryside. As the major industries moved from local and family ownership into larger, corporate, conglomerate structures, the involvement of senior management in the community diminished. The centers of economic growth and economic power became less easily accessible and less responsive to the needs of the city. The city is a regional center for medical services, providing the only hospital care for a string of five smaller industrial communities along the river on which the city is located. There are two hospitals in the community both of which have recently developed psychiatric services; there is, however, no mental health center. There are a small number of psychiatrists in private practice but very few in full-time practice, and there is a small child guidance clinic.

The child guidance clinic has a small multidisciplinary staff and offers the only exclusively child-centered psychiatric services in the region. It has an ambiguous relationship with the community at large and with the medical delivery system in particular. There is a mystique surrounding its image. Perceptions by outsiders about how the clinic functions are more often than not based on fantasies, wishes, and fears and, like all such constructions, are not easily modified by facts.

It has long been a firm "fact", for instance, that the clinic is so insulated professionally that it could afford to close for a month in August and a week in the winter. In point of fact, it has not been closed for any period of time for at least ten years. The waiting list is another myth that is also an irritant. There has always been a waiting list, it varies in length; there has never been a long wait for intake, and all services in the community have some kind of a waiting list. None of these facts have modified the perception that there is a lengthy waiting list and that, therefore, referral is pointless, available selectively and only to a chosen few. In fact, the majority of the clinic's caseload is working class and at least one-third of the clinic's billings are to Medicaid. Recently the maximum wait for treatment is up to six months and many cases begin much earlier. The community myth is that the waiting list is endless, negating the usefulness of referral. One of the functions of this myth is the alleviation of community guilt: If the child guidance clinic has a waiting list, this deflects concern about delays, for example, in the assignment of children to special education programs; and, in fact, the loudest protesters about the waiting list are school systems.

Among the serious long-range consequences of these legends are delayed referrals, referrals only when cases reach critical dimensions, or referrals after repeated efforts to find alternative programs in the community. A fourteen year-old boy is referred, for instance, after six years of frustrating failing experiences in school, associated with anger, rage, and depression, but referred when the situation has settled into a state of intense, passive withdrawal associated with the onset of a turbulent adolescence and a family burdened with a sense of despair. These factors, the long history and the family despair, make it unlikely that outpatient treatment will be effective. On the other hand, the clinic is the last resort and there are no alternatives. Some of the rippling effects of this are the extended commitment of limited staff time to difficult and complex cases, limited staff time for preventive work, and considerable staff stress over the conflicting demands of services versus consultation.

The clinic and its staff is seen as both indispensible and inadequate for its task. It is the principal referral source for many children of the community, and it is seen as elitist, superior, and somehow peripheral and out of the mainstream.

The defining characteristic of the community, for our purposes, is an impoverishment of mental health resources and a concomitant tendency to dilute, to overextend and to battle against a powerful tendency to try to be all things to all people. The relative scarcity of resources, added to the widespread perception of the clinic as relatively unavailable, has significantly influenced consultation programs.

While different members of the staff have provided consultation and informally still do so, the principal consultant to these two programs has been the director of the clinic, a child psychiatrist, functioning however quite differently in each program. In one he is the agent of the clinic to the school; in the other he wears a different hat, retained as an independent contractor offering his own services and collecting his own fees. This difference is important and will be discussed further. One aspect of his role in his long, twenty-year tenure in the clinic, so that he brings to his role as consultant a wide knowledge of the history of the development and growth of services in the community.

Nonpsychiatric and nonmental health services in the community have felt compelled to develop their own skills, to handle their own problems internally, and to fall back on their own resources. This is reinforced, in the public school, by Public Law 94–142. This law, which mandates education of children with special needs using community resources, raises the threat that schools must pay for their use and perhaps even be financially responsible for treatment. This has inhibited case referral to the extent that only the most difficult cases are referred, often after many efforts by the school system to develop their own program until a point of no return has been reached.

Typical, for instance, is the referral of a somewhat intellectually limited boy with an IQ of 80, and a family history of deprivation, who becomes increasingly withdrawn as he approaches adolescence, passively aggressive and resistant in a learning situation. Because he is not by definition retarded, he cannot be placed in a special class and because of massive family disorganization, the family cannot press for special services. The school has made a range of half-hearted attempts to deal with him, including use of a special reading teacher, pressure on the pediatric clinic to prescribe Ritalin, and limiting the school day. This goes on until his aggression leads to exclusion from the school, at which point he feels hopeless, helpless, and incompetent. And, at this point, a referral is made to the child guidance clinic.

Because of the pressures on the school, on the one hand, to provide questionably appropriate services and, on the other hand, the imperative need to save money, the school is reluctant even to request consultation, let alone make an early referral.

Consultation on an informal basis is frequent and always related to a specific case. There is a problem in this process. Since school systems are large and since personnel change with each consultation, there is no time or opportunity for the development of a mutually comprehensible language or for the clarification of points of stress so crucial to successful ongoing consultations. The two experiences to be discussed suggest that this creation of a group cohesiveness is crucial to the successful development of a consultation program.

The towns in which the prep school and public school are located are similar suburban cities contiguous to the large industrial core city. Both towns are largely bedroom communities with some industry and both are rather parochial in the sense of their need to maintain control over their own affairs. While there are significant differences which play some role in what happened, there is enough similarity to suggest that the differences in the development of the two programs depend more on the intrinsic nature of the two consultation programs themselves.

PREP SCHOOL

The prep school was a well established and traditional classic boarding academy, physically enclosed, all-male, with limited ties to the community and typical in its denial of problems. If students were having difficulties the problems were ignored or the students were willy-nilly extruded. The appointment of a new headmaster announced a period of startling change. The school moved towards coeducation; the percentage of day students increased among seniors. The drug culture, the political consciousness of the 1960s, and the Vietnam War all eroded the ancient barriers that had protected the school.

The new headmaster was responsible for the establishment of the consultation program. He had been a dean of students at a small college which had a widespread, easily accessible network of mental health services, and he had an explicit interest in developing something similar for the prep school. The consultant was invited into the school because of the headmaster's recognition of the specific needs of individual students.

Although this concern was and remains central, it became evident very early that both the presence of the new consultant and the school's new focus on the student as an individual with problems cast a new light on institutional issues as well. What has developed is a process which accommodates more effectively a seesaw between the student with his or her unique problems and an institution struggling to respond more appropriately to each student and to a changing world. While the consultant's role was established slowly, there have been some very consistent and stable aspects to the consultation program. The same consultant has been coming for over twenty years. He was invited in by the headmaster and asked to remain by his successor; from the start there have been strong links to the headmaster's office. Both institutional and individual decisions are always more acceptable and more effectively implemented when the headmaster is involved in the process. Another invariable element has been time itself. The consultant's time slot has never changed and has become so fixed that a recent unexpected and unusual variation caused universal joshing, sarcasm, and consternation.

Although the goal of providing access to specialized services was clear, what was initially less clear were the inherent obstacles to reaching this goal. Although members of the school staff in critical positions—the chaplain, the class advisor, or others by virtue of special qualities in their relationship to students—believed they knew students who should be referred, these referrals did not materialize or when they did the process was clumsy and more often than not defeating. A depressed student was told by his advisor that perhaps he should see a psychiatrist to discuss his failing grades. Another faculty member asked by the student about the referral expressed doubt as to the need. The student was confused by the conflicting advice, uncertain about the reason for referral and, because of the involvement of two faculty members, skeptical about privacy. He came for one appointment, refused others and at the winter holiday decided not to return to school. This sequence of events was not atypical. The student was often poorly prepared for the referral or not prepared at all, or too many hands participated, generating and conveying conflict and uncertainty.

There was, in addition, no identifiable internal network to support referrals. Students were perceived and treated as somewhat dependent. They could not easily make their own arrangements and were not encouraged to do so; they had no personal transportation available. Leaving the campus involved a system of sanctions and prohibitions, and their day was heavily scheduled, allowing little time for private commitments. While it was frequently true that the process of identification worked well and that faculty could pinpoint students with problms, more often than not referral to the consultant did not work out.

At this point, very early in the development of the program, the consultant was presumed to be available in some sort of isolated office to talk to individual students. In fact, he was isolated in the basement of the school infirmary and surrounded by a phalanx of nurses. Privacy, which is difficult at a small rural school in any event, was virtually impossible because of the gauntlet the student had to negotiate to get to the consultant's office. There were other, less tangible but as real, obstacles. Faculty often blurred the issue when presenting to the students the idea of psychiatric help—"Maybe he can help you with your study habits"—when the concern was with the student's increasingly difficult encounters with peers. They hinted at, or explicitly mentioned, the headmaster's suggestion that the student had better go along with the referral or his stay at school might be at risk. Faculty was often wary of this new presence, as well as negative, resistant, scared or at least in doubt, and by equivocation conveyed this to the student.

The school has a system of periodic class meetings in which faculty discusses students. In addition, major disciplinary matters are handled by a disciplinary committee which has a somewhat public feeling to it, although the sessions are not open. There was, therefore, no strong feeling of confidentiality in the school. Although the consultant assured the students of his confidential stance, students with good reason questioned this. Furthermore, referring faculty often would ask the student how his appointment went or expected feedback from the consultant. Other faculty would learn about the appointment from the powerful network of gossip and would then speak to the student about it.

It became clear that these issues—of privacy, confidentiality, means of referral—had to be confronted and this would require dealing with the faculty directly. Concerns about confidentiality permeated other issues and other decisions. There was the matter of record keeping. Because of a sense of uncertainty about file security and about the eventual fate of students' records, it was decided initially to keep no formal records. The consultant kept his own notes. Later, as a more formal process evolved, the chaplain functioned as recording secretary for cases discussed in the class meetings. Case notes were kept on file cards locked up in the chaplain's office.

This particular responsibility of the chaplain was an outgrowth of historical circumstances. The school's chaplain at the time of the start of the consultation program had a gift for working with problem students, attracted them, and provided a resource for the more atypical members of the community. He was a key referral source, was almost always involved in case issues, and almost automatically became the principal administrative manager of the consultation process. Subsequent chaplains, albeit with very different relationships to the students, continued to assume these responsibilities. Until the faculty members began to feel at ease with the consultant enough to call him on their own, all appointments were made through the chaplains. This is still true in large measure; the chaplain sits in on all case conferences, keeps whatever records are kept, and is generally identified in the system as the entry point to the consultant.

The conference in which the consultant participated on a regular basis began essentially as a case conference but did have to confront institutional concerns. Boarding schools, for instance, have poorly defined but nonetheless explicit and implicit roles as parent substitutes. The problems and consequences of these roles become the consultant's concern very early on. Decisions made regarding these concerns figured substantially in the history of the consultation. Should, for instance, a student be referred to a psychiatrist without explicit parental consent? Since many of the students are either past age 18 or close to it, and since all are in many ways independent of parental control, the question is a genuine one. There are matters of unstable and ambiguous assignment of parental responsibility. Divorce is increasing. Very often the custodial parent is not the tuition-paying parent. Does this give the latter a right to access to information about the student's contact with the psychiatrist? While these questions have never been finally settled, identification of the questions has led to changes in function. For instance, in the past the parents had always signed medical permission forms in advance; these now include permission to refer to the psychiatrist. That is, the student can be referred to the psychiatrist or can request an appointment and the parents do not have to be consulted. And this is clearly spelled out in permission parents are required to sign at the time of admission to the school.

Typically the need for this is first identified in a particular case, generalized and then structured into policy.

A student whose family was Chinese, living in the Far East, made after several verbal threats a serious suicidal gesture. There was no available family in the area and his immediate family, while accessible, could not reach the school until several days later. Hospitalization was urgent. The one facility available required some guarantee of payment. Under the pressure of these circumstances, the school agreed to assume responsibility for these payments. Confronted later with parental resistance to this financial commitment, the school made certain long-term policy decisions. The requirement for anticipatory consent to be given on admission to the school was instituted and a decision was made never to assume responsibility for payment for hospitalization.

The consultant was involved in both this particular case and the resultant policy regarding the hospitalization process. That is, he was asked to see the suicidal student on short notice, advised the hospitalization, urged it upon the school, and was instrumental in arranging for hospitalization and locating the one available facility. In addition, subsequent to this experience, he took part in a series of meetings involving the headmaster and key administrative staff in establishing policy about permissions, payment for fees for hospitals, confidentiality, and parental responsibility.

There have been other decisions arising from this process. For instance, communication with parents by the psychiatrist is not mandated. It is always implemented with the student's consent, and it is required only by specific circumstances, such as a referral for psychotherapy or counseling outside the school.

Since there are limited community resources for referral, the consultant agreed to see students for psychotherapy in his own office. From the start, this never seemed to work out. The students accepted the referral to the consultant and then did not follow through or came only a few times, or constantly demanded schedule changes, asked to see the consultant at the school and then withdrew.

The consultant suggested these problems be discussed at a meeting with administrators. At this meeting it became clear that students were seriously concerned about issues of confidentiality. Faculty had heard this from some students, and the consultant in discussing a treatment recommendation with a student learned from him that this issue was a worrisome one. As the consultant was readily identifiable within the school, he was also perceived as part of the establishment. Despite the consultant's declarations of confidentiality, students were skeptical and resisted involvement. As this became clear, the decision was made never to make a private referral to the consultant.

Reasons for revising this rule have always seemed justifiable and rational. For instance, because of the meagerness of available referral resources and the great distance at which they are located, there were times during the school year when none were available. Occasionally this was used as a reason to refer privately to the consultant. At other times an assessment was made that a short-term crisis intervention was needed and that private referral would take too long and the consultant had available time. In none of these instances was the referral successful, thereby reaffirming the value of the originally established rule.

The increasing focus of the consultation program on developing internal resources and services has, in any event, reduced the frequency of referral. Clearly, one of the functions of the consultation program as it presently exists is the creation within the school itself of the appropriate referral resources, and of a faculty able to assume quasi-therapeutic responsibilities and willing to take on more complex counseling roles.

As a general rule, this was the course of consultant events as they developed. That is, there was a kind of balance between concerns related to the individual student presenting difficulties and more general issues put in focus by a particular student's problem, which could then be discussed as to how they affected the life of the school. Each clinical experience occurs within a context—the student responds to the school, the school to the student—and within this reverberating system points of conflict and stress occur which are then identified either by the consultant or by his contacts within the system.

A severely obsessional student who had been reasonably successful and productive at the school was noted to be increasingly preoccupied with the management of catering services at the school. At first this seemed reasonable enough, catering services never having been adequate to their task or very popular. As his plans for change became more elaborate and complex and he more insistent on their implementation, more and more members of the faculty and administration became involved. The consultant was asked about this casually and learned that the dean of students was aware that other students had expressed irritation and concern about this student. Information presented at a meeting suggested a student who was decompensating and on the verge of a severe psychotic disorganization.

He agreed to see the consultant and the diagnosis was confirmed. He was given a leave of absence, evaluated further at home, and was hospitalized. In this process it was learned that certain faculty members had been concerned for several months as had some students, but they had not shared these concerns.

Several administrative meetings covered some of the issues presented by this case, such as the role of the class chairman as a confidential focal point for faculty with concerns about particular students and the availability of the consultant to discuss student behavior which appeared deviant, in such a way that faculty felt secure that their observations would be taken seriously. Other issues included the school's need to clarify the boundaries of acceptable psychopathology, its willingness to consider each case individually, and its belief that neither a referral to a psychiatrist nor even psychiatric hospitalization necessarily means a permanent exclusion from the school.

There are other examples.

An angry day student was referred because of his repeated violation of minor school rules often ending in self-damaging accidents. In his two initial contacts with the consultant he expressed a clear sense of rage, frustration, and humiliation because of what he perceived as second-class citizenship. This was presented as an observation to both the headmaster and the chaplain, both of whom were aware of this as a longstanding problem for day students. This was discussed with a larger group and efforts were made to create for day students a more viable role in the community.

Over the course of this consultation experience, a complex process has created a kind of dual system. Specific students who come to the attention of the class chairman from faculty, other students, or administration, are discussed at a case conference which includes those faculty members and members of the administration who are involved with the student. Confidentiality is maintained. School issues that arise from the process, or through the general process or change in school, can be referred for discussion to an administrative group chaired by the headmaster and including the consultant, the chaplain, the class chairman, the assistant headmaster and others, as circumstances dictate. In the first part of this process, where the focus is on the individual student, an effort is made to develop a treatment plan for the student. In the second part of the process, there is a conscious focus on formal issues as they affect the life of the school as a whole.

Among the general issues discussed have been the structure of housing at the school with the coming of coeducation; the problems of establishing acceptable limits to the use of drugs, recognizing the almost universal but highly variable use of marijuana; the need for reasonable rules about drinking with the change in the age of majority; and problems of responding appropriately to sexual activity, which is more open with coeducation and with significant changes in the community's response to both heterosexual and homosexual activity.

Trust has been a major factor. It appears that trust has been a function of the length of the particular consultant's commitment to the school, the regular and repetitive nature of the consultation, the headmaster's active role and the conviction of the consultant that the best-working model for consultation is one that recognizes the need to share the expertise of a variety of professions and skills. It was quite clear that the best hope, in this particular setting, for the development of more flexibility and acceptance of the deviant or troubled student depended on increasing faculty sensitivity and awareness. It was also found that the consultant could function most effectively if his assistance were voluntarily sought, if the problems were viewed as shared ones, and if it was recognized that the consultant and the educator brought different but related skills to the problems of the troubled student.

An early effort was made to include all faculty in conferences with the consultant. This was misguided and unrealistic. Some faculty members, for instance, had been at the school for as long as forty years and surely saw no reason for a psychiatrist and were not about to accept one, particularly if they felt they were being lectured at. Others were the central figures for small cliques of students and viewed the identification of clique members by the consulting process as threats to the integrity of their small circle. The full faculty did not attend these conferences, there was resistance and resentment from many of those who did, and the sessions were nonproductive, dull, and sterile. The decision was then made to focus on the individual case and to involve only the appropriate faculty.

From this early decision, diversification in the demands upon the consultant has evolved slowly and has been accompanied by, and has resulted in, numerous changes in the relationship of the consultant to the school. For instance, he is identified by first name by an increasing number of faculty members, many of whom only know him tangentially. There have been other changes in the way faculty relates to him: greater willingness to call the consultant's office in the community; easier sharing of problems; increased attendance of fearful, resistant or doubting staff members at meetings of the consultation program; and a recognition that the consultant can usually contribute to the solution of the problem but neither is nor claims to be omnipotent. In fact, the fantasy of this omnipotence has to be dispelled early if consultation is to work effectively. It can be a serious interference, whether believed by the consultant or by the consultee.

In marked contrast to Gerald Caplan's proposal that a consultant should move in and out of the system quickly, this particular program has clearly been dependent for its success on the continuing presence of the same consultant. In this instance, we believe it was the interplay of several features characterizing the program that made it work. These include: the extension of the program over time; the consistent identity of the particular consultant; and the fact that the need for consultation was felt within the school, consultation was not imposed from without and was actively supported by the headmaster and his immediate staff.

THE PUBLIC SCHOOL

The town in which the Child Guidance Clinic served as a consultant to the public school is also peripheral to and serves as a bedroom community for the central industrial city. It has many of the demographic characteristics of the town where the prep school is situated. Major services, such as medical and hospital care, are provided by the city. There is also the same, thin spreading of mental health services and the same feeling in the public school that services are unavailable, inaccessible and that they must either be provided by the school itself or the whole issue simply evaded.

There are also some differences which must in part account for the different history of consultation program in this setting. The community is much less stable with considerable rapid growth and a very mobile population. This reflects the fact that the town is a suburban community for two other industrial cities where there is much movement of middle-level executive staff. In addition, the town has much readier access to the relative richness of a university center with a medical school, a mental health center, and large psychiatric community. The problem is that medical care tends to be sought in one direction while more mental health and psychiatric facilities are available in another. This often appears to lead to confusion for the consumer and the lack of coordination of care.

The public school system is a relatively large one with five primary schools, a junior high school, and a large high school. It has scattered pockets of special programming, of a fairly high level of sophistication, but in certain areas it provides little and this at a time when services in other systems are growing rapidly. There is, for instance, only one school social worker at the primary level; and the one position at the secondary level is often unfilled. There is considerable discoordination within the school system also. There is no clearly defined pattern, for instance, of referral to community services and no explicit allocated responsibility for making referrals. There is great ambiguity in the power structure so that it is never really clear who is the responsible chief of special services. At times an assistant superintendent who is explicitly against special programming assumed the role; at others a school psychologist with considerable skill as a grants-person seemed to have the job.

The need for consultation came from the state Board of Education which established guidelines for the implementation of the special education law. One of the requirements was for consultation. As so often happens there was a personal connection—the then-Director of Special Services had had an internship at the Clinic. She arranged initially for the clinic to provide the consultation. Funding for consultation came out of special grants so that the system never had to make a specific financial commitment and consultation never appeared as a line item on the local town budget. Contracts between consultants and administration were rare and efforts to develop some means of communication with the superintendent's office were not successful.

In the early stages of the consultation program there was much enthusiasm and much sense that consultation could and should solve many of the problems facing the school in establishing special programs, in identifying children with special problems, in working with parents, and in facilitating processes of referral. Two members of the clinic staff were involved initially and it is clear, in retrospect, that extraordinarily ambitious goals were set. There was a sense of expansiveness and the consultants agreed to a variety of agendas and proposals which made demands for time and skills which were often difficult to satisfy.

At the beginning an effort was made to construct a program which would reach all of the primary level teachers. There were immediate difficulties. No preliminary efforts had been made to secure the explicit support of the individual principals. There were problems in release time, in scheduling meetings, in teachers knowing if the meetings with the consultant were obligatory or voluntary, and great problems in setting an agenda for the meetings which would be meaningful for the classroom teacher. The convening authority, the Department of Special Services, felt that the teachers could learn from the consultant about how to deal with children causing stress for them in the classroom. There was mutual ignorance—the consultants had little knowledge of the classroom situation and the teachers had a wish for quick, clear, and easily formulated answers. There was, as a result, not only mutual ignorance but much mutual frustration. The consultants came out of a clinical setting and were used to the specific case presentation which the teachers were not prepared for, and they also functioned in a field in which quick and easy solutions were not expected. Their willingness to tolerate uncertainty was confusing for the teachers.

The lack of specific principal and superintendent participation was a further hindrance to the development and growth of the consultation program. There were two schools in which the principals were openly supportive and encouraging. In these schools the consultants were invited into classrooms, were asked by teachers to discuss specific problem children, and were often involved in discussions at the principal's office regarding planning for special programming. Expansion of these consultation functions, however, were difficult because of the limited time available and because of the fear of showing favoritism if the consultation was not made available to the schools.

As experience accumulated, a number of efforts were made to remedy these problems. On the one hand, attempts were made to involve administration more effectively. Several meetings for this purpose were held in the superintendent's office. What became evident early on was that the distance between the general system concerns of the administration and the specific clinical skills of the consultants was too great to be bridged easily.

An effort in another direction was to bring the consultant more directly into the classroom and in contact with specific case problems. The school psychologists expressed a need for some outside supervision with complex and confusing testing experiences. One of the consultants served this purpose—the psychologists meeting him at his clinic office.

The principals and teachers who expressed the greatest interest in consultation were at a school in which the system had begun to develop a range of special programs; self-contained small classrooms, resource teachers, a high concentration of limited social work time, special tutoring programs, and special early education program for young children with identified development disabilities. The teachers in these programs showed more interest in the consultation, were open to having visitors and observers, and were open in expressing doubts and concerns about what they were doing. The consultants began to spend more and more time in this one school. Looking back over time, it is evident that what happened was the gradual constriction and consolidation of what had been an overambitious commitment to something that was more manageable and more readily focused and implemented.

When it was most successful, the consultant was asked to observe in selected classrooms; after the school day the full staff met, further case material on the child observed was presented, and it was possible from this material to develop some consensus about programming and to generalize and to apply what was learned to other situations.

A gain in the process of consultation has been the willingness of the teachers and staff in the prekindergarten program to examine a child in depth; that is to understand the child in the context of its life history, its family structure, its behavior in the classroom, as well as trying to grasp and understand developmental changes. This is not an easy process. Early in the consultation when the consultants were meeting with groups of teachers, there was an emphasis on isolated fragments of behavior, context was often ignored, parental role was not understood, a quick solution was demanded and the teachers were frustrated, if not hostile, when this was not provided. It is only as the consultants began to work more consistently with one group of teachers and one school and began to visit in the classroom that a broadening of perspective could occur. This is particularly true in the prekindergarten program where parents were included in the classroom, where history could be obtained, and where efforts were made to observe parent and child together.

The problem for the consultant in this setting was to help the staff recognize when they had reached the limits of their expertise and when it therefore was appropriate to use or to refer to experts or professionals in other settings. The basic pragmatic cast of educational thinking often led to a denial of the value of establishing a valid diagnosis. Distinctions, for instance, between a truly aphasic child and an autistic one were often unclear and the prognostic significance of the difference underestimated. Small evidences of growth and developments in an autistic child will typically be interpreted by school staff very optimistically and in the process the subtler evidences of continuing disturbance such as bizarre language usage or intermittent poor delineation of boundaries will be pushed aside. There seem to be several reasons for this. On the one hand the teachers are very dependent on this kind of change to justify their efforts and program to themselves. Also the problem of referring the child, the difficulties in finding alternate and different resources reinforce the sense that their program has somehow to serve all the needs, and that a referral is useless and pointless.

The consultants believe that one of the continuing tasks is to help staff in the school to establish more realistic goals, be more willing to use the skills of others, and be more receptive to the possible value of other and different approaches either as alternatives or as additions to present programming for the child.

In many ways this process was not unlike what happened in the prep school. The consultant became well known in this setting, staff felt increasingly comfortable with him, and were able to share anxieties and disquiet. There were, of course, significant differences from the prep school. There was not access to policy setting so that real changes could not be implemented and the consultants had no overall impact on school policy and attitudes.

Another difference is that beginning from a position at which it was felt that the consultant would make a significant impact on the system as a whole the guidelines for consultation became narrower and, in this setting, more realistic.

An additional and perhaps even more determining cause for this development is a fiscal one. The school system never did make a financial contribution. As grant funds began to dry up more and more, limits were placed on the consultation program.

In its final form, one consultant met on a regular basis with the teaching staff for a preschool program for children with a variety of developmental and other handicaps in which there was an emphasis on parents-child intervention. Parents participated actively in the educational process, had their own group activities, and were encouraged to work directly with their children in the classroom. This program was also supported by grants, received little service support from the local system, and survived in large measure because it was favorably viewed by the State Department of Education. There was no available school social work and the staff have developed their own testing tools. They feel that referral is difficult, as it is for all the reasons outlined, and for this reason have focused on the growth of their own observation skills and what they view as their own diagnostic as well as, in some ways, therapeutic capabilities. The role of the consultant in this setting is to support the wish to become more skilled observers while at the same time trying to help them recognize when it is necessary to turn to and use outside expertise, limited as this is.

This is much more difficult for a public school than it is for the prep school. There is a much stronger sense in the public school that it must be "all things to all men" than there is in the prep school. This may in part be due to Public Law 94-142 which requires payment by the public school for services it requests from the community. However, this is probably only part of the explanation. Another reason is the lack of administrative support for the function of consultation. One of the goals of consultation is to help the system define its appropriate role—in this instance, defining the appropriate educational limits for the nonnormative child—then it follows that it must also help the system use its community resources creatively. If there is little encouragement on the part of the administration for this process then it is difficult for line staff to use consultants to help establish both these parameters and these linkages.

This paper describes the different history of two consultation programs of the same community but in a similar setting, focusing on the nature of these settings as they might account for the very different experiences they had with mental health consultation. The critical differential seems to be the identifiable support and participation of administration; the nature of the financial commitment to and responsibility for consultation; and whether the requirements for consultation is felt internally or imposed from the outside.

14

Staff Consultation
in a Public School System

Lee H. Willer

There is perhaps no more useful a place for a child psychiatrist to work than in the kindergarten through ninth grade school area as a consultant. It is a two-way situation in that while offering assistance there are rewards for the physician in seeing vast numbers of children through the eyes of caring and intelligent people. In the office or clinic, no matter how devoted, the clinician can see only a relative handful of patients whereas in the school area working through the teachers, large numbers of youngsters can be reached and helped.

Requests for consultation will come in a variety of forms. Help will be sought in dealing with particular children with emotional problems that overwhelm the resources of the teachers. Assistance may also be sought for the elaboration of group dynamics. It may be requested on the basis of an emergency which is ill-defined but when understood reveals a substantive need to rethink concepts and approaches to the children.

I suspect that when all requests are sifted, we come up with a felt need in the faculty for information about both normal emotional growth and development and deviations from the so-called norm. It is further clear that little of this area of a substantive nature has been incorporated into the training of teachers over the years. This still comes as a surprise to me when I meet with a group. I have a built-in expectation that teachers would be thoroughly grounded in

---

general psychology with particular reference to childhood growth and development. If there have been courses they have been *pro forma* and too often not given in a way or with sufficient intensity or depth that the student teacher would have visceral awareness of the material that could be carried to the classroom for integration into his approach to the students in his charge.

The school hierarchy, on the other hand, sensing this tries too often to plug in a teaching module to fill the gap in the teacher's information and understanding. Too often, the module relies on understanding confined to a unidimensional cognitive approach which *de facto* denies the dynamic and complicated nature of the work with the children. I suspect this is revealed in the junior high schools of many of our communities. Schools that were created to deal with a particular age group with inherent developmental tasks turn into holding areas that don't seem to be of much use to anyone . . . and are certainly distressing for the teachers. A variety of tactics are used to teach the children rather than capitalize on the psychological step the child is going through. In effect, devices are used to impose a system on the child's psyche rather than to be responsive to its intrinsic substance and curiosity during the preadolescent and adolescent era.

ENTRY INTO THE SYSTEM

Invitation to the consultant will come through the hierarchy. This does not mean, of course, that the stimulus for the request originated in the administrative staff. I believe it is sensible for the consultant to be aware of the personalities and group dynamic forces in action in the school to be considered.

Using all of his tact, diplomacy and sensitivity, the consultant should clarify in his mind the exact origins of the request. It usually begins because someone is made anxious by a child. Sometimes the request may originate with a group of teachers who have a primary interest in expanding their skill and understanding. It is further clear that the administration wishes to be responsive to the needs of its staff. However, it may well be that the request for consultation means that the administrative staff has not been able to meet the needs of the staff. In schools where there are stresses of budget, ethnic problems, and bad buildings compounding the usual school problems, the consultant can become vulnerable to drawing fire and causing subsurface feelings to gel in rapid fashion by premature or ill-advised opinion giving. This may happen regardless of how well-intended the invitation was or was the consultant's comments.

There must be a period of getting to know each other, involving all members of the situation so that the forces at work can be clearly viewed in the consultant's mind. Further, it is well if the staff is aware that there is open communication among everyone and that conspiratorial cells will not be useful.

The school administration must be reassured that its authority is not being jeopardized by the new consultant who, because of his expertise, could represent a threat to the administrator's adequacy.

In any institution, there is an interplay between the boss and the staff that involves narcissistic gratification for the boss. He gives to his staff, and indeed the consultant may well be a gift he gives to his staff, in the expectation that they will be grateful to him. However, the consultant by his presence may interfere with the narcissistic feeling of the boss if his expertise is more helpful than that of the boss in particular areas that are troublesome to the staff.

One fellow made his discomfort manifest by a variety of tactics once the seminar had reached a full and ongoing attendance. He would schedule concurrent meetings for one or another of the people in the group. Later when it became apparent to him that active choices were being made by his staff to be in the seminar he began to openly grouse about the need for his professionals to really need ongoing education of this sort. When this became apparent it was incumbent upon the consultant to arrange some sort of rapproachement. There is a gamut of approaches, the easiest being a meeting to discuss what seems to be going on. This, of course, requires tact and diplomacy of a high order. In a particular situation it was remarkable that the director had put together such a mature and sophisticated staff. He had given them reign to do what made sense and they had fulfilled his wish. My presence seemed to be a boomerang for him. Indeed, he didn't know how good he was. It was obvious that he thought my ongoing presence was an indictment of his selection process. I informed him that I really was the product of his skill in selecting the staff he did. Things did become remarkably easier between us as well as between him and the seminar group.

In some situations the boss may well be the sort that splits his staff. They may fear him.

A very bright head of a school system that dealt with students' psychological problems was brought into a school system beset by emotional and educational problems and complicated by a major population change. The individual had impeccable educational credentials and had had a significant portion of his training directed by a creative and forceful personality, a person who felt it appropriate to intrude upon the work of his teachers in order to assist their development. The new head of department in our local system had learned his lessons well. He attempted to indoctrinate his staff with ideas that gave little allowance for the maturity and levels of conceptual ability.

The result was that his staff felt oppressed, and since he was specially brought in, he had the additional weight of the administrative hierarchy behind him. Unwittingly, he polarized the staff sufficiently to make the environment become conflicted and tense.

The consultant in this case can very easily be tempted into a rescue mission. This possibility must be recognized by the consultant and not acted upon lest his role be vitiated by internecine warfare.

Not only was the charismatic and forceful personality inappropriate with this particular staff but it would have driven them from their jobs. Many of them had master's degrees and doctorates and were not material for the system in which the new director had been raised. In this particular instance I was able to make use of the inherent good sense of the staff who had come to the point of open rebellion. I differentiated between models of approach in the psychologies. Rather than there being a confrontation between a strong leader and equally strong staff, they were able to conceptualize the problem as one in which there was a clash of models. With this as an instrument they were able to resolve their differences without too much more contention. In this particular instance the differing was between a more comprehensive psychodynamic model and one in which there was the extensive use of so-to-speak "transference cure." This last was not really appropriate for the bulk of the youngsters in the particular school system. When this was sorted out as the issue things did become more civilized.

School consultation is most effective if there is first a series of meetings with administrative staff for them to define what they need, want, then a review of what the consultant observes about the situation in the field, and lastly, a discussion about the consultant's theoretical model and approach in dealing with what he sees. In other words, I feel that administrators and teachers both should know what they are buying. I find it best to have these meetings separately, first with the headmaster or principal, and then with the staff, and finally, perhaps with both together so there is as little ambiguity as possible and everyone agrees about what the consultant should do. Further, the contract should be renewed at least yearly. This means a measured pace involving several weeks. The consultant must be deliberate and not hurried.

FACULTY PRESSURES AND PROCESSES

The teaching profession is in the same predicament that medicine faces with regard to an understanding of psychology. It would be well if the teaching of this material could be accomplished in college, but we are up against the same inevitable clocks of development in our teachers that we are aware of in our medical students. It is the rare medical student who has the emotional maturity to consider in a visceral sense the concepts of psychology. Most often we achieve, if we're lucky, an intellectual tolerance. This may be understood if we accept that the final resolution of adolescence is not considered truly completed until ages 27 to 30. The teachers we work with, of course, are products of the same developmental clockwork. In view of this, I believe there is no other place for this training than on the job where the school system can maintain a quality control for some measure of internal consistency and coherence in approaching the children in their charge. Happily, teachers are not as rigidly determined to have cognitive control as are medical students.

It has been my experience that teachers, when confronted with some of the modules relevant to mental health material, become uneasy. They have difficulty in articulating that they feel much of the material as inappropriate because it is an imposition rather than a sensitivity to the needs of the children. I suspect that the capacity crowds at museums these days have perhaps less to do with the state of our economy than with the desire to be in touch with authentic experiences. It is in this realm of authenticity that the consultant can be of most help in assisting teachers to sort out their concerns about the relevance of material. It is here that the consultant can offer a theoretical as well as factual model for teachers to start to use in screening data with reference to their mental health course material as well as in their observation of the children.

The difficulty for teachers studying psychology is the tradition of the cognitive and behavioral perspectives versus the dynamic viewpoint. Repeatedly, for example, teachers remark that when a student has difficulty at home before coming to school it will be obvious in the class. Teachers who use the reward system involving gold stars and such are then used unwittingly by the children. The child not earning his gold star will link up the teacher psychologically with the seemingly punitive parents. It makes more sense, I think, to abandon the reward and punishment system and instead take note of what is going on in whatever way the teacher feels appropriate. In this way the child knows he is in contact with someone who understands him and what is going on with him. When this is discussed, the teachers respond almost with relief, many of them having felt that the reward system was spurious but not having been sure why. The concept of conditional love, which can be malignant in child development, should be reviewed in such discussion. The child gets the feeling that if he doesn't conform to adult expectations he will be hated.

If the model is to be useable it should be a representation of the complexity of the child. This means, I believe, that it cannot be limited to a reductionist construction but must involve an attempt at ordering the experiences that bring about the child's behavior (motivation), from internally as well as externally determined sources. The motivations can be described as they impact upon people and things but the manifestations should not be confused with etiology by the device of correlation. Rather the interaction of internal and external sets must be kept in mind. Additionally, the social setting, the organic-neurophysiologic entity, as well as the genetic makeup of the youngster should be capable of synthesis into a representation of the child that can be of use to the teacher. As Allan Stone remarked, he could not accept that "the race that produced Shakespeare could be reduced to a conditioned reflex" to explain its functioning (1978). The medical model that we use must be expanded to encompass both time and setting as we view our patients. The model should include a sense of causality, family context, and a psycho-educational plan.

I suspect there is more to be gained in the mental health area from the teaching of good literature and history with reference to notable personalities than from a mandated mental health course which enforces concepts of thinking that is vaguely appropriate for particular individuals in a classroom. The goals of mental health and self-development through education reach a confluence in emotionally understanding the people of history and literature.

I have in mind, for example, a young patient of mine who was being taught in school how to sort decisions and values by use of a hypothetical situation. The question posed was how to stop a student from shoplifting. The teacher, following the curriculum seemed to be left with a variety of choices for helping the miscreant which the class was to consider. The patient heard all of this but dismissed it out of his greater concern over why the teacher thought they were a class of thieves.

The point here is one familiar to all of us in the psychological fields of medicine. It is not unusual for individuals to personalize issues to the detriment of the subject matter. This is something of which teachers are well aware. As a consultant I have found that often my job has been to help them examine and deal with this awareness. What I am talking about is a fine line between teaching in a disciplined way within a subject area and imposing rigid and inhibitory outlines that would defeat the process of education.

There is, furthermore, a distinction to be made between understanding and knowing. To my mind, knowing is a level beyond understanding. To me it indicates an integration of subject matter so that it is part of the fabric of the individual. The distinction here is between a concert pianist and a parlor performer. The first makes use of his instrument to speak and the latter uses the instrument to make sound.

George Miller states, "Our lucky ones [students] come out with something that was never taught—how to meet the intellectual crises of the moment" (1981). I would add here—not merely the intellectual but also the emotional crises of the moment.

It is usual to divide the consultant's job into various segments depending upon with whom he works . . . that is, the child, teacher, the hierarchy, and so forth. My preference is to work directly with the teachers. I prefer not to have consultations involving the children directly, but prefer that the teachers give their perceptions. The first reason I prefer this tactic is that the numbers of children requiring assistance are well beyond the clinical resources available to most school systems. Secondly, developing the teachers' psychological sophistication, in my opinion, is one of the prime purposes of our consultative functions. Many problems, such as transient situation adjustment matters, can be dealt with by sophisticated teachers without hardening the matter for the child. Further, differing character styles can be described and dealt with through the teachers' increased sensitivity without getting into protracted evaluations and so forth. Lastly, as clinicians we are aware that significant numbers of parents will be unavailable in efforts to assist their children or will not permit psychological intervention. The school and its teachers may be the only avenue of help for these youngsters.

The teacher in the school setting is the ultimate instrument of our work with the children. The analogy of the psychiatric trainee is appropriate here, the difference being that we expect the years of training of our clinical students to be apparent as quickly as possible so that we can proceed with the treatment process. The teacher, on the other hand, must be offered a model and information about approaches to the problem so that the developmental thrusts of the so-called normals can be capitalized on and the aberrant spotted.

TROUBLED CHILDREN

The aberrant child should be spotted for a variety of reasons, not the least being so that the teacher doesn't break his heart trying to reach a particular child and end up feeling guilty and "writing off" the child with a self-protective barricade to defend his self-esteem. The child's needs, no matter how demanding, should be considered so as to determine what can be accomplished within the school setting. How far can the resources of the school, both in material and personnel, be stretched before the child skews the environment to the detriment of the other children? Referral should be made to clinical personnel out of the school when the resources are no longer adaptable.

The guidelines for referral might be that first, the teachers' efforts and classroom direction are skewed from their academic course increasingly to the needs of a particular child. Secondly, the active involvement of the parents is required as in conventional treatment of a youngster. Hopefully, referral to a clinic will offer the child the full range of clinical services, including those geared for supportive and maintenance work as well as those which can reasonably be expected to provide thorough investigations of the individual's psychological disturbance with an expectation of relief, as is generally thought of in clinical settings. It is not uncommon for school people to want to help beyond all reasonable limits. It is of no use to point out that there is a distinction to be made between the posture of helping and proper substantive assistance to a child.

The recent development of a variety of laws concerned with the care and protection of children mandates a role for many of us, including the schools. It is public knowldge that some of the law requiring the so-called mainstreaming of children with a variety of disorders, including those of psychiatric nature, will lead the schools to seek third-party reimbursement. In effect, the school will be asked to replace the outpatient child guidance center or outpatient clinic. These days, with the open accessibility of medical records, there is apprehension in the clinics resulting in most records being reduced to vague banalities in order to shield the patients. I must confess to not knowing how this will be dealt with in the educational hierarchy, though many schools have always passed on the "real truth" orally while writing down innocuous comments.

Schools these days are so much under public pressure, they are often not very willing to become involved with parents in conventional child therapy modes. Any youngster with an organically-based learning problem cannot escape the emotional repercussions of this problem. For example, one dyslexic youngster was given tutoring in reading and writing by the school. Simultaneously, his mother continued to work with him in her own style to compensate for her guilt about feeling she had damaged him. This joint approach can impede his maturation and autonomy. It is with this in mind that I would prefer to have the child referred to a separate facility that can deal with the reading problem and the family rather than confound the academic environment with more burdens than it has to at this point.

USE OF SEMINARS BY THE CONSULTANT

Since the consultation is being requested in a setting geared to the cognitive sphere, I find it is helpful to present a series of seminars, starting with growth and development of the child using a variety of articles from the literature, followed by a series of seminars on group process. My model is a psychodynamic one and the teachers seem to find it of value. The seminars also give the participants an opportunity to know one another, as well as to know from where the consultant is coming. In reviewing growth and development material, as well as some of the deviations resulting in pathology, the teachers will bring in material from their classrooms.

One of the teachers had a home room in the home economics classroom. She had several children who showed the dynamic as well as the developmental flaws of the delinquent. She had not been able to get the youngsters to come to school with enough regularity to say anything about getting there on time. As she heard the materials in the seminar about the mother–child relationship, she wondered what would happen if she baked some bread in the morning. I urged her to give it a try since it seemed a creative solution and would speak directly to the youngsters if our concept of a depressive core in these youngsters was valid. She did this and noted that the children not only came to school regularly but arrived before she got there, waiting to work with her in the bread-baking process. This device was sufficient to get a positive working relationship going with these children which permitted further involvements in the school.

Teachers are aware of the narrowness of the cognitive approach to understanding the child. The problem is the seeming absence of other models to place alongside it and expand it. By definition the cognitive approach must exclude the unconscious, unless they happen to be English teachers or disposed in the direction of literature, in which case more often than not they can articulate unconscious and symbolic issues and symbols. Borrowing from Winnicott (1964), the teachers are gradually confronted with the distinction of the "true" from the "false self." By understanding children's growth and development, rather than fighting what is natural in development, the teachers can develop ways of capitalizing upon it as in the case of the bread-baking teacher. It is by letting the youngsters know they are being sensitively and empathetically viewed, rather than giving them slogans by which to relate to the teacher, that the child can grow as his own person. Some of our most difficult patients are those who are very bright and throw up an intellectual smoke screen that in some cases can delude the therapist into feeling that he is working properly with the patient only to find that the patient has cynically learned his lessons and merely parrots the therapist's words and thoughts to him. In order to avoid this, teachers must have a visceral awareness of the other dimensions of the human psyche beyond the cognitive apparatus. Formal teaching by the consultant can contribute to their feeling confidence and direction from their intuitions.

Teachers studying the growth and development continuum see the variety of tasks they have before them, only one of which happens to be teaching academic material. They all know this but in context of seeing the developing child within a psychodynamic model, the pieces begin to fit together. The teacher moves beyond his manifest role, presenting an ego-ideal or role model. He gives the child a figure to work with in modifying his value system from that of his parents.

Teachers get drawn into the developing emotions and fantasies of students. He or she may well become a fantasy derivative from early Oedipal material the child may be reworking. Generally the young woman teacher seems to have an easier time with the crush of the boy. She intuitively conceives of the Oedipal displacement. Most young male teachers in my experience also see this but when a burgeoning adolescent female is coming to grips with Oedipal issues, under the guise of preadolescent or adolescent sexuality, it is not unusual to hear from the men about flirting and erotic pressure which is being resisted. There are, of course, rare examples of male teachers who succumb, with the ensuing unfortunate outcomes for both the teacher in the form of guilt and the trauma and overstimulation for the girl which produces later sequillae.

A woman patient revealed the following in her anamnesis. As a child she had been assaulted by an adolescent boy. This led to emotional and behavioral difficulties in subsequent years. As a junior in high school she became enamored of a particular male teacher. In the course of a tutorial he succumbed to her approaches. They both were appalled. In reconstructing the events from the patient it is clear she had been acting out feelings derived from her trauma among other items. The teacher on the other hand was having personal difficulties at home. The mix of the two was most unfortunate. He left the teaching profession in which he had considerable talent. The patient seemed to have a further need to detoxify the experience by having repeated encounters with men some years her senior. She did develop a reputation among the school staff of being seductive, as she reports it. This sort of gross stress reaction is familiar to all of us who have worked with children, boys as well as girls who have been seduced. (This applies to both heterosexual as well as homosexual activities.) The need to repeat the event to master the stimulus is well known.

By raising the developmental aspects of the child to the teacher's awareness, with normal and aberrant the consultant also helps the teachers to confront emotional issues which may well be uncomfortable within themselves. In other words, known developmental issues are removed from unconsciously determining feelings by access to clear consciousness. At the very least, intellectual defenses are reinforced to guard against overt or covert acting-out.

The teacher can be a substitute for the parent, an enforcer of social rules, or a friend. He also may be an enemy to the family value system and unwittingly threaten that system, not by any active deed but rather by his ordering of data and the enlarged view he may present of the world and the human condition. How the teacher deals with this may determine if the child will continue to grow or be fixed in an archaic world. Additionally, with the conceptualizations of Kohut, Kernberg, and others with reference to "the self," there is little question that the profundity of the teacher's role in child development within the "group" as represented by the classroom deserves much more attention.

CONSIDERATIONS OF GROUP PHENOMENONOLOGY

Ultimately the teacher is a group leader. It is this last role that should place group dynamic material in a prominent position in early dealings with the teachers. As a group leader the teacher is the cement that glues the classroom members together.

I was asked to consult with a teacher who was a member of the seminar with reference to his classroom. He was having a difficult discipline problem. From the seminar he thought that he knew what the problem was but wanted me to visit the classroom and given an opinion. He wanted me to see the structure of the room. It had been divided by screens and mobile blackboards and bulletin boards into carrels. At no time could more than two children see him in the classroom. The purpose was to give each youngster as much privacy to concentrate in as possible. However, not being able to see the teacher removed the glue that held the class together. I suggested that he follow his inclinations in removing the partitions and in making sure that however the class was set up, he be plainly visible to all constantly. This ended the problem in the classroom.

The concept of group dynamics is in the minds of many teachers but dimly viewed. It is for this reason that a formal seminar in group theory is a valuable adjunct, I think, to any consultant's program in a school system.

It is sensible to have a voluntary staff training group available for the teachers who are interested. I do not feel it is wise or appropriate for the group to run on for more than about 13 to 15 sessions during the year. Here I differ from what seems to be a trend among my colleagues in group training. It is my observation that to run a group for a complete year on a weekly basis is in effect a commitment to treatment. There is the danger of casehardening if material is evoked prematurely or unwisely in a short service group. In a small staff, if a group is run intensely there is the danger of unconsciously taking out stirred up feelings on youngsters in class. These opinions come from observations in institutions such as schools and clinics as well as from individual contacts with teachers and clinicians in other roles. There is a danger of a truncated group becoming, in effect, an emotive experience which does not seem to be particularly useful.

As a *de facto* group leader, the teacher makes use of not only one-to-one interactions with the child but of group dynamics as an instrument in dealing with the individual child. If the group is viewed as a horde, sight of the individual child is lost. At all times the child is the focus of interest. Children know of the teacher's sensitivity, and I suspect that in classrooms where there is difficulty we could find a lack of awareness on the teacher's part. Factors that enhance or destroy group cohesiveness are worthwhile bringing to the fore. In other words, thinking that is familiar to us in clinical work with groups has application in the classroom.

A crowd as an unorganized group contrasts with the characteristics of a stable group (Freud, 1921) in structure, continuity, purpose and values, and communication codes. To enhance group cohesion, common needs must be satisfied such as protection and affection. Positive affective ties, shared interests and ideals, plus an atmosphere of equality and justice, are significant. Group ceremonials help. For example, the class with an internal student government arrangement in which there are periodic meetings to foster planned activities such as a class party or play. Not only will the activity of the class as a unit be useful, but the process by which the job gets accomplished will add structure, no matter how bent Robert's Rules of Order become.

A common enemy is useful to cement a group. The classic example here is the intramural and interschool activities. The uniform of the team, a T-shirt or a patch indicating membership in a group with a common foe, no matter how friendly, encourages esprit. This is not to be a remedy for other problems in a group or in its leader, but it does enhance the ties in a group that are vulnerable despite the best efforts of the teacher. Dangers to group cohesion are found where there is uninhibited expression of drives, undue egocentricity, jealousy, and competition among the members. Beyond this and perhaps more importantly is the interaction between the group leader–teacher and the children. There is an enormous variety of joking, teasing, challenging, and punishing that is inevitable on the part of the teacher. However, when this reveals a teacher who is too self-involved and/or exhibitionistic, and the needs of the children are sacrificed to the needs of the adult there will be difficulty that demands confrontation and relief.

Classroom learning materials should not be overlooked in discussing group phenomena with our consultees. Generally speaking, the more fluid the materials the greater is the invitation to regression in the vulnerable youngsters. In a class that is prone to regression, it is well to suggest that more solid materials be used. In the early grades when the children are temporarily vulnerable to regression, rather than having activities requiring paint, clay, or glue, I would suggest construction paper, wood, and pencils, or crayons. This concept applies not only to academic materials but also to food available in dining areas. It has been observed that the meatballs from a spaghetti dinner can be used as Ping Pong balls by youngsters in a regressive surge.

Division of space can be critical, as in the example above, describing the room divided into carrels. Shop classes with multiple benches breaking up open area tend to inhibit group interaction in contrast to what we in group therapy are familiar with, namely the open circle with no impediments to interaction. Beyond the classroom space, we are called upon to look at the so-called open classroom. In contrast to enhancing group interaction, if in this case there is a disruptive group in one teacher's area (it is no news that each class seems to have its own characteristics, apart from the influence of the teacher), then efforts should be made to limit the interaction lest the teachers' best efforts be subverted to controlling the interactions among the groups and children within the groups. The consultant may then be called upon to suggest either architectural changes or changes in the group composition if there is to be attention to the main task of the school. Generally speaking, the less the physical obstruction between class members the more animated the interaction. This, of course, assumes an average mix of children from active to passive in their energy discharge.

For example, in a new school that was brilliantly designed it became quickly apparent that with a change in population the new mix of children was not really appropriate for this open structure. The teachers, who were superior, were exhausting themselves in maintaining a minimal amount of order. The difficulty was that late-latency children were placed in proximity to a class of younger children with the resultant mix being weighted on the side of regression. The teachers were reluctant to make changes in the architect's design, since it was ideal and suited their earlier wish. In contrast again to the example of the class in chaos because of lack of visibility of the teacher due to too many barriers, we had to reverse our field here and suggest barriers and some closing of the open space to reduce the interaction with the other class. In effect we vitiated some of the design of the building but had more peace, quiet, and less exhaustion in the staff.

Sometimes teachers say that a class seems to be a tinder box with explosive outbursts by one or more members. A number of factors must be considered. First and foremost is the concept of contagion. Contagion depends upon the need of the group to maintain its integrity; that is to say, a group must maintain itself rather than fragment. We must look to the status of the initiator. Is he a bully who overwhelms the class by his aggression or perhaps a child with explosive, unpredictable outbursts that terrify the other youngsters? In some situations the initiator may be a passive child who has the capacity to unwittingly foment action by being a victim. The variety of remedial approaches available here includes the dramatic intrusion of the adult to isolate the instigator. Removal of the child should be the last remedy. Contagion further depends upon the affinity of the action to the group code.

In some areas children band together in protective clusters, and this will disrupt the school setting involving Black, Oriental, Mexican or other groups. This is a problem that requires a larger remedy than the classroom teacher can provide. Sociocultural factors may overwhelm the best efforts of a school and require political–community changes. The physical and psychological exhaustion of teachers in this arena is well known. The political and social effort may require community organization and support of the beleagured school or perhaps a different school program and goal geared to the particular wishes and needs of the community. Consultants need to acknowledge these issues without nihilism or hopelessness, and to continue to focus on the areas in which teachers can and should direct their energies.

The group code is always more or less respnsive to the teacher's countertransference. The degree of response depends on a variety of factors within the teacher as well as the hierarchy of the school, or indeed the system. If there is an atmosphere of equality and justice and the teacher is available to the youngster, the classroom can be calmed. Equality here does not mean that each child is treated alike, of course. Equality in this instance refers to an awareness of each child as befits his needs at a particular time. If the teacher can be sensitive to his charges in this fashion, the children seem to relax knowing that if they have particular problems the teacher can be counted on to be with them. If there is a congruence of needs from several children, they can wait if the teacher sends a signal that they will receive attention as quickly as possible. In other words, if needs can't be dealt with immediately then there is at least the temporary promise of gratification. If the teacher's resilience is stretched then discretion is the better part of valor, and there should be a request for aides in the room.

Lastly, in dealing with a group, feeding is a group bonding instrument that should not be overlooked. The morning coffee klatch is a social exercise in most groups. We should use this awareness with our school children, particularly grade school children. A ten o'clock or ten-thirty feeding of crackers and milk should be considered if resources permit. Although we are not in the school to make milk sops of the children, a token feeding can be seen as a direct communication from the teacher to the children of his or her feeling about the children. In a most primitive sense, food is love. It cannot be a *pro forma* thing, however. If the teacher has highly ambivalent feelings about the children then it will boomerang as a tranquilizing device.

In the best of all possible worlds the teacher should not be placed in the position of the custodian or policeman. But there are teachers who feel they have to take on the children in the fashion of marine seargeants or, contrariwise, as psychoanalysts. It would be ideal if the teacher could be available to his students in a positive environment provided by a benign ogre. In order for the teacher–student or therapist-patient relationship to be successful the positive must be maintained at almost any cost. If the teacher lines up with the superego or the id, he immediately loses his role in the positive transference. Instances of alignment with the id are numerous and are seen in situations where the teacher is a pal. In the short run, there is an alliance on a primitive level, but the child ultimately becomes frightened or at least wary. It is a situation in which the child feels vulnerable and without protection, indeed, even sacrificed. This was reported when academicians essentially urged youngsters to join in political excess and street activism, as in the student upheavals of the late 1960s and early 1970s.

If the positive transference is lost, the struggle with the child becomes just as if it were anywhere else. The child is deprived of an environment in which he can see himself and what the teacher has to offer because he is so embroiled in his struggles. Without the positive transference the teacher is as helpless as a therapist in a similar situation. The child should at all times feel free to talk about his difficulties in the presence of the teacher and not be in the position of defending himself against what he considers a part of his difficulties. This does not mean that the teacher assumes the role of therapist but that he gives the child a sense that he is aware of the youngster as a person. If the child's difficulties transcend what the teacher is able to deal with, then a referral can be made with the expectation that it will succeed rather than, as is too often the case, a child being referred too late, when the teacher is at his wits' end and feeling punitive or reliatory to the youngster. This referral can have little chance of success.

THE SPECIAL PROBLEM OF SEX EDUCATION

The topic of sex education in schools seems to be with us on a grand scale with the rates of illegitimacy ever increasing. I suspect we are being simplistic in our approach to the problem. We are equating the fact of an illegitimate pregnancy with lack of sexual information. Those of us in the field of child psychiatry are frequently confronted with pregnant teenagers. I don't recall cases in which there was a lack of information or, more importantly, a lack of available sources of information. Most often it seems that the youngsters who get themselves pregnant have another agenda which, unfortunately, seems to be transferred to the genital apparatus. It is obvious when these youngsters are seen with their babies that we are dealing not with parents but with children who are attempting to gratify archaic needs . . . identifying with the baby in being taken care of. Most often these seem to be depressed girls with feelings of emptiness who speak of their wish to be held and cuddled.

The coital act is not where the educational need is. To treat this as a cognitive problem is to evade the issue and further the youngsters' estrangement from people who might be of assistance. The problem is displaced then with institutional agreement, to the problem of sex education. I agree with Winnicott (1965) here that it would be best if biology were taught in biology classes with biologists, and that the rest of the faculty be alert, as hopefully the parents should be, to questions about sexual material, these questions to be responded to as the adults' creativity allows. To bring in outside experts and lecturers, is to vitiate the role of trust that has been built up by the teachers. If there is a need for outside experts then it probably means that the teachers themselves are having a problem in addressing the area and perhaps they should be worked with so that they can cope with the material as it evolves from their charges. In this way we would avoid the imposition of materials at a time when the child is not ready for it.

SUMMARY

Teachers as a group are good observers and reporters. As communication and concepts are elaborated they are quite able to describe in their terms what we as clinicians can translate into our clinical concepts. My approach with them is to review youngsters they are concerned about, using their data. If it is more than an occasional situational problem the child is reponding to, then I urge use of clinical resources, via the guidance department, to a proper apparatus out of the school.

The teacher should not be the one to make the referral unless he is in an unusually strong position with the family. It can contaminate the relationship with the child if parents balk and get angry about directives to get help. Here again the guidance people or others in the school hierarchy should be the ones.

The psychotic, the severely depressed, or the acting out youngster, as well as the rest of the gamut of pathologies seen in the clinics, I feel require more than a classroom teacher can offer in a curative way. I do believe the wish to cure gets confused with a need to contain and to be comfortable enough to get some academics accomplished. Using the principles of group dynamics as well as increased understanding of the growth and development model, each teacher will use his own creativity to reach the children.

Overall I don't believe we, as consultants, can or should tell our consultees what to do, any more than we generally tell our patients what to do. The more these people understand the more creative in problem solving they seem to be. Furthermore, they are able to set reasonable limits on their efforts which service to avoid end-stage hostility to the child.

Finally, I would emphasize the importance of open contact with the administrative hierarchy to maintain an environment in which the teachers feel actively supported and encouraged to use themselves fully. We should present them with alternatives and altered ways of viewing problems. We most frequently offer them the option of recognition of affects and ways of coping with these affects in contrast to mere intellectual awareness.

BIBLIOGRAPHY

Stone A: Remarks at the scientific session on violence (Boston Psychoanalytic Society: Boston, MA) July 1, 1978.
"What is an Educated Person." New York *Times*, May 18, 1980, p 22E.
Winnicott DW: *The Child, The Family, and the Outside World* (Penguin Books: Middlesex, England) 1964, pp 216–220.
Winnicott DW: Ego distortion in terms of true-self false-self. *The Maturational Processes and the Facilitating Environment* (International Universities Press: New York) 1965, pp 140–152.

APOLOGIA

During the past thirty years in the process of learning, writing and teaching I have worked and reworked my thinking with reference to group theory and practice. Particular words and ideas are no longer ascribable by me, and therefore I would like to express my debt to the following authors and their literature. If I have omitted a reference, it is not out of lack of gratitude but the blurring as to origin of material which is now organic to me. For the knowledge I am indebted to:

Abrams J: Seminars and supervision at St. Elizabeth's Hospital, Washington, DC, 1953.

Freud S: *Group Psychology and the Analysis of the Ego*, stand. ed., vol 18 (Hogarth Press: London) 1921.

Scheidlinger S: Seminar at the Judge Baker Guidance Center, 1955.

Scheidlinger S: *Psychoanalysis and Group Behavior* (WW Norton and Co: New York) 1952.

Slavson SR: A textbook in analytic group psychotherapy (International Universities Press: New York) 1964.

Special Perspectives

15

The Pediatric Perspective

Hugh C. Thompson

Pediatricians vary in their perceptions of child psychiatrists and of the value of diagnosis and treatment by child psychiatrists. They also differ as to problems which they will refer for consultations. This chapter discusses the reasons for these differences and presents a brief review of the literature, as well as opinions of the author and a selected group of practitioners and acedemicians as to what problems should have psychiatric consultation. Poor school performance and adjustment is mentioned. The choice of consultation and practice setting, as well as the use of other mental health professionals, is discussed. Lastly, the chapter outlines obligations of both the referring physician and the consultant, regarding use of child psychiatrists, and causes of patients' failure to get maximum benefit from a consultation.

VARYING PERCEPTIONS OF PEDIATRICIANS

The attitude of pediatricians toward the use of child psychiatrists is the result of several influences. One is their personal orientation before entering a medical career. Family, friends, personal physicians, and the media play a part. A favorable personal or family experience with a psychiatrist creates a positive bias. Unfavorable biases are reflected in such statements as: "Psychiatrists are unscientific"; "They spend a great deal of time with little result other than expense"; "Psychiatrists themselves need psychiatric help"; "Psychiatrists are only for the wealthy"; "Psychiatrists are for those who are crazy, are in a mental hospital, or should be in an institution."

Second is the amount of training in pediatric psychiatry received in medical school. This varies greatly. Older physicians may have had little contact with any type of psychiatrist outside of a few lectures, a visit to a state hospital or an occasional afternoon in an adult psychiatric clinic. On the other hand, more fortunate students may have had a stimulating child psychiatrist make daily or weekly ward and outpatient rounds during their pediatric clerkships, or may have taken an elective course in the area.

A third influence is contact with child psychiatrists during pediatric residency. Some services require a psychiatric rotation. In others, there may not be a child psychiatrist on the regular staff, so young pediatricians enter practice with little knowledge of the subsepecialty.

Fourth is the available resources in the community. A pediatrician practicing in a small city with no child psychiatrist within a hundred miles will refer rarely, whereas another in a city with a medical school, child guidance clinic, and several child psychiatrists in private practice will often call for help.

The last determining factor is the pediatrician's personal experience with the available mental health resources in the community. A child guidance clinic which holds its staff conferences at hours when the pediatrician is most busy in his office, or which does not invite him to these conferences and sends no written or telephone reports for many months, if at all, will get few referrals. On the other hand, the psychiatrist who reports by phone after the first visit and sends good written reports promptly and periodically will get many.

RECOMMENDATIONS FOR PSYCHIATRIC CONSULTATION IN PEDIATRIC LITERATURE

Nine current pediatric textbooks likely to be easily accessible to pediatricians, family physicians, house staffs, and medical students differ considerably in their discussions of consultations with child psychiatrists.

Two texts have detailed comments. Harper and Richmond in Rudolph (1977) give the major indications for referral, stressing not only patient manifestations of major disturbance, but also disturbed patient–doctor relationships and physician uncertainty as to his own competence to treat the disturbed patient. They also mention the confusion created by the varying roles of mental health professionals.

Prugh and Kelly in *Current Pediatric Diagnosis and Treatment* (Kempe et al., 1978) state that home environment, demonstration of age-inappropriate behavior, intensity or frequency of symptoms, the child's inner suffering, and intractable behavior may all dictate referral to a psychiatrist.

In addition, Hoekleman et al. (1978) offer good suggestions for consultations in general, without specifying referrals to psychiatrists. Kaye, Oski, and Barness (1978) state, "Only after the primary physician has thoroughly explored questions about the child's development or problems in his total development, may he turn to a child psychiatrist or other mental health specialist."

All texts mention referral to child psychiatrists or mental health facilities for specific problems such as autism or suicide attempts, but differ markedly in their emphasis and specificity.

A search of journals commonly available to primary physicians uncovered two published in the late 1960s. Schwab and Brown discuss uses and abuses of psychiatric consultation, especially in hospital practice. Among the faults the primary physician should be careful to avoid are failure to pay attention to nurses' comments, to refer some dying patients, or to recognize patient and family anxiety. They also condemn using referral as a last resort. The authors urge that psychiatrists obtain a comprehensive view of the entire case by careful chart review, use the consultation for teaching, and not write lengthy consultation notes filled with jargon.

Moskowitz points out that a positive attitude toward psychiatrists will help to achieve a successful consultation. Referral may be made if the primary physician is annoyed or dissatisfied with the patient or family or with his own inability to solve the problem. The physician must be sure that the resources he suggests are available and must not overestimate to the family what may be achieved. The child patient is to be included in discussions about the referral so that he or she understands what might be discussed in the psychiatric consultation. Soliciting his or her consent enables the patient to save face without having unreal expectations.

SITUATIONS WHERE PSYCHIATRIC REFERRAL
IS DEFINITELY INDICATED

There are a group of problems which, the author believes, should definitely be referred to a child psychiatrist for consultation and possible treatment. Fortunately, these are rarely seen in a general pediatric practice. Their implications are so devastating for normal social functioning that the general pediatrician, even if well-grounded in behavior disorders, is wise not to assume their care unaided. These problems are listed alphabetically and not in the order of importance. Some may overlap with others.

1. Anorexia nervosa
2. Autistic behavior in the young, or psychotic behavior in the older child
3. Character disorders (the amoral individuals often labeled as sociopath, often resistant to any treatment)

   4. Gender identity disorcers (e.g., the very feminine boy)
   5. Incest
   6. Suicide or homicide attempts or gestures.

SITUATIONS WHERE CONSULTATION DEPENDS ON THE SEVERITY OF THE SYMPTOMS AND ON FAMILY ENVIRONMENT AND ATTITUDES

   Referral to a child psychiatrist should be made if symptoms are severe and if management by a pediatrician or other professional has been unsatisfactory. Some situations in which they may occur include:

   1. Alcohol or drug abuse
   2. Anxiety, fear, hysteria, hypochondria
   3. Behavior uncharacteristic of child (e.g., destructiveness or agitation in a usual quiet, easy-going child)
   4. Chronic illness (e.g., diabetes or asthma where emotional factors may actually trigger attacks)
   5. Child abuse
   6. Cruelty, disobedience, destructiveness, lying, stealing, truancy
   7. Depression
   8. Divorce of parents
   9. Persistent encopresis (soiling) in older children
   10. Emotional illness in close family
   11. Hyperactivity or attention deficit disorders
   12. Marked failure to socialize
   13. Pregnancy in early teen years
   14. Runaways
   15. School phobia

   It is recognized that primary care physicians and mental health professionals will differ in estimating their own abilities to handle the above situations. In the past several decades, there has been increasing emphasis on behavioral pediatrics in residency training so that in the future, practitioners will have sufficient expertise both to anticipate and to prevent some of the problems as well as to manage more of them. There will remain, however, a hard core of patients in whom good results are not obtained, and these should be acknowledged by the pediatrician and referred before the patient suffers permanent scarring which a more sophisticated professional might have prevented.

SCHOOL DIFFICULTIES

Before referral to a psychiatrist is made for poor intellectual or social functioning in school, there should be a careful developmental workup. This includes speech and language evaluation, neurological, vision and intelligence testing, and knowledge of the home and family. There will be left a small group of children for whom school difficulties seem to have emotional causes beyond the ability of the pediatrician or school resources to assist. These children should be seen by a child psychiatrist.

QUESTIONNAIRES REGARDING REFERRAL
CUSTOMS OF PEDIATRICIANS

So that this chapter would be more than just one pediatrician's opinion, a questionnaire regarding representative problems which might be referred to a child psychiatrist was circulated to 15 pediatric academicians on the University of Arizona faculty and to 20 Arizona pediatricians in office or hospital-based practice. The 35 pediatricians covered a wide age span, sixteen subspecialities, several practice settings (solo, single-specialty group, multispecialty group, HMO, neighborhood health center, full-time hospital and military hospital). Two cities of a 500 thousand to 1 million and three cities of 20 to 50 thousand in population (two of them over 100 miles from a child psychiatrist) were represented.

As problems of less than extreme severity may be referred to a variety of resources, those questioned were asked their personal preferences regarding referral to a psychiatrist's private office, a child guidance clinic, other mental health facilities, school counseling services, a behaviorally oriented pediatrician, or a child psychologist.

Physicians were asked to answer as if each problem were severe. Part of the covering letter, the questionnaire, and important segments of the results are given in the appendix. Thirty-four responses were received. All but one (No. 14) of the twenty-two problems would be referred by a majority of respondents. Autistic behavior, incest, and anorexia nervosa would be referred by thirty-three of the thirty-four respondents. Suicide gestures/attempts, alcoholism, or substance abuse and depression by thirty-two.

The private office of a child psychiatrist was the single referral choice of twenty-three respondents for autistic behavior, of twenty-one for suicide gestures/attempts, of twenty for hallucinations, of nineteen for depression, and of fourteen for anorexia nervosa, of twelve for hysteria and of eleven for encopresis. The psychiatrist's office was the single referral choice of no more than seven respondents for the remainder of the problems.

Several respondents gave more than one choice for a considerable number of problems, without designating a preference for one over another. The number of respondents who did this for each problem is shown in column M (multiple). Comments made by twenty-five of the thirty-four respondents indicated that personal judgment as to the competence of the consultant, the finances of the family, and the available community resources determined the choice of consultants for such problems.

Where a referral site other than the private office of a child psychiatrist received a substantial number of votes for any problem, that site and the number of votes it received is noted in column O (other).

As the sample is small and nonrandomly selected, no statistical significance is attached to the results.

CHOICE OF CONSULTANT AND REFERRAL SETTING

The proper choice of a consultant and referral setting may greatly influence the success. There are several practice settings with different characteristics.

Child guidance clinics have the advantage of being able to conduct various kinds of testing on the premises. They also have several levels of professionals skilled in particular areas. Where indicated, group therapy sessions can be easily arranged. Sliding fee schedules permit a full range of services to patients regardless of the family's financial resources. Most clinics are partially funded by government, United Way, or other charities.

Child guidance clinics also have drawbacks. Lesser trained persons may have most of the patient contact, with the psychiatrist often limiting input to the initial staff conference and infrequent followup sessions with the therapist, and not seeing the actual patient or family. The referring pediatrician is apt to draw a parallel between such service and the performance of major surgery by a resident, with the senior surgeon only looking in at times during the procedure.

Family counseling agencies and other mental health clinics which serve adults and children have the advantages of child guidance clinics and also treat the entire family. This is often important with disturbed children whose parents may be the persons most in need of help. Such clinics may or may not have the full battery of testing services at hand. Their professionals may not be as well-grounded in pediatric problems as those in a child guidance clinic.

University clinics have the advantage of being headed by highly qualified child psychiatrists chosen for ability to teach, do research and give patient care. They should have a complete range of support services. Their basic function, however, is teaching, so that patient contact will often largely be with trainees under varying degrees of supervision.

The private office of the child psychiatrist has the virtue of offering maximum attention from the caretaker with greatest sophistication and expertise. Many psychiatrists work with other professionals to whom they delegate responsibilities for data collection and testing. The psychiatrist in the private office may appear to the patient to offer the highest degree of confidentiality. Some families feel that clinic records will be available to many people. At the same time, the costs may be greater and the burden of payment falls more heavily on the family. Public funds are not available in many cases and some insurance policies do not cover psychiatric care.

OTHER MENTAL HEALTH PROFESSIONALS

Other mental health professionals, child psychologists, psychiatric and other social workers, school counselors, and behaviorally oriented pediatricians are also available as consultants. A primary care physician often does not know the extent of their training and expertise, but their approach to patients and reports may seem quite similar to those of the child psychiatrists. What kind of case should be referred directly to each one of these very useful individuals? Is their training really sufficient for the problem? Will they request consultation from a child psychiatrist if the situation demands it? These are difficult questions to answer. The author has had both excellent and poor experiences with the use of all of the above. If the patient's situation is complex and has long range, serious potential, the author chooses the consultant with the greatest expertise.

DETERRENTS TO REFERRAL TO PSYCHIATRISTS AND TO ACHIEVING MAXIMUM BENEFIT FROM CONSULTATION

Family objections are a major deterrent to obtaining consultations. Some objections are unreasonable, others very valid. To some people, there is still a stigma attached to consultation with psychiatrists: "People will think he is crazy." There may be a fear that a major emotional illness will be uncovered or that the parents have been guilty of neglect or that their own emotional problems may be revealed. A new and unknown caretaker may be unsatisfactory. Inconvenience, time, and expense are involved. Psychiatrists are notoriously reputed by some lay persons to advise many visits, all of them of long duration. They are said to charge high fees and not to achieve "cures." After all, there is no appendix to remove or penicillin injection to be given for a strep throat. Besides, "everyone knows that children outgrow these things."

Interestingly enough, many mothers say it is the father who will not allow a psychiatric consultation for the child. This is sometimes true, but can also be an excuse for the parent who would bear the major brunt of the inconvenience. When the patient is an older child, he or she is apt to resist because of encroachment on leisure time and a failure to see him or herself as different or inferior, especially in the emotional area.

To answer these objections, the pediatrician or family physician must take the time to give a thorough explanation of the serious long-term implications of untreated mental illness and the value of prevention. He should also correct false impressions mentioned above. Both parents and patient should have separate explanations at their levels of understanding. Comparing the overall expense to a short hospitalzation may help to put the cost in perspective, as well as pointing out that psychiatric care may be a much better long-term investment than orthodontia, a year in college, or even a family vacation. Contracting initially only for an evaluation may overcome the objectives. The decision about therapy can be left until later. It can be emphasized that a finding of no major psychopathology from the psychiatrist will be as reassuring as a biopsy report of a benign, not malignant, tumor. If psychiatric therapy is undertaken, the family should have realistic expectations as to what may be accomplished.

An occasional deterrent to obtaining psychiatric consultation is difficulty in getting an appointment in the near future. This may be because what appears to the family or even the referring physician as an emergency seems otherwise to the psychiatrist who expects that work-up may take weeks and therapy months or even years.

Lack of communication between physicians is a frequent deterrent to maximum benefit from psychiatric consultation. As with any other referral, the primary physician should give the psychiatrist all available information about the patient, the family, and environment. It is safe to say that this seldom occurs.

By the same token, psychiatrists or mental health clinics often fail to report either promptly by telephone or later in detail. The referring physician is entitled to pertinent history, reasons for investigations, findings, plans for therapy, and the results. Communication should continue throughout the course of the treatment. At times, families have told the author that the psychiatrist had terminated therapy some time earlier because "there was nothing wrong." The child's problem was obviously still present and no report had been received from the consultant. It is difficult to know whether a psychiatrist's failure to communicate is caused by a feeling that everything connected with his patient relationship is so confidential that it can not be revealed even to another concerned physician without a breach in confidentiality. The failure to communicate could also be a part of maintaining a "mystique," laziness, or just poor medical practice. It has been the author's experience that patients and parents seldom object to even the most personal details being told to another health-care professional, if the reasons are clearly and simply explained.

SUMMARY

Consultation with child psychiatrists is viewed quite individually by pediatricians depending on their background and experience. Some problems by their nature clearly demand consultation with a psychiatrist, while others can be handled by other mental health professionals. Some problems should be referred if the severity is marked. Settings in which psychiatrists practice have different advantages and drawbacks. Problems of obtaining a consultation of maximum value to the patient are shared by the family, patient, primary physician, and consultant.

BIBLIOGRAPHY

De Angeles: *Pediatric Primary Care*, 2nd ed. (Little Brown & Co: Boston) 1979.
Green and Haggerty: *Ambulatory Pediatrics*, 2nd ed. (WB Saunders Co: Philadelphia, London, Toronto) 1977.
Harper and Richmond (in Rudolph).
Hoekleman, Blatman, Brunell, Friedman, and Seidel: *Principles of Pediatrics— Health Care of the Young* (McGraw-Hill Book Co: New York) 1978.
Hughes: *Synopsis of Pediatrics*, 5th ed. (CV Mosby: St Louis) 1980.
Kaye, Oski, and Barness: *Core Textbook of Pediatrics* (JB Lippincott: Philadelphia, Toronto) 1978.
Kempe, Silver, and O'Brien: *Current Pediatric Diagnosis and Treatment*, 5th ed. (Lange Medical Publications: Los Altos, CA) 1978.
Moskowitz JA: The pediatrician calls for psychiatric referral. *Clin Pediatr* 7: 733, 1968.
Rudolph and Einhorn (eds.): *Pediatrics*, 16th ed. (Appleton–Century–Crofts: New York) 1977.
Schwab JJ and Brown J: Uses and abuses of psychiatric consultation. *JAMA* 205:65, 1968.
Smith WB: *Introduction to Clinical Pediatrics*, 2nd ed. (Saunders Co: Philadelphia, London, Toronto) 1977.
Vaughn, McKay, and Behrman (eds.): *Nelson's Textbook of Pediatrics*, 11th ed. (Saunders: Philadelphia, London, Toronto) 1979.

APPENDIX I

Pertinent Material from Covering Letter Sent with Questionnaire

Because a pediatrician's perspective on referral to a psychiatrist is so varied, dependent on early home orientation toward the specialty, medical school, residency training, community resources, and personal experience, I am sending a questionnaire to a small selected group of practitioners and academicians with differing ages, practice settings, and subspecialty interests. The results will be incorporated in the chapter so that the latter will not solely portray one individual's bias. No statistical implications will be drawn.

Please take the few minutes required to answer the questions asked and return it to me promptly. *Whenever problems in the questionnaire have a wide range of severity from insignificant to very major, please answer as if the problem were severe.* Feel free to add any comments, positive or negative, regarding consultations with or by child psychiatrists.

APPENDIX II

Questionnaire and Results

Please check the YES or NO column to show if you would usually refer the following problems for consultation. If you would refer, indicate to which facility or professional:

A. Private office of child psychiatrist
B. Child guidance clinic
C. Other mental health clinic
D. School counseling service
E. Behaviorally-oriented pediatrician
F. Child psychologist

	Would usually refer		If yes, would refer to		
	Yes	No	A*	M**	O***
1. Autistic behavior	33	1	23	2	0
2. School failure emotionally triggered	27	7	2	6	F8
3. Runaway	26	8	2	4	B7
4. Incest	33	1	10	5	C9
5. Destructiveness	22	12	4	7	E5
6. Pregnancy under 15 years	19	14	0	2	E9
7. Hallucinations	29	5	20	3	

		Would usually refer		If yes, would refer to		
		Yes	No	A*	M**	O***
8.	Severe mental illness in family	20	13	5	6	
9.	Resistant unresponsive encopresis	30	4	11	3	E9
10.	Chronic illness with emotionally triggered non-compliance	21	13	5	8	
11.	Parental discord disturbing child	26	8	3	6	C8
12.	Cruel behavior by patient	26	8	6	8	
13.	Suicide gestures/attempts	32	2	21	6	
14.	Trichotillomania	12	21	7	0	
15.	Hyperactivity and a disturbed family	25	9	2	4	E10
16.	Alcoholism or substance abuse	32	2	4	6	C11
17.	Hysteria	25	9	10	6	
18.	School phobia	20	14	3	7	E8
19.	Persistent stealing in older child	31	3	6	5	F9
20.	Anorexia nervosa	33	1	14	9	E9
21.	Child abuse	28	6	3	5	C8
22.	Depression	32	2	19	9	

*Numbers in this column show number of respondents giving private psychiatric office as primary choice.

**Number of respondents giving more than one referral choice without designating preference for one.

***Referral choice *other than* A and number of votes received.

16

The Ghetto Child

Virginia N. Wilking

The problem in considering the consultation process under special circumstances with special groups lies in the need to include the usual while focusing on the unusual. Children and their families seen in consultation in the ghettos, the inner cities, and in burnt out urban areas are children like other children. Their developmental lines extend in the same directions as those of other children and their relationships reflect dependency and independency in familiar ways. Similarly, consultants walk and talk in familiar fashion and do not take wings and fly. In the face of the sameness, and indeed, because of it, one becomes aware of the differences and their implications. Clinical staffs working in the most conventional of settings are limited by their experience in one way; those working in farout settings are limited in another. It is to be hoped that staffs can make the adjustment, if moved; we know that patients cannot do so easily. Consultation is an active process and takes active participation under known conditions.

The differences lie in the specific nature of the outer environment as well as in attitudes. The differences are most obvious when moving back and forth between different settings but it is possible to be less aware of the similarities. Thus patients and families in different settings approach consultation with the same feelings of dread, of hope, and of anger, and deal with the same ranges of resistance within themselves. They deal with the same lethargy, the same degrees of helpfulness, the same kinds of human error in the human services environment.

"There is no one here by that name."
"That is not on this floor."
"Can I call them for you?"
                    and
"I'm so sorry; the letter says the 7th
but she meant the 8th."

A mother who responds to the suggestion of a clinic visit with her child by saying "But I am not able to come in during the day *at all*," may be unsure and resistant in any setting in addition to being busy. Certain families may see these obstacles, internal and external, as unique to their own system and confuse the internal and external natures of the reality facing them. Only experience and the wisdom of a Solomon would help them to differentiate the inner from the outer, the specific from the general.

Clinical settings are shaped by the environment in which they are made. The clinical settings in the halls of academe are often hard to find because of choices offered between buildings A and B, the hall to the right or to the left, and room numbers running from 105 to 115 with 113 omitted. An approach to a city hospital, where an unmarked building has a closed-off door with a small sign saying "around the corner" may be characteristic but not reassuring.

Whatever the bricks and mortar, whatever the specifics of place and people, consultation in any setting is always an action with the implication that there is something unique in the way the act is carried out. Seventeenth-century England was as great a time for consultation as our own, and the *Oxford English Dictionary* (1961) deals with consultation at length. The emphasis is on action and not on any particular process by which information is obtained.

The skilled practitioner as a consulter gives professional advice, beginning by "presuming rather casually then consultedly" and proceeding to put "their last consulted, devised enterprise in execution" (Ibid.). The last, in best seventeenth-century prose, is quite applicable to the final purpose of consultation.

The consultation process need not involve a detailed knowledge of the family and child, but it is a tenet of consultation that one learns from, and then gives back to, those from whom one has learned; the less you know about a child, a chief complaint, a present illness, a family and a community, the more there is to learn. In psychiatric consultation with a child and family one learns and hopefully understands and then, as a consulter gives back the understanding. For a consulter of a different race or social background, the learning demands an early recognition of ignorance about cultural detail, coupled with a clinical sense that at certain points the differentiation must be made between cultural differences and insanity, cultural goals and compulsive obsessive neurosis, streetwise behavior and loss of impulse control.

There is no distance at all between a seventeenth century clergyman consulting with himself in order to plumb a spiritual depth and a beleagured child psychiatrist trying, in consultation, to divine the nature of the problem with which he is presented by understanding the child and the family against the background of their surroundings: those *geographical*—house, street, neighborhood; *those temporal*—age and stage, duration of symptoms, milestones, and family history; *those abstract*—what is said, what is meant, what is. Synthesis is implicit in the act of consultation, an act through which consideration is given to what is known. In a series of steps history taking and observation become formulation, diagnosis and planning. "Presuming rather casually than consultedly" (Ibid.), as previously noted.

The mechanics of consultation are in the message. The phrases, "seeing a child," "seeing the family," "talking with them" (soon to be remembered as "they didn't tell me anything") describe those actions which constitute the experience of child and family seen in consultation.

It is the beauty of the word *consultation* that action is implicit in its use. Evaluation, the more limiting word, more often used, has a more passive connotation and is without commitment to action, whereas with consultation, there is "a consultative, knowing act" (Ibid.).

SETTING

The action in this instance is being carried on in the Child Psychiatry Clinics of the Division of Child Psychiatry, Harlem Hospital Center, on Lenox Avenue in the center of Harlem. Our procedures reflect our experiences—good, bad, and indifferent.

REFERRAL FOR CONSULTATION: REFERRAL PROCESS

The first stages of engagement, the preliminaries of consultation, involve the referral process which, in the majority of cases is initiated by individuals other than the family. There are few referrals from private doctors, many from other hospital clinics. Referrals from other clinics may have originated in schools, which also make their referrals directly to child psychiatry. The innocuous statement, "The mother is extremely interested in her child and is asking for this help," often bodes ill and represents reaction formation, obscuring two years of determined efforts to make the mother say she is asking. There are referrals from the family court, usually through a staff member assigned to family court one day a week. There are referrals from day care centers, and there

Table 1. Referrals to the Division of Child Psychiatry Harlem Hospital Center—January 1 through February 28, 1981

Referral source	Developmental psychiatry clinic (birth–5 years)	Child psychiatry clinic (6–11 years)	Adolescents psychiatry clinic (12–15 years)	Treatment program for court related children (±10–15 years)
Public school		22	9	
Pediatric clinics	5	3	2	
Pediatric ward		3		
Self-referral	2	10	3	
Woman's center (abuse)	1			
Crisis intervention (abuse)	1	1		
Adult psychiatry	2	5		
Family agency		1	1	
Family court				5
Child psychiatry clinics		1	1	
Psychiatric emergency room			1	
Total	79			

are referrals from the pediatric award often beginning with the statement, "This is a child who needs followup," or even more familiarly, "Discharged before being seen."

These are the generalities. A review of the referral sources of children and adolescents seen at different child psychiatry clinics gives the particulars (Table 1).

Our process involves letters, telephone calls, and walk-ins. Referrals, whatever the original physical form, are recorded on a referral sheet, and the patient remains a figment of the referral process until the first appointment, when he or she crosses a border of the process and becomes a case. The new referrals are reviewed weekly and planned for assignments are made and appointments given. If the original referral source suggests danger and urgency the referral becomes a child psychiatry emergency consultation and follows a slightly different route with the same cast of characters. The naming or renaming of the nature of the situation is an important part of the response. Somewhat different rules apply in emergencies. Family defenses are down and the need for action, already part of consultation, is heavily underlined.

In addition to the statement made by letter, by telephone, or in person, there are sometimes further reports from the school or court or information from a hospital chart, sometimes reports are sent from special education programs and committees on the handicapped. Usually, releases for these reports are obtained the first time the family comes in.

THE CONSULTATION

In the consultation, the consultant(s) themselves finally see the child and family, whether the consultation is carried on by one or by several persons individually or by several acting as a team at the same time and in the same place. Consultation carried on by a team accustomed to working together can be a very satisfactory experience for child, family and staff, providing time for family observations, time for individual meetings, time for group and individual meetings.

The unit of time can extend from one hour-and-a-half in an afternoon to several visits planned, cancelled, and rescheduled. Because this is a medical setting, a child psychiatrist or resident under supervision is always part of the consultation, but it may also be essential to have the skills of a social worker or psychologist at hand. The child may have contact with many agencies and the psychiatrist may be unclear about who is managing the case and a competent social worker may be needed to enter the maze and offer the bewildered psychiatrist the thread that will rescue him or her from the bureaucratic Minator. An IQ can be estimated and organic features described, but the details of the class placement and the basis for understanding a child's fears may demand the skills of the psychologist, and extensive testing.

The least common denominator may be the child psychiatrist, common in this setting to all cases at intervals. The mother of one of our patients, when speaking of his father, could also have been describing the psychiatrist's presence: "I like it this way; permanent but not constant."

The consultation starts with a casual glance into the waiting room from a distance and then a more direct and inquiring glance, and introductions with the inclusion of the child or adolescent in the introductions. In Harlem, the glance must sweep the room like radar: "Is he with you?" "No, he's just a friend." "Are they yours?" "Yes, it's my grands." As previously quoted "presuming rather casually then consultedly" (*New Oxford Dictionary*, 1961).

The habit of pulling the family along in the first stage of the consultation is probably a good one. It requires stamina, a certain amount of space, and a degree of authority. Part of the history can be taken in a group situation, given sensitivity to dangerous areas, but this kind of overview of a family is just that. It is a valuable adjunct, identifying siblings, hangers-on, generations and generation gaps, as well as making family attitudes and interrelationships clear.

The review of the chief complaint with a tactful softening of certain hard edges sets the scene for parent (or guardian), child, and other family members as well. Needless to say, this would be grossly inappropriate where the complaint must be emphasized and put in clear relief. Younger staff sometimes think they should maintain an attitude of "we see that in our work," where an acknowledgement of the shocking, and a heightening of the seriousness of the situation, is far more appropriate. A young resident, obtaining the family history of a seven-year-old boy who talked of dying, asked his guardian about his aunt's death and was told she had gone out the window. "How did that happen?" "I pushed her" was the reply. The resident continued calmly—and inappropriately— with the history-taking without further comment.

A patient's developmental milestones, school performance, history of accidents, illnesses and hospitalizations provide considerable information. Questions can be used to follow-up: "And then—?" "And when was he—?" "Does his father still come by?" The stereotypes of single parent homes will not do in the face of the evidence of a new baby and adequate male identification, and the presumption that the child of a clearly impaired mother has had nothing is equally mistaken. (Jamal is four years old. His mother's hangovers are monumental; she seems to pay him little attention. His sister has been seen holding him over the edge of the fire escape, but Jamal is still a splendid child, developmentally whole at four years.)

The history may suggest what you might expect, but the knowing comes from observation of the child and his or her interactions with the familiar family members and the unfamiliar room (objects, wooden building blocks, small wooden fences, toy cars, scrap paper, pencils) and the doctor's eye. The mental status can be telescoped by catching a sentence here and there. "I don't want to go to the elevator with them," is a full sentence indicating good cognitive function, awareness, ego strengths, and overtones of the oppositional. Another full sentence like that from a five-year-old, and there are fewer diagnostic problems and no need to ask who is president, although color identification could be tried out. At age seven, right or left handedness can be observed. A drawing serves as Bender, Goodenough, Rorschach, and Childrens' Apperception Test, while games explore neurological functioning.

This can be done within a family interview but some of the serious questions to be asked should be tried first in private. One ten-year-old said he didn't like talking in the family group with father, brother, and two sisters because, he said, "My father gets so suspicious."

There can be an economy of effort in all of this but the basic questions should be asked, "Do you worry?" and "What makes you angry?" "Have you been sick?" "Who was?" "Were they very sick?" Children coming with clear indication of their feelings should not be asked, "Do you get angry?" or "Did you mind when your mother died?" Here assumptions can be made and a child enabled to answer a question such as, "Which way did you feel—angry or sad?" "When did it hurt most?" "Why did she do that? It is hard to understand." And most importantly, "What do you think?" "What would help?"

Classic "wondering" belongs later on in treatment or in therapeutic intervention carried on as part of longer term consultation. Simple declarative sentences are better initially: "I think," where appropriate, or the ever useful "It seems as if . . . ." The beginning of interpretation, "Could this be it?" can be said to the child; he or she should be reassured that this is all that need be said to the family. The establishment of a tacit understanding is the consultant's version of the Anna Freud seduction and implies a promise of help although the child cannot always understand the cost. A joint interview with child, principal family member, and other staff who are involved ends the sessions or session, with other family members added or subtracted as counted up on a giant abacus. Causes of difficulties can be mentioned, including the several factors involved, the pain inherent in what has been said recognized, and plans evolved. There must be continuity between complaint, causes, and the kind of surcease that can be expected, with the possibility considered that the efforts needed for change are too great to be made. The consultant must say what has to be said with certainty—if the certainty is there—as to cause, effect and the attempt at cure. But he or she must expect to say it more than once and, to be believable, must make it clear that he or she understands there may be proper reluctance to accept the view held and the recommendation offered. Alternatives should be discussed, their relative worth documented, and an agreement to disagree reached if possible.

If there is no certainty an absolute decision should be postponed. Pepy's Diary for May 19, 1665, noted a decision "not to do anything suddenly, but consult my pillow."

It is sometimes possible to end at this point. The identification of a problem is wholly satisfactory, the discussion of the problem reverberates, a spring wound too tight unwinds, movement in a certain direction is checked almost imperceptibly.

When a family cannot tolerate even the beginning, and often it does not, the consultation that is begun is left hanging. Sometimes the family is lost to the clinic because we cannot make certain followup efforts except in emergencies. At other times the family fights off the clinic as it would any other maurauding band. If the family is strengthened by the consultative effort, the refusal to respond may be therapeutic in itself. This is possible, but in the face of some of the symptoms with which the clinics are presented, unlikely, and the child remains at risk although not all of the risks are equal.

EVALUATION OF CONSULTATION

More usually the consultation is most effective as a beginning. Psychotherapy is proposed, family members are seen, various groups are mobilized, referrals to special education classes are initiated or supported, and medication is given. Followup visits can be seen as a treatment of choice or used as an alternate plan when regular visits cannot be maintained. These irregular visits when made even at three month intervals are usually referred to as "having treatment" and "seeing a doctor." Eagle-eyed guidance counselors ignorant of this therapeutic relationship ask for the details of treatment sessions and suggestions are made by school social workers for a more disciplined approach to behavior modification.

The therapeutic residual left over from these visits as well as from more orthodox forms of treatment must be measured in the Child Psychiatry Clinics at Harlem and elsewhere. The urge *to do* fulfills the implications of consultation and to act is natural to the professional and nonprofessional denizens of mental health settings in disadvantaged areas, but there needs to be a measured and deliberate approach to the action taken. Unfortunately, in our setting the continual demands reinforce the tendency to continue to act using familiar but general guides: "Will the action do harm?" "Is it possible?" and "Is it soundly based on what is known?" do well as a beginning, but specifics must follow. There used to be a game where children would circle another child and cry "What is your name, what is your father's name, where do you go to school?" The questions are to the point. We must continually ask ourselves, "Who exactly is this child? What are his particular needs?"

CONCLUSIONS

It is obvious, in the abstract, that there are biological givens and environmental interactions, that there is nature and there is nurture and that every child has a specific envelope which determines the nature of diffusion from internal to external environment and vice versa (Plant, 1950). In the ghetto and in consultation with a black child, staff and patients alike—white staff, black staff, and black families—are necessarily living within their immediate decade, trailing after them victories and defeats, some shared, some not, from the past. If white staff members are respectful of black families, black families will shift the emphasis in the kind of respect they give recommendations made by white staff. Prejudice is not overcome but fear and anger at least are held in abeyance. Racial issues are not usually brought out in consultation unless there is a breakdown in one kind of communication and substitution of another at the top of the lungs. The discussion of color comes out with the familiarity and the lowering of defenses in the course of treatment.

On the other hand, the patient's age and stage relate to the general. This is theory, born out by experience. In actuality, if experience with consultation in Harlem is reviewed, it can be seen that children in Harlem are as specific to their time and place as other children are to their's—no more, no less. And it can be suggested that their time and place involve:

1. Less security for families and thus less for children
2. More families who succumb to pressures in various and flamboyant ways, leaving children in nonfamilies with emotionally depleted caretakers
3. More violence around the corner, more overtones of violence, more families in which a family member has died violently
4. More explosive feelings with escalation of problems
5. Strengths but at various levels: There may be only survival, which does not support the developmental process in full
6. Fewer families standing up to the rigors of full involvement with child psychiatry clinics. Many families take only part of what is offered
7. Negative feelings and hostility expressed directly. (If not too destructive of the process, the open expression of feelings can allow more rapid therapeutic intervention)
8. More losses per child per family

In addition doctors share in the privations of ghetto medicine:

1. Professionals who stay become more, not less available and committed to their patients but still maintain some professional distance
2. Staff in these settings remain aware of families' strengths and prize them but are extremely alert to danger
3. Political pressures and administrative neglect make doctors realistically pessimistic at times. These privations and the resentments they cause are shared with patients:
   Disturbed adults in the lobbies
   Elevators not working
   Confusion about entrances
   Cuts in staff, reducing amenities
   Stealing of equipment
   Garbage on hospital sidewalks
4. Hospital staff members make themselves more responsible for desperate families, and for those in which the mother or caretaker is mentally ill
5. Mental health professionals struggle with the awareness that more children in our setting will go into placement away from home than in others. The reluctance to act arbitrarily or prematurely sometimes allows staff to miss the appropriate time for intervention. And more abused children are seen

What is specific environmentally is very specific and determines a certain ambiance, but the attributes determined by biological determinants are equally specific and are seen in that cultural ambiance as well. As Gertrude Stein was reported to have said, "When you get there, there is no there there." The consultant continues here and there, creatures of his or her time, eager "to consult one's feelings, to have regard for them in forming a determination (*New Oxford Dictionary*, 1961).

REFERENCES

New Oxford Dictionary, vol 2 (Oxford Clarendon Press: New York) 1961, pp 884–885.
Plant, JS: *The Envelope* (New York Commonwealth Fund: New York) 1950.

17

Consultation in Disasters— Refugees

Raquel Cohen

The emergence of mental health consultation in relocation settings offers a new opportunity in child psychiatry. Mental health specialists are beginning to be more visible and more welcomed within relocation camps and other programs for displaced persons to the extent that they now have an enlarged base of knowledge dealing with uprooted and displaced individuals who may be fleeing political or natural disasters. It is the intent of this chapter to formalize the documentation of child-psychiatric consultants working in relocation camps and thereby add to the data base of this new field in child psychiatry. A *consultant* is herein defined as a child psychiatrist with consultation skills who is asked to participate inside an organized relocation system and assist the staff in finding adequate approaches to deal with families and their children or unaccompanied children. The consultant is further defined to be both aware of and sensitive to crosscultural issues presented in these types of groupings. This is especially true when a refugee population migrates from a country other than its homeland.

Camp will be defined as the temporary geographical site where individuals will be given shelter, food, medical care, and recreational opportunities. This setting is organized and managed by the government—federal, state, or local. It is a transitional setup and the staff's goal is to resettle the population as rapidly as feasible into the communities.

Camp staff, herein referred to as *consultees*, are workers who have specific responsibilities and tasks to perform in order to negotiate the objective of re-locating the refugees/victims. How the consultee discharges these responsibilities is dependent on both his sensitivity and knowledge of human behavior under stress and his awareness of problem-solving techniques using mental health prin-ciples. The emotions, attitudes, and behavior reactions of these consultees can either facilitate or hinder the coping, adaptability, and acculturation of the anguished refugee/victims.

Refugees/victims are herein defined to be individuals in life transitions. They are displaced adults and children who are victims of forceful migration or disaster. They suffer from the most traumatic, dehumanizing, and painful cir-cumstances that can befall a population. They have been moved by foot or transported by vehicles across long distances, generally without explanation, preparation or planning. The circumstances that accompany these trips can be uneventful or as traumatic as capsizing, losing a parent (escaping from Saigon, 1975) or being bitten by dogs (Mariel, 1980).

Emergency relocation procedures are defined to be the resettlement ac-tivities practiced by a group of camp workers whose job is to find a sponsor for every refugee or a housing site for every victim of disaster.

The psychiatric consultant needs to be aware of the following areas of knowledge affecting the children and their resettlement experiences:

1. Antecedents
    a. circumstances in which family units left home
    b. experience of travel
    c. identifying characteristics of family/child
        1. economic
        2. social status
        3. employment skills
        4. physical health of all members
        5. mental health of all members
2. Conditions of entering the transitional, temporary location (camp)
3. Coping and adaptation approaches to the camp conditions over time
4. Circumstances and conditions of leaving the transitional setting (camp)

Some of the above issues merit special discussion. The antecedent condi-tions that surround the experience of the relocation of the child have a bearing on the child's social and psychological reactions to the camp. The crisis climate of most camps does not lend itself to being sensitive to the needs of frightened, anxious, vulnerable children. Particular children will be noticed and singled out because of their "acting out" behavior (infraction of rules, destruction of prop-erty, excessive use of medical facilities).

The consultant was asked to advise how to handle the situation of Henry, a ten-year-old Haitian refugee who kept stealing food from the camp kitchen. In spite of the fact that all meals were provided for the families, Henry was caught several times in the process of hiding and carrying out food. On mental status examination it was found that Henry was an anxious child who had lost his father on the boat trip to the United States and who believed he would have to provide for the future of his mother and four younger siblings. The camp staff was assisted to understand the meaning of the behavior and help Henry with his need to mourn his father's death, allay his anxiety for the future, and help the mother to rely less on him as "the head of the household."

As the family and child become comfortable with the camp routine, the different phases of adaptation to the relocation will proceed. A portion of the population (approximately ten percent) will begin to show early patterns of maladaptation. Many of the signs and symptoms can be considered and classified under the DSM III diagnostic categories of conduct disorder, reactive disorder, depressive disorder and posttraumatic disorder.

Disorders of sleep, eating, bowel, and bladder appear regularly in young children. The clash between cultural child-rearing customs and camp life shows its most dramatic impact at these stages.

Juan, a seven-year-old boy, only son of an older couple who had lost their home after an earthquake, was refusing to be separated from his mother. He couldn't be persuaded to get undressed to go to bed at night and wanted to sleep on the floor of his parents' temporary camp shelter in a camp setting. He refused to play with other children and was preoccupied with noises and the weather. It was helpful to explain to the consultee the concept of cumulative trauma and its effects on the child's ego.

Issues of attitudes, prejudices among ethnic groups (U.S. staff and refugee), and expectations of how children should be disciplined and reared surface quickly. Regression in habit, maturity, or behavior of children under stress (such as loss of bladder and/or sphincter control) adds a complex dimension to the problems of the child in his interaction with the new environment.

Patterns of acculturation also emerge during this stage of adjustment to the camp. Different rates of adaptation will occur and influence the interaction between different members of the same family. Also, processes of acculturation differ. Some families show patterns of withdrawal; they turn inward, tend to reject the norms of the camp, are unable or unwilling to ask for advice or guidance from the host population. Other families reach out continuously and develop healthy, interdependent bonds with individuals around them.

BACKGROUND

Although acknowledging the importance of and need to document the history of refugee migration and recent disaster-assistance programs, the system established by the United States to deal with refugees/victims, and the many governmental and voluntary agencies that assist them, this chapter will focus on the role, skill, and procedures that are needed by the child psychiatrist who chooses to become a consultant to a camp professional staff. Several appropriate techniques will be described and categorized so that the work of the consultant with displaced individuals, and children in particular, can be conceptualized.

Among the historical and experiential processes that are cited in mental health literature, the following are singled out to delineate those which a consultant must understand to work with refugee populations:

1. Adaptation (Hamburg, 1967)
2. Acculturation (Szapocznik, 1978)
3. Value systems (Kluckhohn, 1961)
4. Coping mechanisms and their relation to:
    a. culture, ethnicity, roles, status (Padilla, 1980)
    b. age of child and developmental states (Freud, 1965)
    c. health (integrity of CNS) and vulnerability (Nagera, 1981)
5. Social support systems (Caplan, 1974)
6. Maternal and child bonding theories (Bowlby, 1969)

RATIONALE

It is hoped that this chapter can assist the child psychiatrist to plan and implement a mental health program within a refugee camp.

First, attention is directed to the conditions within the setting of the camp where the consultant will participate and share his expertise. Then procedures and techniques are prescribed that will be helpful to the consultant in developing a cooperative, coprofessional role with camp staff (Cohen, 1973). Finally, guidelines are developed to map out the specific areas, both concrete and conceptual, in which the consultant might participate and intervene.

The central assumption is: Planned and programmed incorporation of mental health principles within a refugee/victim camp is necessary not only for a child's healthier adaptation and eventual successful relocation, but also to support and enrich the consultee's function.

There are some effects of successful consultation which will enhance the psychological well-being of the consultee and help prevent the serious problem of burn-out that is pervasive in this type of work.

SETTING

The camp exists within a socially chaotic environment in which there is a sense of emergency at all times.

The following factors contribute to this crisis climate:

1. There is minimal time to gather data to investigate the reliability of data
2. Staff members and policy change constantly
3. Decisions are made rapidly with little regard for clear concepts, objectives, or tasks
4. The staff and client populations are stressed, irritable, and tired

Change is the essence of the camp setting. There is fluctuation in all levels of personnel, regulations, policies, and standards. As a result, the camp organizational structure is loose and a strong sense of identity is lacking. Also, the inconsistency that exists adds to problems of miscommunication and misinterpretation. The psychiatric consultant to the camp must be particularly sensitive to all information about change. This environment of the refugee camp is characteristic of all rapidly formed, transitory settings for displaced or uprooted populations.

TECHNIQUES AVAILABLE TO THE PSYCHIATRIC CONSULTANT IN REFUGEE CAMPS

Consultation

The mental health consultation is a technique that is helpful in relocation camps to assist agency staff. The following conceptual principles underlying consultation in these camps are noteworthy to identify:

Focus: Consultation in relocation camps can be defined to exist for

a.   personality or conduct disorders of the refugee/victim;
b.   emotional disorders of the refugee/victim; and
c.   staff interpersonal relations.

Level of responsibility: The camp staff members who meet with a consultant do not give up responsibility for the outcome of the individual's resettlement program nor for his mental health adaptation. The freedom of the camp worker to accept or reject what the consultant says enables him to take quickly as his own any idea that appears to him in the current situation.

Quality of relationship: The basic relationship between consultant and consultee is collaborative. There are no bureaucratic hierarchy levels between them; instead, they work as two colleagues who join their efforts to problem solve. A coordinative relationship is fostered by the consultant's usually being a member of another profession and entering the camp for a specific time frame.

Site: Consultation is usually offered during meetings which take place in response to the consultee's awareness of problems with children. It takes place in the camp setting.

Time of commitment: Consultation is expected to continue until the camp closes. Through the period that camp programs exist, many types of consultation objectives can be identified. For example, a consultant can be dealing with a case consultation and also consulting on some major policy problem at the same time.

Content: The consultant responds to that segment of the consultee's issue which the latter presents, but he does *not* seek to remedy other areas of inadequacies in the consultee's expertise or some of the camp programs which are working ineffectively. The consultant must, therefore, be prepared for continuous changes of focus, in regard to both the content and scope of consultation problems and the identity and hierarchical position of his consultees within the continuously shifting organizational structure of the camp.

Objective: Consultation has both an immediate goal—to help the consultee understand the underlying causes of the problem he is trying to solve—and a long-term goal to increase the consultee's capacity to master other types of problems. This increased sense of confidence will tend to foster the consultee's feelings of self-esteem and personal worth which will, in turn, strengthen his job performance. Although the focus of the process is on the work issues and not on the personal problems of the consultee, the consultant does observe the feelings of the consultee and respects his privacy and confidentiality.

A young male staff member asked for consultation in dealing with a female, sixteen-year-old Cuban refugee living in one of the federal camps. The problem that he identified in dealing with the adolescent was that she kept breaking the curfew established by the authorities. He wanted to help her so that she would not be punished. As he described her behavior, it was clear that he was containing his anger at her rebelliousness but was not aware of it. The consultant didn't deal with these feelings but empathized with the difficulty of dealing with adolescents and proceeded to focus on the methodology to antici-pate her behavior and set limits within the cross-cultural communication bar-riers. The problem of cross-culture is a constant theme in most refugee camps where staff or one culture is expected to live among and assist traumatized popu-lations of another culture.

Limits of consultation: Since a relocation camp setting rarely provides the psychiatric consultant with a clear set of expectations for defining the role to which he has been accustomed in his traditional clinical work, he must develop a new conceptual map that he carries within him into this field.

This conceptual map must indicate the limits of the consultant's profes-sional domain. Although his role may not be prestructured, he is not, in fact, free to do anything that comes into his head or to respond completely to all requests from consultees.

He is constrained by the policies, both formal and informal, of the camp setting. These policies do *not* allow him to move on to other major areas of camp problems which may not have a clear connection with the mental health of a refugee or victim but which he believes might improve the quality of life in the camp.

A consultant was asked to help a group of camp staff to deal with the aggressive acting out behavior among young Cuban males living in a barracks within a federal refugee camp. The consultant met with the group in the bar-racks and was able to realize that the design of the living arrangements precluded any possibility of privacy, fostering instead a need to "protect" areas belonging to each adolescent. Although these issues were discussed, the consultant had no access or power to change the physical living accommodations in the barracks.

He is also constrained by the camp's laws and regulations as well as by its formal patterns of communication and authority. His intervention is not likely to be welcome if he takes sides in informal power struggles among staff, or if he suddenly disrupts the orderly process of decision-making that the official, bureaucratic system has developed in the camp.

Types of mental health consultation: The consultant is aided by a system which allows him to categorize each situation, process the flow, and predict what the most promising methods of dealing with it are likely to be. There are many useful ways of classifying mental health consultation for this purpose. The most classic distinctions are made by Caplan (1968) and are based upon two major divisions:

1. Between a primary focus of the consultant on an individual case problem and attention to an administrative problem related to a program or policy of the camp.
2. Between a primary focus of the consultant in giving specialized opinions and recommendations in regard to the program difficulty and, attempting to improve the problem-solving capacity of the consultee through the handling of a case problem.

Refugee/victim-centered case consultation: This is a traditional type of consultation where the consultant is asked for his opinion, diagnosis, and assessment of personality problems of an individual refugee. In addition, the consultant might recommend a plan for the most effective approach to resettling the refugee/victim.

The primary goal of the consultation is for the consultant to communicate a method to the consultee indicating how the refugee/victim can be helped. A subsidiary goal is that the consultee will use his experience with this case to improve his knowledge and skills in working with other refugees and will be prepared to handle comparable future problems.

A staff member asked the consultant to help him deal with a nine-year-old Vietnamese orphan who kept returning to a family that had befriended him enroute to the camp. He had been housed with a foster family chosen by the authorities. As the situation was analyzed, it showed that the foster family was a close-meshed one with one infant and a toddler. The "friendly" family consisted of parents and two adolescents. When the consultant obtained a detailed history of how the orphan spent his day he learned that the child had to accommodate his activities to the baby's schedule. This caused many difficulties between him and his foster mother. Advice and suggestions were given by the consultant on how the needs of the child could be balanced with the household routine.

Consultee-centered case consultation: The consultant focuses his attention on trying to understand the nature of the work difficulties for a consultee with regard to a refugee/victim and on helping him to remedy these difficulties.

The consultee's difficulties may be due to:

1. Lack of knowledge about the type of problem presented by the refugee
2. Lack of skill in making use of such knowledge
3. Lack of self-confidence in utilizing his knowledge and skills
4. Lack of professional objectivity due to subjective emotional complications

The consultant may assist the consultee to increase his knowledge or skills; he may support and reassure him to increase his self-confidence; and/or he may help him increase his professional objectivity so as to reduce the distortion in his perception of the refugee's condition.

The hope is always that improvement in professional functioning will enable the consultee to solve the problem of the refugee/victim and that this improvement will be maintained in the future in relation to individuals with similar difficulties. The aim of this type of consultation is frankly to educate the consultee, using problems with a current individual lever and learning opportunity.

Mary, a ten-year-old girl who was housed in a temporary shelter following a tornado, was brought to the medical unit for diagnosis of continued vomiting. As she was being evaluated, the child became more anxious. She lost control of her bladder and urinated on the floor. This strange behavior upset the examining physician who called in a psychiatric consultant. The consultant focused on explaining to the physician the situation in which Mary had been found under the collapsed porch of her home, after spending part of the night alone. Understanding how posttraumatic situations affect children, produce regressive behavior and weaken acquired bodily control functions assisted the consultee in dealing with his patient. The consultant was able to sort out pathology, traumatic reactions to past events and adaptive mechanisms to continuous stress.

Program-centered administrative consultation: The work problem in this type of consultation is in planning and administration of the camp and the concern is how to develop a new program or improve an existing one. The consultant helps by using his knowledge of administration and social systems, of mental health theory and practice, and of problem development in other areas in order to collect and analyze data about camp issues. He suggests short-term and long-term solutions for the administrative human problems of the camp organization.

The primary goal for the consultant is to prescribe an effective course of action in planning the program.

The recreational director of a camp complained to a consultant that he was unable to interest a group of adolescent refugees in attending organized activities. As the issues and schedules were analyzed, it became clear that attending these events produced a conflict for the refugees who wanted to be first in line to eat at the cafeteria. The recreational activities were at the end of the day and overlapped with the time when waiting lines to enter the cafeteria congregated. The adolescents preferred to go there than to the recreation, due to their anxiety that food would be exhausted before they arrived.

Consultee-centered administrative consultation: This is similar to consultee-centered case consultation. However, the focus is on problems of programming and camp organization instead of problems with a particular refugee/victim.

In addition to lack of knowledge, skills, self-confidence, and objectivity, the consultee's problem may be the result of personnel conflicts—poor leadership, authority problems, lack of staff role definitions, communication blocks and so forth. The consultant's goal is to understand and help remedy these working conflicts. His successes will enable the consultee to develop and implement plans to accomplish the mission of the camp.

Some literature on consultation (Berlin, 1964; Cohen, 1964) uses the restricted definition that denotes a process of interaction between two professional persons, the consultant who is a specialist and the consultee who invokes the consultant's help in regard to current work problems. This differs from the broader understanding of consultation and support activities which defines the consultant to be included in the organizational and administrative responsibility for program and clients.

This latter model is more appropriate for the aims of the consultant working in a relocation camp. Observing many aspects of human behavior is necessary for the psychiatric consultant to understand the refugee. His active participation requires an understanding of the following: 1) the living conditions within the unfamiliar setting of a refugee/victim camp; 2) the community environments in which the refugee will resettle; and 3) the changes involved for the refugee in the final activities of resettlement and physical transportation to his sponsor, community house or employment area.

Psychological assistance may make the difference between success and failure for a refugee/victim. Therefore, it is essential for the consultant to have different levels of responsibility and involvement. This is exemplified by the following description:

A consultant who was working with the leaders of a city that had been destroyed by an earthquake was asked to participate in a series of meetings to plan the care of a large number of refugees housed in two camps. The activities to be planned included housing, feeding, child health care, and placement of housekeeping and recreational facilities. The consultant participated with all the human service systems affecting this population. After acquiring first-hand knowledge of the problems faced by the service organizations and the needs of the victims, the consultant was able to introduce psychological concepts into the design program service plans.

Collaboration

Another technique utilized by the child psychiatrist in the refugee camp is collaboration. In collaboration, the consultant participates with the consultee in understanding, investigating and analyzing the problems of the child refugee.

A counselor in a camp asked the consultant to assist him in dealing with a fourteen year-old Cuban refugee male who had three episodes of convulsion. The goal of differential diagnosis was to establish whether these attacks were organic or functional. The EEG appeared normal. The consultant interviewed the youth and learned that in Cuba his family believed in witchcraft. He had come alone to the United States and felt so lonely, frustrated and depressed in the camp that he believed he had been "punished by the devil." When he became overwhelmed by his feelings he also became frightened at the thought that the "spirits were in his body." The consultee participated with the consultant to change some of the boy's situations and to help him adapt to the difficulties of living in camp.

The responsibility for the refugee/victim is shared between the consultant and consultee, each of whom is expected by the other and by the refugee to carry out certain procedures. These procedures may be carried out by the consultant who will act both directly with the child and indirectly with the consultee. For instance, the child psychiatrist may evaluate the child refugee/victim in his living setting, recommend that the refugee/victim come for counseling, prescribe medication and, subsequently, discuss the case with the consultee. On the other hand, the plan of action may be sequential and may have several phases in terms of assisting the refugee/victim through the tasks that he must complete before resettlement. The child psychiatrist and consultee working in the transitional camp setting maintain continuous contact with each other during the duration of the operations and share the responsibility for successful outcome.

There are important differences between this pattern of professional interaction and the traditional type of consultation. In collaboration, the consultant determines his behavior primarily on the basis of his evaluation and diagnostic assessment of the refugee/victim, for whom he accepts direct responsibility. He works together with his colleague, the consultee, who will examine other aspects of refugee/victim life and who will participate in seeing that whatever procedure is recommended will be carried out.

Although the consultant may communicate his procedures, there are some areas of diagnostic content that are confidential and should *not* be shared with the consultee. This distinction between classic consultation and collaboration within the refugee camp setting is noteworthy.

It is possible in a relocation camp to combine consultation and collaboration elements. However, the following problems can occur in combining the two techniques: 1) miscommunication, 2) barriers in interpretation, 3) overstepping the boundaries of the task of the consultee, and 4) scapegoating. The behavior of a consultant who over-identifies with the refugee/victim's plight highlights issues of miscommunication and misinterpretation of cues given by staff, leading to overstepping the boundaries of the psychiatric consultant.

A consultant was asked to accompany a camp counselor to the building that housed adolescents who had broken a camp regulation. The camp setting was staffed by paramilitary personnel and the building served as jail for the camp. One of the adolescents who had been caught hit one of the guards and was handcuffed to his bed pending investigation. The counselor was interested in finding out what had happened and in using his expertise to help the youngster regain control.

He started asking questions of the guards and turned to the consultant to ask him to interpret the issues to the military personnel. The consultant became incensed and believed that he was being manipulated to sanction this type of punishment. He berated both the counselor and the guards for their lack of sensitivity and went to see the director of the camp, accusing the camp counselor of allowing a refugee to be handcuffed.

After an investigation, it was found out that the camp personnel had followed policy and were trying to help contain a very dangerous situation. The consultant had very few facts before he became emotionally overwhelmed.

Education

Consultation has an aspect of education directed to helping the consultee with his current work problems in relation to a specific refugee/victim or his program. The consultee uses consultation to add to his personal knowledge and to reduce areas of misunderstanding in order that he may deal more effectively in the future with a similar problem.

It is this educational aspect of consultation that makes it an important refugee/victim resettlement method. A goal is to spread the application of the psychiatric consultant's mental health knowledge to the many agencies that will continue working with refugee migration/resettlement.

Education as a specialized professional activity needs to be conceptualized as an indirect methodology. This indirect methodology has important merits in a relocation camp, including the widespread effect of the resettlement agencies on large numbers of refugees/victims. In order to use the limited time of the consultant effectively in helping the consultees deal with the problems of a refugee/victim, the child psychiatrist needs to design specific boundaries with the maximum educational carryover.

OPERATIONAL GUIDELINES

The focus of this section is to provide consultants with common guidelines and language necessary in order to work with consultees. These consultees have the responsibility of planning, initiating, and making the resettlement program of refugees/victims operational.

A key concern for the consultant is to match the activity rhythm and professional tone of the camp worker. This tone reflects crisis, emergency, and immediacy of need.

Steps to Developing Mental Health Consultation in a Refugee Camp

1. *Proximity and Reputation*: A fundamental principle in developing a positive relationship with camp personnel and gaining trust and credibility is to create proximity and establish the reputation of being trustworthy, competent, and interested in helping without infringing on the rights of the staff or endangering their approaches and programs in the camp (Caplan, 1968).

2. *Offer Collaborative Services*: Initial contact can be established by the offer of collaborative services to the refugees/victims referred for psychiatric diagnostic evaluation. Such referrals when accepted can be used as a cue to the needs of the camp workers. Each case is carefully observed to assess the problems that the individual presents. The consultant then offers to share information and assist in the problem resolution with the appropriate worker.

3. *Initiate Simple Report System*: The rights of the refugee/victim to confidentiality and competent diagnosis and treatment can be safeguarded even while relationships with the other staff are being built during the initial period. This means, however, sending an immediate written communication, followed by subsequent information on the progress and management, to the appropriate camp staff. Language must be simple and understandable. These reports can also provide opportunities for mental health workers to participate in daily meetings with as many staff persons as possible, thus initiating relationships and beginning to build a picture of the social system and culture of the camp. The opportunities to disseminate knowledge, support therapeutic attitudes, and assist in developing good team morale exist every time a consultant has to report his findings.

4. *Personal Contact with Authority Figure*: Another important principle is for the consultant to realize the importance of making personal contact with the top authoritative figure of the camp as soon after his entry as possible. The purpose of this contact is to obtain sanction for his exploratory and negotiatory operations in the camp. This is particularly important if the consultant is invited informally by a middle-management member of the staff.

5. *Explore Organized Patterns of Camp*: The mental health consultant should explore the organizational pattern and system of the camp in order to recognize its authority and communication network. He should be careful not to accept a distorted point of view by using information contributed by some people and missing others. In his explorations the consultant should learn about the camp's mission of transitional living as well as about the relief procedures, relocation values, and traditions of its workers.

The consultant can then ascertain whether he can make a contribution that might simultaneously help fulfill the objectives of the resettlement program. Insofar as this is possible, he will foster the building of a relationship of mutual trust and respect that may form a basis for collaboration. He should actively begin to know the camp staff and help this staff get to know him. He should clarify the nature of his expert assistance. He also must clearly express his readiness and availability to work with the camp in pursuit of mutual or compatible goals.

The active exploration of the camp organization was used by a consultant to widen his base of sanction and intervention. When he was asked to assist with a program of daily activities for the refugees, he asked to meet with a group of camp teachers. The consultant had not participated in the educational sector of the camp program, even though many adaptation problems were exhibited by children who were learning English as a second language. He expressed an interest in observing the classroom situation. During his interaction with the teachers he shared his knowledge of the relation of stress and emotions to learning. The teachers became aware of many puzzling experiences they had had with the refugees and asked for further consultation.

This process may provide the opportunity to discuss a wider range of topics, including policies and problems faced daily by the camp personnel. It might also open discussion to areas of staff interest in collaborating to pursue the resettlement goals.

6. *Establish Communication Patterns*: The establishment of communication patterns within the conflicting, fragmented, and distorted network of a camp setting is not an uncomplicated process. The communication link person

who has the power to transmit important information is a gatekeeper as well as a messenger of information across units in the camp. The director of the camp is obviously concerned with area surveillance and legal control. He needs to satisfy himself that the activities of the consultant are not going to undermine his position within the operations of the camp before he will allow messages to pass freely. Until he is satisfied, however, he is likely to exert control and to be highly selective in deciding what type of meetings and communications are to be allowed between individuals. At the beginning, he may permit consultation requests for senior and trusted staff only. Serendipity opportunities allow, at times, for crossing barriers to communication. The following example highlights this occurrence:

As a camp program was winding down, the need to place 150 unaccompanied minors into the community became an urgent matter to the camp director. He called a meeting of all the chiefs of services to develop a plan of action. The consultant to this camp invited himself along with the chief of mental health services. During the discussion it became evident that the manner in which decisions were going to be made would have an important mental health implication. The consultant offered his opinions and suggestions. He had only been allowed to participate in the so-called "mental health program" before this meeting. When the director became aware of the many psychological ramifications of the planning and how it would affect all the components of the camp program, he urged all his service chiefs to confer with the consultant in regard to their programs.

Conflicts of Interest

Conflict of value priorities between the consultant and the staff of a refugee/victim camp can easily occur. Each of the camp workers has responsibilities and may feel that a mental health consultant could encroach on his territory or oblige him to change his way of operating. It may be, in fact, that the consultant will fill functions that no staff person is equipped to undertake, and that he may help them to do better and more easily what they were already doing. However, unless the consultant learns what each has been doing and carefully defines his own role so as not to overlap with their work—and unless he succeeds in communicating this clearly to them—it is likely that some camp staff will either overtly or covertly oppose his entry into the system. The fragmentation and multiple governmental and private resettlement agencies that are part of relocation camp programs make it difficult to constantly keep in mind everybody's task.

Distortions of Perception and Expectation

Some of the distortions of camp personnel perception and expectation will be traditional or cultural; that is, they will be shared by most of the camp staff and will be based on common professional ideologies including their feelings about the cultural background of the refugees/victims. Their perception of the consultant as a person coming from a different background that may clash with the values of the camp staff or is insensitive to refugee ethnic background can promote barriers to communication.

These culturally based stereotypes are, of course, likely to be compounded by individual emotional reactions to and misperceptions of the consultant. This is especially true when the consultant is working within a climate of heightened tension and unrest characteristic of relocation camps, where the normal defensive structure of individuals responsible for solving severe problems may already be weakened.

An essential task of a consultant is to be aware of the irrational perceptual stereotypes utilized by tired, overwhelmed camp staff and existing within the crisis climate of relocation camps. He learns about them from behavioral cues, by being sensitive to the implied meaning of words and actions of the camp staff, and particularly by being aware of any defensive maneuvers toward him. He should allow the staff full freedom to manipulate him, to reveal their stereotype fears, to test and confirm their suspicions, and also to exhibit ways of excluding him. To counteract these behaviors, the consultant should then take steps to dissipate the distortions and replace them with opportunities for the consultee to examine him. He should do this by taking an active role in educating camp staff about his own value system, his feelings about religion and skin color, and his respect for the individuality of human beings regardless of background.

The consultant must be alert to both the manifest and latent content of communication. The need for camp staff to repeatedly test out fearful stereotypes must continuously be met by the consultant's methods to invalidate these stereotypes. He must talk directly and give both verbal and nonverbal messages to clear the air and establish realistic interactions.

Developing a Common Language

The removal of distortions of perception between consultant and consultee in the camp enhances an opportunity for better communication. The communication can be effective, however, only when the two sides share common values, philosophy, and language. This is a serious problem in camp settings due to the many variables already identified. The consultant must make a special effort to learn the specific modes of communication in the camp setting. This relates not only to vocabulary but also to behavior such as gestures, comfort distance between people, and levels of formality or informality practiced by military, civilian, voluntary, and religious agencies.

The consultant must constantly search for feedback from his consultees to ascertain that they have understood his point of view. Likewise, he must check to see that he has understood their verbal and nonverbal communication.

A black American consultant was having difficulties convincing an Irish camp guard chosen from the National Reserve, who was dealing with a Vietnamese family, that he could advise him in how to deal with the passive-aggressive behavior of a fourteen-year-old girl. The consultant was aware of the racial prejudice involved and had to tell the guard about his own experiences in Vietnam where he had been sensitized to understand the behavior of the refugees. After he "earned" credibility with the guard, they were able to focus on how to understand the girl who was not obeying the M.P. controls.

Ground Rules for Collaboration

Ground rules for collaboration include the need to work out and maintain consensus of objectives. The nature of the consultant's operation within the camp and the problems with which he is dealing varies with the type and status of the individual or organization, that is seeking help.

The consultant must continuously ensure that his current role, as identified by the power-authority structure, is clearly defined. This role clarity will help the camp staff know what kinds of situations are appropriate to discuss with him and what they may expect from the collaboration.

These ground rules should include a clear awareness of the social sanction for this joint activity, especially as camps continually and rapidly change directors. There must also be guidelines for contacting the consultant. For example, a) who is and is not allowed to contact the consultant, b) where, c) in what situation, d) for how long, e) how often, f) through which group, g) for what purpose, h) what the consultant can be expected to do, i) what he must do, and j) what he will not do.

Successive Stages of Camp Specialist's Role

At the beginning of his contact with a camp, the consultant may be a relatively unknown and unsanctioned visitor whose operations are confined to helping a single group of staff members with a particular refugee/victim. The specialist may observe or examine in order to make a diagnosis, prescribe treatment, or refer to another component of the health or medical health delivery system inside or outside of the camp. The specialist is strictly a case evaluator.

At a second stage, the consultant may have received permission from the camp director to explore the possibility of more extensive collaboration. He may be invited to meet with staff and increase their knowledge of mental health matters by giving them short lectures, by leading discussion or by directing half-hour seminars. During such rapid, focused interactions, the psychiatric consultant will learn about the intense work problems and severe difficulties the staff encounters with the refugees/victims. Camp staff will discover whether the expert's attitude is relevant to their immediate concerns and whether he is willing and able to assist them with their urgent problems. During this stage, the consultant serves as an emergency expert whose role is that of staff instant educator.

During the third stage, the specialist may be invited on an occasional or a regular basis to talk with individuals or groups of the staff about specific refugees/victims. He will be expected to screen each refugee and make referrals to other clinics for investigation and treatment, or else he may be expected to offer advice on appropriate management within the camp. The consultant's role clearly includes full consultation during this phase.

The consultant may also be expected to act as a collaborator in certain cases and to treat some of the refugees/victims himself, either during his visit to the camp or in some other clinic in the community.

In addition, the consultant is likely to be asked to deliver messages about refugees/victims who are being treated in his clinic or other hospitals and to provide reports from his colleagues to the camp staff about the progress of these cases. During this stage, the consultant plays a liaison role.

REFERENCES

Berlin IN: Learning mental health consultation: History and problems. *Ment Hyg* 48:257–266, 1964.

Bowlby J: *Attachment and Loss* (Basic Books: New York) 1969.

Caplan J: *The Theory and Practice of Mental Consultation* (Basic Books: New York) 1968.

Caplan J: *Support Systems in Community Mental Health* (Behavioral Publications: New York) 1974.

Cohen RE: The collaborative coprofessional: Developing a new mental health role. *Hosp Comm Psychiat* 24(4):242–246, 1973.

Cohen RE: Working with schools. *American Handbook of Psychiatry*, vol 2 (Basic Books, Inc: New York), pp 216–217, 1974.

Freud A: *Normality and Pathology in Childhood* (Int Univ Press, Inc: New York) 1965.

Hamburg D and Adams J: A perspective on coping behavior. *Arch Gen Psych* 17:227–284, 1967.

Kluckhohn FR and Strodtbeck FL: *Variations in Value Orientation* (Harper & Row: New York) 1961.
Nagera H: *The Developmental Approach to Childhood Psychopathology* (J Aronson: New York) 1981.
Padilla MP (ed.): *Acculturation–Theory, Models, and Some New Findings* (Westview Press) 1980.
Szapocznik J, Scopetta M, Kurtines W, and Ananalde M: Theory and measurement of acculturation. *Interamer J Psychol* 12:113–130, 1978.

Special problems

18

Consultation and Mental Retardation

Henry H. Work

"No one ever told me."

"I have taken my child to many people, but I never got a clear answer."

Such plaintive statements, unfortunately not uncommon, are typical responses to an individual consultation about a retarded child. Society's attitudes about retardation are modified from time to time and in culture to culture, but they still express the constancy of despair and demand the best in consultation skills. In addition, unfortunately, the consultation skills that are needed to assist those who care for a retarded child are almost global in character.

The arrival of a retarded child in a family, the presence of a "different" child in a family, the concerns of a community about the presence of a retarded child in its midst, or the problems of an entire school system in dealing with a number of slow learners in classes can become the signal for a consultation. Like other mental health consultations both the fears of the individual and the sense of failure on the part of the consultee demand assistance. Retardation suggests that not only is something missing in an individual, but there is a loss for everyone associated with that individual. Thus the demand for help on the part of the consultee is obvious. Yet at the same time it is often difficult for parents, teachers, and others to seek out assistance in a manner similar to ordinary medical consultation.

An anencephalic child survived in a new-born nursery for 53 days. During that time the staff was beset with revulsion at the sight of the child, inability to talk with the parents, and guilt about their own sense of failure. Ultimately, physicians for other patients felt that their patients were getting poor care and pressured the pediatrician for the anencephalic child to seek the advice of an outside psychiatric consultant. He was able to talk with the staff, parents, and physician to gain understanding, permit ventilation, and allow the care in the nursery to go on.

The general guidelines for consultation to individuals or groups are appropriate to this field. The fact that retarded individuals are often slow in development suggests that one of the major focuses of consultation is to the parents of the retarded child. Referrals, therefore, to a psychiatrist come frequently from a pediatrician baffled by the concerns of the parents about the fact of retardation. Since true consultation involves the relationship between the consultee and the consultant, the latter must be aware not only of the clinical facts surrounding the child who is the focus of the consultation, but of the anxieties of the colleague as well as the anxieties of the parents involved.

Consultation normally involves advice without necessarily consent. Consultation in the field of retardation involves advice which is often hard to emotionally understand and is often unwanted. Therefore, the art of consultation in this field depends on the standard relationships between consultant and consultee with an additional burden of carrying a message that may have the implications of long-term care, pessimism, or futility.

Whereas in many medical consultations the pain of the individual leads to a search for diagnosis, the presence of the intolerable thing called "retardation" often suggests that the patient is about to be dumped rather than remedies sought.

A pediatrician sought advice about his responsibility to the parents of a two-year-old whose developmental milestones had been consistently slow. The child, attractive and seemingly pleasant, had not sat until ten months, had not walked until 20 months and was not talking. The anxieties of the parents about speech finally overtook their belief that the child was normal because his appearance was normal. The pediatrician unfortunately had taken a "he'll grow out of it" attitude and felt that now he was faced with a situation that demanded professional intervention. The consultant, however, rather than intervening, assisted the pediatrician in leading the parents through the developmental milestones carefully and repeatedly until they too were able to sense and understand the potential delay. A basis was established for continued consultation related to the anticipated slowness of change in the child.

It is not infrequent that a consultant who sees a retarded child and discusses the situation with the parents and other colleagues gets a request a year or two later from another consultant for the earlier findings. It is obvious that the parent, dissatisfied with the first consultation, has gone on for more. This may be only one of a succession of such consultations. We are accustomed to think of this in terms of the "shopping" phenomenon and attribute to the parents (or other professionals) the concept of seeking a more comfortable diagnosis. Overlooked is the fact that each of these consultations may be mishandled by ignoring the specific concerns of the parent and others, concerns based not only on the diagnosis but on the meaning of the life-long sentence which is included in the diagnosis.

It, therefore, becomes very important in initiating a consultation focused around a child (and in mental retardation, consultations are nearly always focused around a child or a group of children) to develop a long-range plan. The plan includes not only the observation of the individual and an understanding of the diagnosis but also an understanding of the specific need for the consultation. If the latter includes resistance by parents to knowing the diagnosis, this must be included. It may represent the fact that a clear diagnosis has been frequently given to the parents but each time in slightly different terms. The task, then, is the elucidation of this confusion. Although there has been a translation of the consultation result to the consultee on a direct level it may not have included an understanding of the needs of the referring doctor.

Consultation to pediatricians is often hampered by misjudging, on both sides, of the knowledge levels of the individuals involved. Many pediatricians, having themselves struggled with trying to assist parents directly, become frustrated and seem to be turning to a consultant for a relief of their own frustration. Consultations from schools often come about for similar reasons. Teachers may well understand the special education problems of the retarded but have difficulty with the parents who are pressuring them to pour more learning into the head of the child than he or she can absorb.

A school system referred a ten-year-old boy to a special class which seemed appropriate to his moderate retardation and school failure. The father became incensed. He felt that if the school had tried harder the child could have made it in a normal class. Earlier he had punished the boy for failing to learn and now he wished to take the school system to court. The referral for help focused initially on the boy, moved to the parents, and then involved the school system whose anxieties had been aroused by the attack on them. An understanding of the underlying antagonisms was necessary before anything could be done to be of assistance to the child, who remained innocently in the middle of this tangled situation.

School consultations carry additional burdens. Such requests epitomize one of the issues of consultation in the field of the retarded; namely, that many people are involved. A teacher who herself is having difficulty with a child must pass a request for consultation along to the principal or other authority and must get the parents' consent and involvement even in the initiation of the consultation. Some of these contingencies suggest that the consultation be much more than a mere description. If carried out, it has to focus not only on the clinical picture of the child but also on the anxiety and concerns of those who are in the caring position.

Too many consultations have foundered when consultants overemphasized the extent of a disease. The consultant is an authority, and power is invested in this authority. On the other hand, the consultee deserves learning and understanding, as well as authority.

Too often the consultant is viewed from outside as a magician, particularly in the field of retardation. Where everyone is aware of a sense of hopelessness, the consultant is turned to in order to restore hope for the life-long process of living with or teaching the retarded. The authority and sense of power of the consultant invokes a hope that directive intervention will occur. True consultation, of course, does not involve direct intervention but, rather, giving advice to others. In the field of retardation the others may be parents, teachers, or community authorities who would prefer directive intervention in care rather than an expectation that they themselves must do something.

How then to use the authority and at the same time be appropriately humble? Although the consultant is called upon for an opinion, the process of doing the consultation involves an invasion into the lives of others. Especially at an institutional level, when the psychiatrist is called on, there is an invasion of the process of care in the institution as well as of the clinical approach to specific problems. In the process of collecting information and determining some scientific facts, the consultant is often caught up in the politics of the issues that abound in the care of the retarded. This can be as true in a family as it is in a large institution.

A psychiatric consultant to a child service agency sensed a warm response from staff members with whom she dealt. The staff, however, expressed frustration and a lack of progress in the treatment of their clients. It took some time for the consultant to be aware that there was an almost active resistance on the part of the child-caring staff, who not only felt that they were imposed on by the professionals but also harbored some very classical stereotypes about the children for whom they were responsible. Not until a large-scale discussion of these issues could be made was it possible to return to a focus on patterns of specific child care.

There is currently a sense that consultants must become much more directly involved in the process surrounding the individual for whom the consultation is requested. Whether the useful magic of authority can be retained in such an approach is not clear. There has to be some sense of detachment or removal in order not to be caught up in the very anxieties that surround a retarded individual. The worries of the parents that the child will never be a member of society, the annoyances of the parents at the failure of the child to learn, or the frustration of teachers and others who are trying to assist the retarded child make it necessary for the consultant to have some detachment. To understand the anxieties is one thing; to get involved in them and overlook realistic needs is another. It is obvious in any discussion of consultation that the authority of the consultant is based both on knowledge and the person having the knowledge. The overuse of this knowledge is easy; humility is difficult to attain.

Therefore, the timing of the arrival of a consultant is critical. The consultant must be aware not merely of the stated problem but of why the consultation is requested at a particular time. The meaning of seemingly specific questions cannot be ignored. The omnipresent "why" applies not only to the immediate question but to understanding that question in time, in family process, and in community process.

One should, therefore, be wary of giving an immediate response. Those who have been through more than one consultation may often demand a quick spot answer. Nothing is more hazardous. The consultant may come fresh to a case which seems to ask simply the diagnostic question, "Doctor, what is the matter with my child?" The question, however, may involve a renegotiation of the process of consultation, as well as a deep understanding of all of the consultant actions that the parents have been through before. At times this may call for a delay by the consultant and a protracted consultation which can assist the parents and others in coming to an appropriate conclusion. A pediatrician, faced with an infant retardate, may spend months in assisting parents to understand the failures of development of the retarded child. Similarly, the process of a later consultation by a psychiatrist (and they are nearly always called in late) may require protracting the consultation process so that everyone shares in the observations and the understanding thereof.

In the field of mental retardation consultants are frequently called in to deal with groups. They may be parent groups; they may be teacher groups; they may be community groups. Critical, therefore, in light of what is said above is an understanding of the process and timing of these particular groups. Consultation at that level involves not merely diagnostic skills, but collaboration, new alliances, and shared knowledge. Getting agreement for a plan of action involves not only getting everybody involved and collaborating but also sharing what knowledge is available and clarifying misconceptions of knowledge as one goes on.

Ultimately, in all consultations there are the hard facts of decision. There is a great temptation on the part of all of us as authorities to forget that decisions are made by others on the basis of good advice and consultation. Until it is recognized that the parents of the child must carry out the decision, based on information from the consultant, the situation will remain unchanged except in the sense that the parent may go on seeking other advice. Telling parents that the child is retarded due to a specific clinical syndrome and should be placed in an institution or should be handled in a particular fashion is not an end. If such advice is given, it has to be followed up. If such advice is to be followed up, it must be understood. If such understanding is to occur, it must also require the consultant's understanding of the practical problems and the resistances to both understanding and action.

The complexities of psychiatric diagnosis, therefore, suggest that failure to finish the process and thus achieve a sense of completeness is a major pitfall. Not sensing underlying feelings leaves the facts of the consultation cold, sterile, and useless. Consultation is not psychotherapy; yet if it does not involve a psychotherapeutic understanding of the issues that prompt the request, then, like any other process of psychotherapy, it will be a failure.

19

Child Psychiatry Consultation: Psychiatric Emergencies in Children and Adolescents

Virginia N. Wilking

The process of consultation changes subtly under different circumstances in different settings and populations. The population seen in psychiatric emergencies in childhood or adolescence is characterized by the needs of the child, family, or society dealing with it. Child psychiatrists seeing children and adolescents under these circumstances can be important agents of that society. However, child psychiatrists are not always at hand. Such consultation should be available and made use of.

A great deal is expected when the consultant is available. He must be ready to take any opportunity offered to bring psychic order out of the chaos that is typical of true psychiatric emergencies. The energies mobilized in the production of the emergency must be used systematically and therapeutically in the service of the ego, as noted by Berlin (1970).

Emergency consultation requires rapid response to psychiatric challenge, making use of basic tenets. Observations are made, a history is taken, an evaluation of patient and family is performed, diagnosis and differential diagnosis are considered, and treatment planning is shaped into disposition under unlikely circumstances in a short period of time.

The heart of the matter may be in the consultation process, but the psychiatric emergency itself provides the body and the framework. An emergency is defined as a "sudden juncture demanding immediate action (i.e., "escape, door, exit, egress, as in *case of fire*" (*Concise Oxford Dictionary*, 1929).

PSYCHIATRIC EMERGENCIES

It is interesting to look at the "have nots" before proceeding to the "haves." Thus, psychiatric emergencies are not listed in the indexes of Kanner's *Child Psychiatry* (1972), Finch (1960), Shaw and Lucas (1970), and *Principles and Practice of Child Psychiatry* (Chess and Harribi, 1978) (except in reference to emergency hospitalization). The cumulative index equivocates and lists psychiatric emergency in children under such entries as Child Services, Child Psychiatry, Crisis Intervention, Emergency, Mental Health, and Psychiatry.

The pediatric literature may either fail to mention psychiatric or even psychological emergencies or redefine them in a pediatric image. Thus, Gray (1980), in discussing pediatric emergencies refers to "psychological problems" without specifying their nature. *The Pediatric Clinics of North America* in their 1979 volume on pediatric emergencies chose only papers on suicide, child abuse, and incest. Jacobs (1978) recasts almost all so-called psychiatric emergencies as social pediatric emergencies in a territorial foray.

Kliman in his *Psychological Emergencies of Childhood* (1968) does not have the word *emergency* indexed. Chapter 5 is headed "Minor Emergencies," which include the first day of school, the first summer at camp, moving to a new home, and when an older family member moves. The emphasis is *crisis*, although the word used is *emergency*, and the themes involved are the tremendous ones of death, loss, and separation, all a familiar part of the human condition. The difference comes in the timing and the way in which the emergency is handled. The events referred to in Chapter 6 "Overstimulating and Horrifying Experiences," are those in which children are exposed to the primal scene, parental suicide, parental murder, as well as brutality, terror, and abandonment, and clearly constitute emergencies. However, the intervention comes after the emergency and is not concurrent with it.

Kahn in *Psychiatric Emergencies in Pediatrics* (1980) writes carefully on the events that constitute or rather involve emergency but cover emergencies without discussing the consultation process. Definitions of psychiatric emergencies in childhood and adolescence are useful overall, although they may tell one little clinically. They tell one little more about the settings and the most about the author. They deserve listing, reading, and use in defining the problem for oneself. From the breadth of the definitions listed in Table 1 it is clear that there is an "elephant," and different authors in their experiences have taken hold of different parts of the "beast" for their reports.

However, there is general agreement that a psychiatric emergency exists when someone says it does and that there is reason to see patient and family as an emergency when anyone says there is reason to do so. In fact, there is sometimes further differentiation between psychiatric emergencies created by fiat and "true emergencies," although these were not defined further when mentioned by Kenyon (1962), Chodorkoff et al. (1962), and Steinhauer et al. (1971). It is not a function of answering a cry of "wolf" but a matter of the *extremity of need* in patient, family, and community to which the consultant must respond. However, it will continue to be true that although all psychiatric emergencies are equal, and some are more equal than others.

Whatever the theory, disruption of state and degree of discomfort are recognized and the need for action implied. The pace differs as well as the nature of the awareness of internal and external environment and the pressure being actively brought to bear on these two environments. There also is a difference between the implication of an immediate action in consideration of the first day of school and the suicidal state.

All observers acknowledge some change in internal state that gives rise to changes in the external state, although they may not emphasize the sequence. The changes are seen as occurring abruptly but against the background of chronic problems whose history is easily obtained. Simmons (1966) describes the vivid contrast between the present and a previous state in adolescents seen in psychiatric emergencies but stresses the chronicity of the problems. This paradox remains a constant: chronic problems are made acute, and acute problems turn out to be chronic. The change in internal state is seen as occurring abruptly in response to an external stress, most often slippage in the quantity and quality of family supports, particularly for the younger child.

Different elements of the psychiatric emergency are given different weight in the definitions in terms of the state of the patient, the psychodynamics, or the degree of alarm in the referring agency. Mattsson and associates' (1967) definition of "a condition of emotional distress in a child which family feels incapable of handling" seems most suitable to psychiatric emergencies as they present in children and adolescents on a day-to-day basis.

Clues to the nature of psychiatric emergencies lie in the definition and, therefore, to an extent in the "eye of the beholder." Sullivan (1958) sees the family as a psychological unit, as do Burks and Hoekstra (1964). Work (1966) sees psychiatric emergencies as created by the children for their families, and Dickman and Steinhauer (1981) view emergencies as reflections of upset of the steady state and developmental crises with the child chosen by the family as problem carrier. Berlin (1970) and Simmons (1966) emphasize the internal state

Table 1. Definitions of Psychiatric Emergencies

Atkins and Rose (1962): Minor problem one day, major psychiatric problem the next.

Berlin (1970): Acute internal disequilibrium.

Burks and Hoekstra (1964): Extent of emergency determination by referring source.

Caplan (1961): Crises of any individual manifesting upset of equilibrium.

Dickman and Steinhauer (1981): Rapid development squeezed into so short a period that the existing defenses are overwhelmed or upset in the steady state.

Jacobs (1978): Crisis situation which reflects acute temporary state, or acute temporary state of tension in which a sudden increase in anxiety gives rise to a feeling of disaster.

Kenyon (1962): (1) Any patient sent as such. (2) Accepted as such after prior consultation. (3) All cases considered too urgent to wait.

Klein and Lindemann (1961): Emotional predicament encompasses individual crisis situation and emotional hazard.

Mattsson et al. (1967): A condition of sufficient emotional distress in a child which he, his family, or the referral source feels incapable of handling even a few hours.

Steinhauer et al. (1971): Any urgent request for immediate psychiatric intervention.

Ungerleider (1960): Situation demanding prompt attention, whatever reason.

Work (1966): (1) Child created crisis for his parents. (2) Act weighted by community.

---

but in relation to the family, and Morrison (1969) works with family in an emergency seen as an acute family crisis.

Table 2 lists the major symptoms noted on referral. The reasons for referral given by different authors represent a wealth of experience. Where the reasons are most similar they reflect the most basic and most terrible of disruptions in the inner and outer self of family and child. When the reasons differ they are more idiosyncratic. Sullivan (Ibid.) in writing about psychological aspects of pediatric practice and acute psychiatric emergencies, begins his discussion with intractable crying, Jacobs (1978), discussing social pediatric emergencies, runs through death and adoption to learning, while Kenyon (1962), Burks and Hoekstra (1965), and Work (1966), Mattsson et al. (1967), Wilking (1967), Morrison (1979), and Steinhauer et al. (1971) all include threatened or attempted suicide and threatened violence or assaultive destructive behavior as reflecting a common experience. Most authors include acute anxiety in one form or another as a manifestation rather than a dynamic. Most included some bizarre, dramatic, or psychotic behavior in addition to a form of sexually aligned symptomatology. Jacobs (1978), Kahn (1980), and Dickman and Steinhauer (1981) combine cause and effect, the container and the thing contained, in their list of symptoms.

There is no hint in these definitions of psychiatric emergencies or the major reasons behind the reasons for referrals in acute psychiatric emergency, no glimpse of the "wheels within the wheels," the family relationships within relationships. The acute situation is set into motion by crucial events, and at a given point in time these factors seem omnipresent and do not help to differentiate one emergency from another, although they reflect the stuff of which the lives of the patients and their families are made. The background simply comes to the foreground, viz, conflict with parents, physical illness, or the loss of a love object, as noted by Mattsson and coworkers (1967). Interference in the function of a parent is listed by Kenyon (1962) and relocation, financial crisis, and major alteration in lifestyle are added by Dickman and Steinhauer (1981) and Caplan (1961).

Table 3 indicates the crucial events, precipitating factors, and stresses of particular importance. The umbrella of family crises can be raised over many of these events. Mattsson (1967) has the percent identified as major in his series of 140 cases.

There are infinite variations on a relatively small number of themes that can be reduced to the lowest common denominator of *loss*: loss of love, loss of security, loss of sense of self, loss of place, all-too-common neurotic strands, as well as those tacked into place during developmental process, unraveling at points of past or present developmental crisis. Still, it is helpful to note which loss which family will touch on or which loss becomes obvious as important in bringing about the emotional predicament (1961) with which the consultant is faced.

Further variations are introduced by the degree of urgency with which the psychiatric emergency is presented. To a great extent, the urgency reflects the alarm raised in the referring source, but the level of alarm depends on the degree to which the symptoms have been raised—suicidal threat or gesture. Sullivan (1958) links the symptoms, seen as a reaction to internal and external

**Table 2. Major Behavioral Symptoms and Chief Complaints in Children
and Adolescents Referred as Acute Psychiatric Emergencies**

Burks and Hoekstra (1964)
  Bizarre suicide
  Disabling, somatic
  Acute, school
  Suicide
  Sexual acting out
  Drunkenness
  Fire Setting
  Homicide

Dickman and Steinhauer (1981)
  School refusal
  Running away
  Drug abuse
  Teenage pregnancy
  Toilet training
  Learning to read
  Puberty

Jacobs (1978)
  Child abuse
  Incest (sexual assault and rape)
  Abnormal birth
  death/death and dying
  Adoption (separation, divorce)
  Learning failure

Kahn (1980)
  Hospitalism
  Acute symptoms

Kahn (1980) (continued)
  Coping with chronic illness
  Acute anxiety
  Aggression and violence
  Grief, depression, suicide
  Child abuse
  Dying
  Rape
  Psychotic
  Drug abuse

Kenyon (1962)
  Threatened violence
  Poor school attendance
  Antisocial behavior (nonviolent)
  Disturbed sleep
  Disturbed elimination
  Fits of depression
  Threatened or attempted suicide
  General backwardness
  Masturbation
  Somatic symptoms

Mattsson et al. (1967)
  Suicidal
  Assaultive, destructive
  Anxiety, fears
  Bizarreness
  School refusal
  Truancy, runaway

stress, with the psychological unit of the family while noting the important
interrelation of constitutional and environmental factors. In every child psychiatry consultation in psychiatric emergencies, there must be this recognition of
the child or adolescent in himself with recognition of the "givens" and the
maturational or biologic factors, developmental history, and past experience.

Emergencies are no respectors of symptoms or diagnoses, although a high
percentage of psychoses and of absolute number of suicidal threats and attempts
is seen. Proper labeling is not as useful as recognition of the actuality of the

Table 2.
(Continued)

Morrison (1969)
  Sexual promiscuity
  Running away
  Bizarre behavior
  Incest–sexual assault
  Drug intoxication
  Fire setting
  Killed pet
  Truancy
  Behavior disorder
  Adolescent turmoil
  Hysterical conversion
  Depression
  Suicide attempt threatened
  Mental retardation

Schowalter and Solnit (1966)
  Acute hallucinations
  School phobia
  Psychotic
  Suicidal

Steinhauer et al. (1971)
  Suicidal
  Homicidal
  Aggressive
  Depression, anxiety
  Sexual, dramatic
  Bizarreness

Sullivan (1958)
  Intractable crying
  Feeding problem
  Separation, acute anxiety attack
  Trauma to parent, to child
  Psychotic episode (drug induced)

Wilking (1967)
  Acute psychotic
  Fire setting
  School phobia
  Acute anxiety
  Homicidal
  Related to sexual acting our or
    abuse
  Depression
  Rage
  Running away
  Suicidal

Work (1966)
  Suicide
  Homicide
  Fire setting
  Sexual attack
  School phobias
  Acute anxiety
  Grief and bereavement

emergency. All of the usual clinical skills are needed: the first lies in the recognition and response to the emergency. The other skills needed in consultation are used in rapid succession in dealing with situations fraught with miserable patients, bewildered and angry families, patient police on their way off-duty, and unhappy colleagues all demanding instant resolution. As noted originally, the heart of the matter in child psychiatry consultation in acute psychiatric emergencies lies in the consultation itself, and we consider that next against the background already discovered.

**Table 3. Precipitating Factors or Critical Events Seen in the Referral
of Children and Adolescents as Psychiatric Emergencies**

*Atkins and Rose (1962) (referred to
    admission)*
Severely disturbed child in family dis-
integrating when community rises "up
in arms"

Burks and Hoekstra (1964)
1. Child seen as sick
2. Child seen as bad (one dramatic
    event in child with disturbed family
    making poor social adjustment)

Caplan (1961)
1. Loss of significant relationships
2. Introduction of new individual
    into social orbit
3. Transition in social status

Dickman and Steinhauer (1981)
1. Parental illness
2. Prental loss
3. Marital dysfunction
4. Introduction of stepparent or
    sibling
5. Relocation, financial crisis
6. Major alteration in lifestyle
7. Child abuse

Kenyon (1962)
1. Exclusion from school
2. Exaggeration of symptoms
3. Acute anorexia, treatment
    problems
4. Suicidal threat by parent
5. Parental illness or threat
6. Miscellaneous

Mattsson et al. (1967)
1. Conflict with parent
2. Physical illness
3. Sexual conflicts
4. Loss of love object
5. Intoxication
6. Pregnancy
7. Grief reaction
8. Sexual molestation

Simmons (1966)
1. Subjective distress (internal
    change)
2. Chronic problems, acute flam-
    boyant episode
3. Psychological disturbance in pa-
    tient with increase in manifesta-
    tions of physical illness

CONSULTATION

Looney (1979) reports on his experience in responding to the emergencies
inherent in setting up a camp for an expanding population of 20 thousand Vietnamese within 24 hours. Others have responded to the needs of children who
have been the victims of mass kidnapping and natural disasters.

Kliman (1968) studied the effect of President Kennedy's assassination on
children, beginning with several children seen just after his death with the nation

still in a state of emergency. The information available about the children's reactions to that tragedy is helpful in relation to dealing with children exposed to other tragedies.

Other consultants have made home visits in the face of a psychiatric emergency. The nature of the symptoms and the relationship of the symptoms and child to family dynamics are particularly clear with the child in his own room and even in his own bed surrounded by family (Welsch, 1965). The consultant first as an observer and listener, then as a participant, begins at the beginning in that care with the bed as a "territory."

The Division of Child Psychiatry of Harlem Hospital Center has had child psychiatry emergency consultation available as a program separate from its clinics and its pediatric ward consultation and liaison service for the last ten years. Unfortunately, its statistics are highly inaccurate. There is an emergency register in which the names of the children and adolescents referred to child psychiatry (or seen in the adult psychiatry emergency room) are entered. Thus, all psychiatric emergencies (including those involving children and adolescents through 15 years of age) should be recorded with name, date seen, birth date, age, referring source, major symptoms, reason for referral, and disposition. In addition, child psychiatry emergency consultation statistics reflect the number of visits made by the family and others and the number of staff involved on each visit. These statistics are broken down by developmental age: birth through 5 years; child (6 through 11 years); and adolescent (12 through 15 years). The case is followed as an emergency until declared otherwise unless referred out of the hospital for psychiatric admission, for placement, or for return to a clinic or resource already responsible. If the family continues in child psychiatry, the case is formally made a case in the child psychiatry clinic appropriate to the child's age. The staff from this clinic will already have been involved in the emergency, and the urgency that staff brings to emergencies militates against proper record keeping.

Because of our small number of trainees and the relatively few patients seen at night (averaging zero to three per month), regular coverage on nights, weekends, and holidays is carried on through child psychiatry telephone consultation with general psychiatry residents from the psychiatric emergency room and crisis intervention service.

The system allows for the referral of psychiatric emergencies from pediatric ambulatory clinic, emergencies more urgent than most on the pediatric ward, emergencies occurring on the wards of other hospital services, and recurring emergencies in patients and families already being seen in one of the four child psychiatry clinics (developmental, child, adolescent, and treatment program) or in any of three child psychiatry psychiatric day treatment programs (therapeutic nursery, child and adolescent psychiatric day treatment program, and the Harlem center for child study). In our setting a great deal of time goes into warding off and preventing psychiatric emergencies, in our own patients and in families who usually function with very little margin for error.

In one family after six months of wear and tear and in the face of increasing urgency, a senior child psychiatrist and a social worker arranged to make a home visit with the police, whose help had been asked in bringing Mrs. M., the mother of a 4-year-old boy in the therapeutic nursery, into the hospital emergency room for psychiatric examination because she was "dangerous to herself." The mother was known to be nine months' pregnant but was not being followed up in a prenatal clinic. The baby's father, a spirit healer, was actively trying to cure his wife of "snakes" and denied her pregnancy. In her conflict and anxiety, this very dependent woman called her social worker and made suicide threats, at the same time giving history of vaginal bleeding. The family did not respond to the doorbell. The police were willing to break down the door but the child psychiatry staff preferred to make further attempts at telephone communication. This was unsuccessful. They returned the next day with two more policemen who decided they were not legally empowered to enter without a warrant. The next day, a new child psychiatry team went to the apartment with still another two policemen and the therapeutic nursery child worker. All came to the emergency room peaceably, although the stepfather was still repeating "snakes." Mrs. M. had emergency transfusions and a caesarean section for a complete placenta previa. The baby was delivered satisfactorily, and the father stated he had made the delivery possible by "killing the snakes."

The adult psychiatry consultation service, the city special sources, and children and pediatric staff spent endless hours in consultation with continued time spent with father, mother, and children. The family then continued under the "watchful eye" of the developmental psychiatry clinic.

Consultation was carried out at cribside. J.B., 2½ years old with a 2% burn, was restrained in his crib for urine collection. His mother and two young siblings had died in the same fire that brought J. to the hospital. The father was not known and no other family member was immediately available. The understandable alarm of the pediatric staff added to the urgency of the situation. A senior child psychiatry consultant with the child psychiatry resident and child psychiatrist assigned part-time to the ward were able to be of immediate help to the child and residents (child psychiatry and pediatric). There was explicit recognition of the child, his name, his strength (in simply being there), and his anxiety at wondering where his mother was. His anxiety was increased by his restraints and his awareness that something was being done to his penis. This was relieved to a degree by raising his head to allow him to see his penis still extant and visible through the transparent plastic urine collection bag. The child psychiatry consultation continued in small therapeutic steps after this beginning. Pediatric staff were directly involved. Although anxiety cannot be dissipated under these circumstances, it seemed to be contained when it was clear that the child had support.

Major Symptoms

In 1967 Wilking (1967) noted the following major symptoms in child psychiatric emergencies: fire setting, acute psychotic behavior, acute anxiety, homicidal behavior, suicidal behavior, behavior related to sexual behavior (rape), depression, rage, running away, school phobia (refusal, reluctance), to which should be added in 1982: child abuse, substance abuse, community alarm, parental behavior, (depression, paranoia, psychosis).

We asked directors of other hospital services to regard rape, child abuse, suicide attempts, drug ingestion, severe burns, and pregnancy in girls younger than 14 years as automatic referrals to child psychiatry.

The following lists examples of problems in major areas and briefly describes what occurred in the consultation:

Acute psychotic behavior: H.Y., a ten-year-old girl, was brought in by her mother, who was concerned by H.'s problems with sleeping. H. agreed she was up at night but complained that her 6-month-old sibling woke her; her mother said that H. woke the baby. Mrs. Y. acknowledged a relation between H.'s behavior and the baby's birth but denied its importance. In addition, she called H.'s auditory and visual hallucinations "her stories."

The initial consultation was with a child psychiatry resident. Subsequent early emergency consultation included a social worker. In view of H.'s ambivalence about the baby, hospitalization and medication were suggested but rejected. Mrs. Y. was able to admit to basic differences in H. as long as she was in control. H. was transferred to the child psychiatric clinic for regular appointments. Conversations continued about "little men in the washing machine."

Acute anxiety: R.P., a fifteen-year-old boy, was seen at the monthly consultation at the pediatric primary care clinic. He came without his mother and described symptoms of depression, micropsia, and auditory hallucinations that were increasing in severity.

The initial consultation was with a senior child psychiatrist, who introduced R. to a child psychiatry resident the next day. An attempt was made to establish relationship with R., but his distance remained. His mother was elusive.

The resident favored joining the family in an attempt to make contact. Symptoms continued. Medication was accepted but was not taken. H.'s referral two months later was unsuccessful.

Homicidal behavior: *D.L., an eight-year-old girl, was brought to child psychiatry with her mother and two siblings by the worker from special services for children for family therapy in an emergency situation. D. was described by the worker as the butt of her mother's anger. Mrs. L. agreed, saying D. was impossible and wanting her "put away." She said D. had been seen holding the two-year-old over the balcony of the high-rise apartment. After D.'s placement, the mother failed her appointments as she had in the past, until she returned with complaints about her six-year-old boy, who was "now going bad like D."*

D. and her family were seen with the welfare worker, our social worker, and a child psychiatrist. D.'s affect was determinedly flat and she shrugged off her mother's complaints. When seen alone, she talked freely and denied feelings about her younger sibling, but also made it clear that she felt she was getting little from her mother who would leave her in charge of the baby and then blame her for problems and threaten her. She used consultation to get herself "out" with having to say she wanted to go. Everyone agreed that the girl was caught in an unsatisfactory situation, and D. was placed the next day.

Suicidal behavior: *G.R., a six-year-old boy, was referred from school, since his foster mother had not brought him in as requested three days before. G. made suicide threats at school and said he wanted to be dead. When the school secretary said, "Be my guest," he drove a paper knife into his ear. G. had been admitted to a pediatric ward for workup of a major motor seizure one month before and had been receiving medication. He had lived with his aunt and uncle since birth, although his mother was in the neighborhood. He spent weekends with his father. The family was upwardly mobile. Hospitalization was discussed for provision of therapeutic milieu and because of G.'s impulsivity, but was rejected.*

The first consultation was with a child psychiatry resident. The aunt (foster mother) was seen with G. and separately. She was puzzled and concerned but silently distant. G. was extremely hyperactive, as he had been since birth. He had excellent IQ function, active fantasy, and strong superego.

He said he literally felt so bad "he wanted to die." A successful beginning to a therapeutic relationship showed that he tested the limits of the consultant, but was able to relax slightly. He paid little attention to his father and mother. He settled into treatment care immediately and before being asked. The social worker was available to the aunt.

Sexual assault/abuse: *L.M., a fifteen-year-old boy, was sent from the pediatric clinic after a report was submitted of child abuse–sexual abuse of two half-brothers over a two- to three-year period. L. came to this country at age 10 years from the Caribbean to join his father, stepmother, two siblings, and a third half-brother and became directly involved in sex play at the time he "joined" the family. L.'s mother had run away with another man when L. was one year old. L. was only a fair student. He had a close relationship with his father but little with his stepmother. He seemed to have little to do with little boys and was generally somewhat withdrawn.*

The family—the father, stepmother, L., and three little boys—was seen in a dramatic consultation. They were all shocked; the little boys were uncomfortable but adjusted quickly. L. was denying any problem and the father was trying to understand the legal situation (although there was none). Relief was experienced by all during the consultation. There was recognition of the mother's concern that she had not known the father's anger and love for his son, and the boy's sudden understanding that he was still really part of the family. L. was accepted for treatment.

Depression: *P.Q., a fourteen-year-old girl, was referred by an abortion clinic. She was pregnant (three months) and was threatening to kill herself if an abortion was not done immediately. The obstetrician had refused because of no parental consent. She said her mother had died the year before and her father five years earlier. P. was living with her brother, which was "a lot of fun." An obstetrics–gynecology social worker had found P.'s mother living in Brooklyn; she gave permission for the abortion. P. was referred to another psychiatric clinic.*

Three consultations with child psychiatrists centered on P.'s degree of depression. P. was somewhat sexually provocative, refused to talk, and was angry. There also were too many contacts. An abortion was performed and P. was sent back to her mother.

Substance abuse: *K.T., a three-and-one-half-year-old boy, was seen as an emergency on the pediatric ward as a childhood schizophrenic with sudden-onset findings of disturbance of gait and speech and bizarre movements. It was finally discovered that the boy had access to his grandmother's Thorazine.*

The consultation consisted largely of observing K., who was somewhat confused; he walked naked on a board and spoke unintelligibly. The pediatric staff had the opportunity to observe changes in behavior and see symptoms disappear.

Agency alarm: *W.V., a fourteen-year-old boy, was brought with his 74-year-old father to the pediatric emergency department for referral to psychiatric emergency by a concerned community worker from a mental retardation center, "for admission because of sexual acting out, which was making him a problem in his day program."*

A child psychiatrist was called to psychiatric emergency, where the patient had been sent after clearance in pediatrics. Examination revealed a moderately-to-mildly retarded adolescent, with speech limited to two- to three-word sentences. His IQ was 50. He showed pleasure in himself and lit up when asked about girls. He was acting silly and was beginning to test the limits of the psychiatrist. A call was made to the center suggesting that a plan be made or reviewed, including a change in medication. W. returned to the center. The community worker, patient, and father were slightly tired but agreeable.

Parental depression: *A mother and her three-year-old child were referred by the adult psychiatry clinic. The mother had been depressed since the birth of her baby and was now failing her clinic appointments. Her dynamics were unclear except by supposition.*

The mother came once for consultation with her son. There were classic signs of severe depression, and the infant's responses were limited. The child was subdued, with limited language. The mother was able to show some concern about the child's speech but failed her next appointment. A home visit was made by the child psychiatrist and social worker. The mother was found in bed with the two children with the lights off and the television on. She responded to the concern shown about her and accompanied the staff to the hospital. She took minimal part in planning for the care of the children.

Psychotic behavior: *A mother, six-year-old C., and a new infant were referred by a child health station as an emergency because of the mother's instability, failed appointments, and threats to remove hyperactive C. from school. Contact was maintained irregularly with Mrs. A. through the group, child health station, and the Harlem Center for Child Study, which C. attended regularly, mostly alone.*

The first contacts with Mrs. A. were carried on largely in the hall. The entire psychiatry team tracked Mrs. A. as she sped up and down the hall, speaking as if she were under pressure. With the cooperation of the entire team, Mrs. A. slowed down enough to plan for regular returns to the infant–mother interaction group. A plan was effected for C. to be seen in a psychiatric day treatment program. Consultation "on the run" served as a beginning.

An attempt has been made to give the major symptoms, history, and something of the course of the consultation to show the ambiance of these meetings. These brief histories do not give a sense of the care that must be taken in seeing the child or adolescent and the exploration of family, all described in great detail by Schowalter and Solnit (1966), Mattsson et al. (1967), and Morrison (1969; 1979). Morrison follows through from the process by which family is seen initially and the way in which they are followed up. Morrison points at the problems faced without highly trained staff, the danger that the consultant will be drawn into the lifestyle of the family, and the inevitable failures. Where successful, the disciplined approach to crisis intervention reduces the levels of anxiety to manageability and continues in orderly fashion. As Berlin (1970) says, "the urgency of the situation permits the family to agree on several tasks they will mutually undertake to reduce the problem for which they sought help."

Schowalter and Solnit (1966) indicate that the psychiatric emergency consultation takes an average of two-and-one-half hours, which agrees with our experience in those cases when there seems to be any sensible process. The consultation not only actually does take this long but *should* take this long. Consultations compressed beyond a certain point, no matter how sure the diagnostic acumen, leave the family behind and lose their therapeutic thrust. The family's compliance is not an indication that a successful process has taken place. The careful appraisal insisted on by Morrison (1969; 1979) must be aimed at and has its part in the process. Of course, time is of the essence. Schowalter and Solnit (1966) and Dickman and Steinhauer (1981) make a point of the need for flexibility in consultants' schedules, which are often at odds with the demands made on both senior staff and trainees. Morrison (1967; 1969) makes specific suggestions of a way in which some of the practical issues in setting up a child psychiatry emergency service can be met.

There is a shape to the initial consultation but there is also a size, measured in terms of time spent. To meet the inflexible deadlines of emergency transport services and acute child psychiatry ward admission services, the needed time cannot always be spent. The shape of the consultation should "bulge" to initially include all who arrive on the scene, unless the family specifically says no. One staff member, usually the one who has begun with the family, must take charge, using short sentences, avoiding jargon, and repeating for the benefit of individual family members the immediate plan of action by introducing and re-introducing the other staff involved. It is useful to repeat the history, often given by telephone or by another staff member, sometimes using euphemisms, sometimes using directness as a way to relate.

If family members are still unclear as to what has happened, they must be told. If the patient is unclear about who knows what, it must be discussed before legitimate confidences can be respected. Staff members have to establish

**Table 4. The Formal and Systematic Examination of Children
and Adolescents in Consultation**

Freud (1962)

1. Reason for referral (behavior problems, anxieties, inhibition symptoms)
2. Description of child
3. Family background and personal history
4. Possibly significant environmental influence
5. Assessments of developmental
6. Genetic assessments
7. Dynamic and structural assessments
8. Assessments of some general characteristics

Goodman and Sours (1967)

1. Size and appearance
2. Motility
3. Coordination
4. Speech
5. Intellectual function
6. Modes of thinking and perception
7. Emotional

Goodman and Sours (continued)

8. Manner of relating
9. Fantasies
10. Character of play

Shaw and Lucas (1970)

1. Relationship capacity
2. Affect
3. Intellectual capacity
4. Neurological integration
5. Reality testing
6. Motivation
7. Acculturation

Simmons (1966)

1. Appearance
2. Mood and affect
3. Orientation and perception
4. Coping mechanism
5. Neuromuscular integration
6. Thought processes
7. Fantasy
8. Superego
9. Concept

their ways of working and clearly, quickly, and openly in the presence of the family. The family has to be helped to understand that resolution of the crisis and even partial relief of subjective discomfort will depend on *knowing more*. A family history that questions immediate circumstances and past roots is necessary. A full history can be taken quickly. This necessity is accepted more easily in an emergency consultation than on less pressured occasions. The family feels at risk and saves its strength for more important tasks.

Equally, family and patient must understand that the consultants really want to know in their own way and to learn themselves just what happened: what is thought, what is felt, and what is thought to be needed. It is important to start early in the consultation to help the patient and family understand that there are connections between what is said and done, heard and observed. It is important to establish that there is a connection between what has happened and what should be done. All of this is done by tone of voice, by glance, and by attitude as being serious. One can work at the comfortable establishment of the fact of serious concern and serious purpose without embarrassment. It must be *felt* and is then most easily communicated to others.

As the picture emerges, there is time for recapitulation of what has been learned, moving on to a discussion of the shape of the plan, firmly based on what has been learned so that the recommendations, comfortable or uncomfortable to hear, have an internal logic. Options should be discussed by priorities given where they are indicated.

When consultants have asked enough questions and have listened to the answers and it is clear they understand what has happened, anxiety subsides in the face of the supposition that someone knows what has been happening and what is going on.

It is at this point, at the end of the day with deadlines looming, that the temptation to sacrifice clarity and knowing just to get finished may become too much for any consultant. The family may ask "What does that have to do with this?" and the doctor may wonder if he should continue with the history of allergies, operations, and accidents, as well as coping mechanisms, gifts, difficulties, play, sleep, and characteristics of earlier stages of development. The answer to the question is *yes*! It is not just abstract knowledge but immediately useful data, helping to flesh out a picture of a real patient and family. Clarification of the immediate emergency utilizing what has been observed in the first minutes should be formalized by an examination of the patient done at the beginning of the consultation and with the points touched on noted systematically.

Anna Freud (1962) speaks of the preliminary communication on the diagnostic profile and of making up the metapsychological picture with structural, dynamic, economic, genetic, and adaptive data. She states the picture cannot be obtained with the few facts obtained on first contact. This is obviously true but particularly in an emergency it is important to observe and to collect data that pertains to the different developmental areas. These data taken together make up a full examination in a child or adolescent when matched with an intrinsic sense of chronological age and development state. Indeed, the metapsychological picture described by Freud seems almost within reach.

Verbal communication should be attempted, but there is the rich world of nonverbal communication to fall back on with the use of small objects, clay, blocks, drawings, and stones to plumb the fantasy life. Especially in an emergency, it is important to establish the ground rules for confidentiality, checking which information can be shared with whom and identifying any information that cannot be confidential because it is dangerous. Legal issues as to whom the information belongs should be clarified according to the laws of the state. The family and patient must be informed of their rights but invited to trust.

The formulation of the manifest and not so manifest content of the consultation interviews should be briefly discussed in series and in parallel with the patient, family group, and other staff, and thought out clearly for oneself. Words should be rationed. In discussing diagnosis the indication of the diagnostic issues raised and their implications may be all one wishes said, but the saying of it may be far too much. There are very narrow limits as to how much verbal communication can be spliced into dealings with a shocked and frightened family.

The interpretation of the reasons for a psychiatric emergency can be made only in part. The *whys* are almost too close to the bone, even though the questions are asked by family recklessly enough. It is always a matter of individual judgment how much support family members can give one another, how much they will accept, and their ability to use support determines how much can be said even when surely understood.

Sharing information is a basic part of the consultation process. *Formulation* is first a silent process for the consultants with a careful attempt to put into words only what can be used jointly in discussing immediate recommendations. These should proceed almost inevitably from what has then been explained. The treatment plan answers the immediate need. Hopefully the first step is taken at the beginning of a continuous plan and not as a step in itself.

In the emergency situation the question of hospitalization comes to mind early on in the referral but is sometimes not answered until late in the consultation. One-third to one-half of the children and adolescents seen in emergency consultation need psychiatric hospitalization. Short of need, psychiatric hospitalization may sometimes appear to be the treatment of choice, relieving child and family of having to offer help they are ill prepared to offer or to receive. Hospitalization should not be undertaken lightly, but the fact that it is discussed becomes a measure of the seriousness of the situation. The responsibility lies with the consultant, but the decision with the family of a minor.

In certain cases the consultant may feel it is his responsibility to protect the patient from harming himself or others. Only under these circumstances should the minor patient be held and hospitalized against the wishes of parents or guardian as a psychiatric emergency at the time indicated by state mental health law. The consultant must be absolutely convinced as to the medical necessity of taking this step and taking the responsibility for the child away from the guardian. Practically, it almost always results in enormous difficulties. No one is pleased and obviously a great deal of harm can be done in upsetting further the already poorly balanced family. It is not a step we have to take often.

In one case, the step of holding a child as a psychiatric emergency was taken on the pediatric ward, involving the complicated administrative steps of transferring the child formally to the adult inpatient service and then arranging his transfer to a children's psychiatric service. We needed to move with dispatch, as the family was preparing to sign out a nine-year-old boy admitted the day before with drug ingestion as part of a serious suicide attempt.

Examination had shown him poorly oriented with poor reality testing; his diagnosis was acute schizophrenia reaction. At one point, he was found on the floor of his room saying he was dead. The family refused hospitalization, poohpoohed the seriousness of the situation, and removed the child from the floor. The precinct was called and the police began to look for the patient, who was hidden by the family. The family eventually filed into Bellevue, patient and all, well ahead of the police. Still, we were right and the child was a high risk.

The end of the matter of the psychiatric emergency consultation is best when it is a beginning that makes a positive contribution to the mental health of the family. The family can reject the recommendations made on many occasions. Even then Mattsson (1967) and Morrison (1969; 1979) maintain a stubborn belief that doing things right makes it possible to leave the family with something that will act in their behalf and that of their child. The combination of psychiatric emergency and child psychiatry emergency consultation is a force for positive change, effective as a catalyst in ways unseen and unacknowledged.

REFERENCES

Atkins TF and Rose JA. Emergency referrals for institutional admission. *Am J Orthopsychiat* 32:347–348, 1962.

Berlin I. Crisis intervention and short term therapy. *J Am Acad Child Psychiat* 9:595–606, 1970.

Burks HL and Hoekstra M. Psychiatric emergencies in children. *Am J Orthopsychiat* 34:134–137, 1964.

Caplan G. *Prevention of Medical Disorders in Children* (Basic Books, Inc.: New York) 1961.

Chess S and Harribi M. *Principles and Practice of Child Psychiatry* (Plenum Press: New York) 1978.

Chodorkoff J, Bryan GC, Miller E, and O'Brien C. Psychiatric emergencies in children and adolescents. *Am J Orthopsychiat* 32:346–347, 1962.

Curran B. Suicide. *Pediatr Clin North Am* 26:737–746, 1979.

Dickman DL and Steinhauer PD. Role of the family physician in the management of psychological crises in children and their family. *Can Med Assoc J* 124:1566–1570, 1981.

Finch SM. *Fundamentals of Child Psychiatry* (WW Norton and Co., Inc.: New York).

Freud A. Assessment of childhood disturbances. In: *The Psychoanalytic Study of the Child* (Yale University Press) XVII, 149–158, 1962.

Goodman JD and Sours JA. *The Child Mental Status Examination* (Basic Books, Inc.: New York and London) 1967.

Gray C. Children's hospital provides round-the-clock specialist emergency service. *Can Med Assoc J* 122:93–98, 1980.

Group for the Advancement of Psychiatry. *From Diagnosis to Treatment: An Approach to Treatment Planning for the Emotionally Disturbed Child*, Ch. 10, 636–660, 1973.

Jacobs J. Social pediatric emergencies. *Pediatrician* 239–269, 1978.

Kahn A. *Psychiatric Emergencies in Pediatrics* (Year Book Medical Publishers: Chicago) 1980.

Kanner L. *Child Psychiatry* (Charles C Thomas: Springfield, Illinois), Fourth Ed., 1972.

Kenyon FE. Emergencies in child psychiatry. *J Ment Sci* 108:419–426, 1962.

Klein DC and Lindemann E. Preventive intervention in individual and family crisis. In: *Prevention of Mental Disorders in Children* (Basic Books, Inc.: New York) 1961.

Kliman G. *Psychological Emergencies of Childhood* (Grune and Stratton: New York and London) 1968.

Looney J. Consulting to children in crisis. *Child Psychiat Human Dev* 10: 5–14, 1979.

Mattsson A, Hawkins JW, and Seese LR. Child psychiatry emergencies: Clinical characteristics and followup results. *Arch Gen Psychiat* 17:584–592, 1967.

Morrison GC. Therapeutic intervention in a child psychiatric emergency. *J Am Acad Child Psychiat* 8:542–588, 1969.

Morrison GC. Emergency intervention. In: *Basic Handbook of Child Psychiatry*, S. Harrison (ed.) (Basic Books: New York) 1979.

Schowalter JE and Solnit AJ. Child psychiatry consultation in a general hospital emergency room. *Am Acad Child Psychiat* 5:534–549, 1966.

Shaw CR and Lucas AR. *The Psychiatric Disorders of Childhood, Diagnostic Dimensions* (Appleton-Century-Crofts: New York), 2nd Ed., 1970.

Simmons JE. *The Psychiatric Examination of Children* (Lea & Febiger: Philadelphia), 2nd Ed., 1974.

Simmons JQ. The psychatric emergency in adolescence. *Int Psychiat Clin* 3: 37–51, 1966.

Steinhauer PD, Levine SV, and Corta GA. Where have all the children gone: Child psychiatric emergencies in a metropolitan area. *Can Psychiat Assn J* 16:121–127, 1971.

Sullivan AW. Psychologic aspects of pediatric practice: Acute psychiatric illness in children. *NY State J Med* 1665–1671, 1958.

Ungerleider JT. The psychiatric emergency. *Arch Gen Psychiat* 3:593–601, 1960.

Welsch E. Personal communication, 1965.

Wilking, VN. What we do about the psychiatric emergency in children: An intimation of one's duty and the like. Delivered to the Froundation for Mentally Ill Children, Inc., in cooperation with Michigan Society for Mental Health, Detroit, May 1967 (unpublished paper).

Work HH. Psychiatric emergencies in childhood. *Int Psychiat Clin* 3:27–35, GJ Wayne and RR Koegler (eds.) (Little Brown: Boston) 1966.

20

Depressed Children

Elva Poznavski

Depressed children are ubiquitous. They can be found in the private sector of medicine in the practice of psychiatrists, psychologists, pediatricians, and many other medical specialities. They are in school classrooms in all grades from kindergarten on up. The juvenile delinquents psychiatrically assessed at the court's recommendation may have depression as part of their psychopathology.

Depressed children are found in community mental health centers and frequently in psychiatric residential settings for children. They are seen in the wards of pediatric hospitals, both in those hospitals which are community based and in tertiary-care hospitals. They can be encountered in almost every consultative position a psychiatrist may take.

Depression in adolescence is not a controversial issue. The concept that "adolescent turmoil" is normative is beginning to fade (Rutter et al., 1976). Depression in adolescents is being reported now at nearly double the frequency of ten years ago (Gallemore and Wilson, 1972). This dramatic increase is probably largely based on recognition, although a real increase may well have occurred as well. The latter assumption is based on the ever increasing rate of adolescent suicide. Recognition that children aged 12 and under can be depressed is gaining wider recognition. The gap in knowledge is mainly about children in infancy with Spitz's anaclitic depression and children under 6 years of age.

THE PROBLEM OF UNDERRECOGNITION

While depression in adolescents is being more readily identified in all forms, from depressive moods accompanying a variety of psychopathology to the classic manic-depressive or bipolar illness, it is still not widely enough recognized. The problem with the under-diagnosis of depression in prepubertal children is an even more serious problem. In the pediatric wards of medical hospitals the depressed child or adolescent is frequently unnoticed (Poznanski et al., 1979). Medical personnel may complain about a child's poor appetite or lack of cooperation with medical treatment without recognizing an underlying depression. In a study of depression (Poznanski, 1970) in children 12 years and under who were patients in a state residential psychiatric facility, fully one-half of the children who were found by the research psychiatrist evaluation to have a major depressive disorder did not have the word "depression" in their psychiatric diagnosis provided by the clinical service staff. In those children for whom the word was used it was a secondary diagnosis. A primary affective disorder was not diagnosed even in children with all of the cardinal features of an endogenous depression.

Because the degree of underrecognition of depression in children is so common, the reasons for this lack of recognition need to be briefly explored. The first and foremost problem in diagnosis is the willingness to consider that depression can occur in the young. A similar problem occurred in child abuse in that it took the medical profession decades to entertain the possibility that parents would physically abuse their children. Myths of adults can and do hinder understanding children's difficulties. Thus the adult myth of children having a relatively carefree existence has masked the eyes of adult observers from clinically recognizing depression in children.

In the 1960s when depression in children was widely felt to exist in masked forms (Toolan, 1962), some of the clinical case descriptions published at that time included good clinical descriptions of depressed behavior. The problem was labeling it depression. Since depression was not recognized, reasons were given for its absence. For example, depression did not exist in children because they lacked a mature superego, they were incapable of enduring long mood states, and they were incapable of understanding death as a universal and irreversible occurrence. The first and last theoretical concepts are likely still correct, but they do not protect children from experiencing depression.

THE RECOGNITION OF DEPRESSIVE AFFECT

The simple observation of depression in children begins with the acceptance that it can occur. This does not mean that the observer should expect and even anticipate depression in a child simply because the child has had a recent loss or comes from a particularly dreary, depriving background. Depression in children can be directly observed.

Psychiatrists tend to focus on the total gestalt of the child and not to study the child's face. Careful observation of the child's facial expressions is needed. A child's face does not have the deep facial lines characteristic of the faces of adult depressives. Children's faces do reflect sadness, however, which fluctuates less and less with the increasing severity of depression. Their eyes drop and the corners of their mouths turn down. Their posture is often slouched. They frequently have poor eye contact with the interviewer and they speak in a monotone voice with short verbal answers. They rarely bring up topics spontaneously in the interview and passively answer questions with a minimum of words. Communication is replete with pauses, sighs, and incomplete answers. The interview drags even when the interviewer is very active. Their nonverbal behavior resembles the adult depressive's. They differ from the adult in that they rarely complain about being blue, down, or depressed. Some children perceive their own depressed feelings, others do not.

RECOGNITION OF COMMON BEHAVIORS
ACCOMPANYING DEPRESSION

Some of the behaviors of depressed children are missed because they are outside of the usual scope of questions asked by the psychiatrist. For example, children are rarely asked how they sleep. Most parents put their child in bed and assume that sleep soon occurs. The depressed child often goes to sleep with difficulty. The children's descriptions of their own sleep difficulties are easily obtained simply by asking. Children appear to know if they lie awake for a few minutes or a longer time. One even encounters the hypochondriacal youngster who complains it takes a half-hour to go to sleep!

Similarly some depressed children become anorexic. However, they are somewhat less likely to describe their eating pattern than their sleep disturbance since this has frequently been the subject of multiple scoldings by the parents. Overall the vegetative signs of depression in children can be observed but they are less frequent and of generally lesser severity than the vegetative signs observed in adult depressions.

One of the most characteristic behaviors of depressed children is a lessened capacity to have fun. Like many other behaviors associated with depression, the degree of anhedonia often correlates with the severity of the depression. Depressed children rarely complain of anhedonia; rather this is an area which has to be actively explored by the interviewer. If the mother is aware of her child's feelings, she may describe her child's anhedonia even more vividly than the child is able to do. Most children, when asked what they do for fun, easily launch into a discussion of their after-school activities. The inability to have fun may be expressed in a variety of forms. A depressed child may frequently complain of feeling bored. Feeling bored on occasion is quite usual; feeling bored a great deal of the time suggests something is wrong. The way that a child describes his after-school activities is important. Even reserved children express some enthusiasm for play while depressed children sometimes sound as though they go through the motions of play activities like robots, in a mechanical fashion without any enjoyment. Some depressed children, when asked what they do for fun, talk about activities that are realistically unavailable to them. Fun for them is not an everyday reality but a rare event. A depressed child may turn down opportunities for play and doesn't feel like going out when friends ring the doorbell. Just as play is restricted, so is fantasy production decreased. This makes the job of entering the inner world of the child more difficult.

A child's self-esteem is frequently lowered when the child is depressed, just as it is with adults. It is, however, much more difficult to get this information from a child since self-concept is still being developed. Questions in this area have to be phrased in a fairly concrete manner, particularly with younger children. Nevertheless, it is worth asking the child if he thinks he is pretty or good-looking, and if his friends like him. The answers are more honest than might be anticipated since children are generally not imbued with false modesty. Children with low self-esteem sometimes don't like to answer these questions and may give defensive replies. Children hate derogatory nicknames and dislike repeating them, almost as if saying them magically confirms them as truths. Depressed children seem to disproportionately acquire derogatory nicknames.

Again like their adult counterparts, depressed children may feel pathologically guilty. Unlike the adult depressive, the child usually has to be asked about guilt feelings and rarely during an interview speaks spontaneously about feeling excessively guilty. A child's feelings of guilt may relate to realistic events viewed out of proportion to reality or may be totally without a realistic basis. It is not unusual for a child, like an adult, to feel responsible for events which he cannot possibly influence.

Another area outside the range of questions a child is usually asked in a psychiatric assessment is about morbid thoughts, suicide ideas and suicide attempts. Suicidal thinking will be missed if the physician does not consider the possibility, and this is particularly important in a depressed child. These thoughts do occur to children and are more commonplace than is generally assumed. Asking a child whether he has ever contemplated suicide is often more upsetting to the interviewer than to the child.

Most children know the word suicide but feel confident they wouldn't do it. Most adolescents have thought about suicide at some time and have spent more time thinking about it as a possibility than younger children. A depressed child can be preoccupied with suicidal thoughts, and, if asked, may talk about these thoughts and describe what methods of suicide he has contemplated. If a moderately depressed child denies having thought about suicide the likelihood of suppression or denial is high. In this situation the child, like the adult depressive, should be considered an active suicide risk until proved otherwise. Often the child's threat or suicide attempt is handled by the parents by punishment. Under these circumstances it is difficult to get information from the child unless the interviewer knows the situation before seeing the child. The reverse is also frequent where the parents are not aware of their child's suicidal thoughts and actively deny the possiblity of their existence even when told of them by a psychiatrist. One of the most difficult areas in working with depressed children is to convince some parents that their child has suicidal thoughts and may be dangerous to himself.

If a child makes a suicide attempt it is important to get the child's and parents' description of the event. Not all suicide attempts are made by depressed children but may be a manipulative act. Suicide attempts by children have to be taken very seriously because one cannot trust the judgment of a child about what may be lethal. There is considerable speculation that suicide attempts in children are massively unreported. Some accidents and "accidental poisonings" could turn out to be suicide attempts if these incidents were thoroughly investigated.

Morbid thinking can exist in a child with or without suicidal thinking. Sometimes the child will spontaneously express these thoughts but this cannot be relied upon. A child may be realistically concerned about a relative's recent illness or death or express more pathological preoccupations, such as dwelling excessively on the death of a grandparent two years past. The well-known concept that children do not have a mature view of death as a final and irreversible act until about age eleven does not limit the occurrence of morbid thinking in younger children.

Children who are depressed may feel tired during the day even when they have had sufficient sleep. Complaints of excessive fatigue occur frequently in adult depressions. While depressed children have a similar phenomenon and may voluntarily take daytime naps, they rarely complain to the physician of being tired during the day. Again, specific inquiry has to be made.

One characteristic feature of depression in children is hypoactivity. The adult world tends to view children as either normal or hyperactive and hypoactivity may go unrecognized as normal activity. Hypoactivity in depressed children represents the equivalent of psychomotor retardation in adults. Although approximately one-third of hyperactive children have some evidence of depressive affect, hyperactive children usually do not show the full-blown depressive syndrome.

Mild motor restlessness, fidgeting, and so on can occur in childhood depression as an equivalent to psychomotor agitation in adults. Restlessness in children is more commonly related to attention span difficulties than psychomotor agitation, however. It takes careful clinical observation and judgment to delineate these two possibilities. Severe agitation such as pacing can be observed in severely depressed children but is far less common than in adults.

Two more behaviors which are commonly found in depressed children are characteristically assessed in most psychological evaluations of children. These are social withdrawal and a decreased school performance. In both these areas the depressed child moves to a lower level of functioning with the onset of depression. These changes are particularly dramatic in acute depressions. In chronic depressions the child may have always had difficulty making satisfying, age-appropriate peer relationships. This is, however, not unique to the depressed child but commonly found in any emotionally disturbed child. In school the depressed child's performance is typically labeled "not working to capacity." The teachers describe depressed children in a variety of ways, depending on the individual child. Some depressed children are quiet and withdrawn. A few indulge in passive–aggressive behavior. Many depressed children are irritable, and for these youngsters fights and squabbles are easily induced by all too willing classmates. Despite these kinds of behaviors, the depressed child is frequently liked by the teacher, and it would appear that this kind of youngster in some ways has more difficulty relating to peers than to adults.

DEPRESSIVE AFFECT VERSUS DEPRESSIVE SYNDROME

The depressed feelings are a fairly common observation. A depressive syndrome is characterized by a persisting dysphoric mood for two to four weeks plus a cardinal group of accompanying behaviors. The depressive syndrome resembles any other medical syndrome, and it is useful to make a distinction between affect and syndrome in order to introduce some homogeneity to populations of depressed children.

The clinical diagnosis of depression is based on observed behaviors. As with many other disorders, the diagnosis is not based on etiology. Various etiological factors have been implicated in depression, but their exact role and importance have not been delineated. Nevertheless, some of those factors which are suspected to have some relation to depression in childhood will be discussed in the section on differential diagnosis.

General agreement about the diagnostic criteria for childhood depression represents a major step forward in the research on childhood depression. The majority of researchers in childhood depression now accept the adult criteria for depressive disorders as given in *Diagnostic and Statistical Manual of Mental Disorders* (DSM III, 1980). In order to be considered to have a major affective disorder, the patient has to have dysphoria for two weeks or longer and have four or five of the following eight behaviors: (1) appetite or weight change (gain or loss of one pound per week), (2) insomnia or hypersomnia, (3) loss of energy, fatigue, tiredness, (4) psychomotor agitation or retardation, (5) loss of interest or pleasure in usual activities, (6) feelings of self-reproach or excessive guilt, (7) poor concentration or indecisiveness (not associated with formal thought disorder), and (8) recurrent thoughts of death or suicide.

A depressive disorder may be the primary psychiatric diagnosis or secondary to another psychiatric disorder, such as autism, schizophrenia, or organic brain syndromes. Depression is not uncommon in the pediatric wards of general hospitals, particularly in cases of chronic debilitating or fatal diseases and in handicapping medical disorders.

MANIC–DEPRESSIVE ILLNESS IN CHILDREN

Considerable controversy exists as to whether or not the same clinical features of bipolar illness in adults can be seen in children, or whether there is a distinctly juvenile form. Anthony and Scott (1960), in a review of twenty-eight published cases of manic-depressive illness in children, discounted all but three for not satisfying their criteria for prepubertal manic-depressive illness. Nevertheless, they concluded that there is reason to believe that manic-depressive illness may occur in childhood, though they note that psychodynamic features, such as fantasies of omnipotence, are more readily documented than in clinical phenomenological entity.

A major difficulty with the concept of manic-depressive illness in childhood hinges on the concept of a manic state in childhood. While the clinical characteristics of mania in adults have been fairly well delineated, the same criteria when applied to children describe any hyperactive child. Sporadic cases of manic-depressive illness in childhood have been reported by Varsamis and MacDonald (1972) and Warneke (1975), among others. These authors concluded that a juvenile form of manic-depressive illness does occur in some children and that a genetically controlled biochemical vulnerability may be implicated in the etiology.

The criteria for early signs of manic-depressive illness in children vary with different investigators. Davis (1979) proposed five primary criteria for identifying the manic-depressive variant syndrome of childhood: affective storms, family history of significant affective dysfunction, hyperactivity, chronically disturbed personal relationships, and absence of psychotic thought disorders. In a study of children at risk for manic-depressive illness, Kestenbaum (1979) noted three possible predictors of vulnerability: (1) a family history of bipolar illness; (2) clinical symptoms including disturbances in affect, distractibility, impulsiveness, and transient rages; and (3) an intelligence test pattern of verbal abilities greater than perceptual motor performance. A study of relatives of hyperactive children showed a low prevalence of affective disorders, suggesting that hyperkinesis is not related to manic-depressive illness (Stewart and Morrison, 1973). Nevertheless, Thompson and Schindler (1976) hypothesize that a subgroup of hyperactive children may have the equivalent of a manic state in childhood.

THE FAMILIES OF DEPRESSED CHILDREN

Almost all studies of children who are depressed comment on the high incidence of parental depression (Poznanski, 1970; Frommer, 1968). Parental depression can and does occur without their children having dysphoric moods. However, children with a depressive syndrome are twice as likely to have a parent who is depressed. Furthermore, the parental depression tends to coexist with the child's depression although other episodes of depression may exist in the parent's past history.

The high prevalence of parental depression can act as a barrier to recognizing depression in the child and obtaining treatment. The depressed parent tends to relate to the depressed child in one of two psychologically deviant ways. Either the parent denies the depressive pathology in the child, even to the extent of denying suicidal attempts by the child, or the parent overidentifies with the child and attributes all of his or her own depressive thoughts and behaviors to the child. In either situation, realistic empathy with the child's feelings and behavior is not present. It is especially difficult to enlist the parent's cooperation in obtaining help for the child when the parent denies depression in the child.

DIFFERENTIAL DIAGNOSIS OF DEPRESSION IN CHILDREN

1. The diagnosis, *adjustment disorder with a depressed mood* is one of the current psychiatric overused diagnoses. Child psychiatrists tend to use this diagnostic category because it implies the least severe psychopathology in the child despite the fact that often the duration of the child's problem alone may be too great to represent a simple adjustment reaction. There are multiple life stresses in all children who come to a psychiatric clinic, whether they are depressed or not depressed, so that the severity of the psychosocial factors is rarely helpful diagnostically. A crucial factor in the differential diagnosis between an adjustment reaction with a depressed mood and a major affective

disorder is the presence or absence of the accompanying behaviors previously described in the diagnostic criteria of the depressive syndrome.

2. *Childhood schizophrenia.* A schizophrenic child may have depressive
   symptoms. A psychotic child is frequently diagnosed as schizophrenic
   without considering other causes of psychosis in children. Although
   rare, children can be psychotically depressed and have delusions of being unworthy, useless or a burden on others, similar to the psychotically depressed adult.

3. *Grief reaction.* A loss of a parent, sibling or other important person
   can precipitate a grief reaction in a child. If it endures it may become a
   depression. The normal reactions of children to bereavement are less
   clearly described in the literature than those of adults. It appears that
   in response to the death of a parent or sibling, children do demonstrate periods of sadness, though of shorter duration than is characteristic of the adult. Children are likely to show evidence of a disturbance
   in their behavior for a much longer period of time than affective expressions of grief. A wide variety of behavioral disturbances may
   appear, such as temper tantrums, disobedience, truancy, running away
   from home, and accident proneness. Thus, the idea that children show
   "depressive equivalents" rather than demonstrating open depressive
   affect was the first conceptualization of depression in children. While
   the focus currently is on overt depressions in children, the concept of
   "depressive equivalents" may still be valid. It requires a tighter definition than that proposed by Toolan (Caplan and Douglas, 1969), however.

   Caplan and Douglas' study (Puig-Antich et al., 1979) of children with
   depressed moods correlates childhood depression with parent loss.
   Loss in their study was globally defined as separation from the parent
   for any reason, including death, divorce, illness, or desertion. The
   authors studied for a period of one year all children on a waiting list
   for psychotherapy. They found that one-half of the depressed children and one-fourth of the control children had suffered some form of
   parental loss lasting six months or longer before the age of eight.

   The distinction between a grief reaction and a depressive disorder is
   not easy to make. We have no guidelines as to the length of normal bereavement in children. In the final analysis, the clinician has to make a
   judgment based on the total clinical history and current symptomatology.

4. *Organic disease with dysphoric mood.* These children require the consultant to make the distinction between apathy from a physical illness
   and depressive affect. The apathy and fatigue of the medically ill child

is different than in a child with primary depressive disease. The relatives and referring physicians may be eager for a psychiatric diagnosis, particularly if there is difficulty in establishing a medical diagnosis. However, it usually pays the psychiatric consultant to rely on his or her own judgment. The author has had children referred as possible depressed patients who ultimately were diagnosed to have Crohn's disease, Schilder's disease, and leukemia.

5. *Children with pathological separation anxiety.* Children with marked separation anxiety can appear depressed when they are away from their parents, particularly the mother. The mother's presence influences not only the child's mood but many other behaviors of the child, such as the child's social interaction. Observers of children with pathological separation anxiety often find it difficult to distinguish the child with simple separation anxiety from the child with separation anxiety and depression.

6. *Children with learning disabilities and depression.* In a young child it can be very difficult to determine whether learning problems precipitate a secondary depression, or if the child's depression is interfering with learning. If it is possible to obtain a good history from a parent, it is easier to find out which event chronologically occurred first. Generally, a young child's sense of time is too poor to get this information from him. In one sense the question is academic since an improvement in the child's depression, whether primary or secondary, will generally improve the child's school performance.

EVALUATION OF SUICIDE POTENTIAL

A thorough assessment of the child and the family is needed to assess the risk of suicide. Suicide risk cannot be studied in isolation. A general knowledge of the family stability and support system is basic. Since suicidal children rarely come from families without conflicts, it becomes essential to assess how much support is available for the child. Families frequently deny a child's suicide attempt, rationalizing the behavior on other grounds, and solving the crisis by punishing the child. Such families are very defensive and it takes time and skillful intervention to help these parents to face the family conflicts.

A history of a loss of a close friend or meaningful relationship is significant. The fantasy by a child of joining a dead parent in heaven has been reported and does occur clinically although not often. It is difficult to discuss time factors relative to mourning. The author has seen a child actively grieving the loss of a grandparent two years later and another child grieving the loss of a sibling four years later.

If a child has made a suicide threat or attempt, the same information is needed as in adults, such as the events leading up to the threat or attempt, lethality of the method, and previous threats or attempts. The suicide threat may be an impulsive, manipulative act by the child. As with adults, not all suicide threats are made by depressed children. Long-term follow-ups on these children are not available. Therefore, children who make suicidal threats cannot be lightly dismissed until longitudinal data are available. Too often behavior first introduced in the jest of fantasy of an individual has a core of reality not initially recognized by the individual or those around him.

Depressed children, like depressed adults, make suicide attempts and successfully commit suicide. The latter wreaks havoc in the family system for many ensuing years. After a suicide attempt there is often a reduction in the child's depression. If there is continued depression the risk of a repeated attempt is greater. Any child who has made a suicide attempt is at greater risk for another attempt than a child who has never made a suicide attempt.

It is important to stress to the family the necessity of locking up pills, guns, and other hazardous items. This is important symbolically as well as having some reality basis, because it conveys to the youngster that the parents are trying to prevent a recurrence.

REFERRING THE DEPRESSED CHILD FOR TREATMENT

The recognition and diagnosis of depression in a child usually indicates the need for some type of treatment. Whether the child should be referred to an inpatient psychiatric facility or for outpatient treatment depends on the overall manageability of the child in the home and school and the degree of suicide risk. Actively suicidal children should be referred to a psychiatric inpatient unit. A pediatric unit is not a good substitute since it is impossible to enforce suicidal precautions in a general medical hospital.

The majority of depressed children can be treated in outpatient settings. Psychotherapy with these children is not substantially different from psychotherapy with other emotionally disturbed children. Because of the child's reduced verbal productivity, the therapist has to be fairly active. Seeing several depressed children in a row can be fatiguing for the therapist.

Depressed children already in a pediatric unit for medical reasons may respond to increased emotional support from the environment. In addition, individual psychotherapy is often of benefit. A pilot study by Puig-Antich (1979) suggests that the tricyclic antidepressant medications may be of benefit for depressed prepubertal children but more drug trials are needed before more definite recommendations for drug therapy can be made. At this time the *PDR* does not recommend any antidepressant medication for children under 12 years. This includes the tricyclics, MAO inhibitors, and lithium.

REFERENCES

Anthony J and Scott P: Manic-depressive psychosis in childhood. *J Child Psychol*, Psychiatry Allied Descriptions 1:53–72, 1960.

Caplan M and Douglas V: Incidence of parental loss in children with depression moods. *J Child Psychol and Psych* 10:225–232, 1969.

Davis RE: Manic-depressive variant syndrome of childhood: A preliminary report. *Am J Psych* 136:702–705, 1979.

Diagnostic and Statistical Manual of Mental Disorders (3rd ed.), American Psychiatric Association, 1980.

Frommer E: Depressive illness in childhood. *Brit J Psych* 2:117–136, 1968.

Gallemore J and Wilson W: Adolescent maladjustment or affective disorder? *Am J Psych* 129(5):608–612, 1972.

Kestenbaum CJ: Children at risk for manic-depressive illness: Possible predictors. *Am J Psych* 136:702–705, 1979.

Poznanski E, Cook S, and Carrol BJ: A depression rating scale for children. *Pediatr* 64(4):442–450, 1979.

Poznanski E, Cook SC, Carroll B, Corgo H, and Cepada C: Childhood depression: A rating scale (unpublished).

Poznanski E and Zrull J: Childhood depression: Clinical characteristics of overtly depressed children. *Arch Gen Psych* 23:8–15, 1970.

Puig-Antich J, Perel J, Lupatkin W, Chambers W, Shea C, Tabrigi M, and Stiller R: Plasma levels of imipramine (IMI) and dismetrylimipramine (DMI) and clinical response in prepubertal major depressive disorder. *J Am Assoc Child Psych* 18(7):616–627, 1979.

Rutter M, Graham P, Chadwick DFD, and Yule W: Adolescent turmoil: Fact or fiction. *J Child Psychol and Psych* 17:35–56, 1976.

Stewart MA and Morrison JR: Affective disorders among the relatives of hyperactive children. *J Child Psychol and Psych* 14:209–212, 1973.

Thompson RJ and Schindler FH: Embryonic mania. *Child Psych Hum Dev* 6:149–154, 1976.

Toolan J: Depression in children and adolescents. *Am J Orthopsych* 32:404–414, 1962.

Varsamis J and MacDonald SM: Manic-depressive disease in childhood: A case report. *Can Psych Assoc J* 17:279–281, 1972.

Vital Statistics of the United States, vol 2, Mortality United States Department of Health, Education and Welfare, Public Health Service.

Warnecke LA: A case of manic-depressive illness in childhood. *Can Psych Assoc J* 20:195–200, 1975.

21

Child Psychiatric Consultation Concerning Childhood Psychosis

Donald S. Gair

INTRODUCTION

Some of the most urgent calls for child psychiatric consultation arise in reaction to psychotic children. The frantic caller believes either that the child is psychotic or that the child is "impossible," at best incorrigibly recalcitrant, whether or not technically delinquent. Another group of children referred to in this chapter become the subject of consultations sought with concern but less urgency. In these the idea of psychosis is not in the mind of the caller but subsequently becomes prominent in the consultant's differential diagnosis. Those referring this latter group may regard the children as mildly retarded, slightly withdrawn, hyperactive, or suffering from a learning disorder, a behavior problem, or any combination.

In the most desperate referrals, the consultant doesn't often bring bad news since the initial views are already dire. When the consultant sees a child who was referred as psychotic and says that the child is less seriously disturbed, or if a child referred as impossible is then diagnosed as psychotic, the consultant's outlook is generally regarded by those making the referral as somewhat brighter than what was originally thought.

However, when a child referred because of what is seen as a mildly vexing refractoriness to treatment is labeled as psychotic, there may be a strong resistance to the new and more alarming diagnostic thinking. Failure to anticipate this possibility can vitiate any chance of usefulness of the consultation. Not that any disagreement with diagnostic certainty on the part of a referring professional is free of the need for tact, but when the disagreement is in the direction of more seriousness, the issue is intensified. Psychosis is frightening to many people. The less dogmatic the consultant is about diagnostic labels, the better.

Dogmatism is rarely justified in diagnostics. All diagnostic entities are to some extent arbitrary, and this is more so with psychiatric diagnoses. The American Psychiatric Association's *Diagnostic and Statistical Manual III* (1980) has achieved more consistency than did its predecessors. However, the careful guidelines still admit overlap between several diagnoses and in the area of childhood psychosis long-lived barriers to certainty still exist.

However, even were the diagnostic entities crystal clear, specific courses of action for each child would not be. Individual prognoses and therapeutic programs are not precisely dictated by diagnostic labels.

Professional efforts are never more challenged or valuable than when directed at the most difficult problems. Referral for psychiatric consultation of a child thought to be psychotic, or who turns out to be, almost invariably involves very serious problems. Such consultations are either the first ports of entry into professional care or appeals to further expertise from embattled professionals. In both situations the utmost professional skill and judgment of the child psychiatrist are needed to help the child and family achieve normal development in the child.

THERE'S A CHILD BENEATH THE PROBLEM

Fear of Insanity

Even in this age of assumed enlightenment, fear of insanity is virtually universal. It is curious that although the colloquial pejorative, "You're crazy!" is widely used with family, friends, and associates in informal banter, when the idea crystalizes in a responsible adult's mind that a child in a classroom, or camp group, or on a pediatric ward may be "really mental," it usually gives rise to a dread as of the supernatural. The sophisticated possession of assorted labels to apply to children seen as "crazy" does little to change this reaction of fearful awe.

Thus it happens that when children are regarded as psychotic, they tend to become stereotyped as unapproachable by ordinary methods of child-rearing and education. Many teachers without relevant experience remove all discipline and everyday expectations from children so perceived for fear of doing the wrong thing and either damaging or provoking the child (provided they will tolerate a deviant child at all). In like manner, the stabilizing and formative social embrace of many of the important adults essential to all children's development is either totally withdrawn or becomes rigid, narrow, and unresponsive to the full range of the psychotic child's needs and capacities when the fear of psychosis is prominent.

The fear and doubt in the adults in this situation is what underlies the urgency of the calls for consultation. These urgent calls usually include the demand that the consultant help have the child placed somewhere else immediately.

The underlying fear of psychosis and the consequent vulnerability to exclusion of a child with this diagnosis can be dramatically exposed when there is a slight change in symptomatology in a manageable child already identified as psychotic and accepted in a treatment program. This is exemplified in the following:

N.R., a boy identified as an autistic child since age six and in his third year of enrollment at a day school for emotionally disturbed and/or retarded children, returned from Christmas vacation at age thirteen with the new symptom of intermittent sudden utterances and slapping his head. This boy had some communicative speech and was attentive to second and third grade academic exercises without progressive learning but with slowly improving social responsiveness. The new symptom was startling but did not involve physical approach to others nor, in between the outbursts (which lasted several seconds), was there any lessening of his previous responsiveness.

The director of the school panicked, immediately called the parents and said that N. would have to be removed from school. With bluntness born of apprehension, he said to the alarmed parents, when they asked what they could do, "Put him in an institution!" The parents, in turmoil, called the psychiatrist who had worked with N. at the time he had been hospitalized for initial diagnosis and subsequent treatment at ages six to nine. The psychiatrist acted as an emergency consultant.

It happened that the symptom of shouting out had first appeared on N.'s thirteenth birthday, an event on which much positive family attention had been focused. Whatever other factors may have been operating, there was a strong possibility that the emotional impact of the birthday played a part in the onset of the symptom.

The consultant's main efforts were with the director. He was able to help him focus on the developmental implications of the onset of the symptom and to recognize its self-contained nature. The director could then both regard N. sympathetically as manifesting some inner distress and also accept the challenge of dealing with the disruptiveness in a creative way, freed by the consultant's explanation from the threat of danger that his fear had suggested to him. The consultant discussed with the parents and the director the possibility that the symptom was a form of Gilles de la Tourette Syndrome, and arranged for various symptomatic remedies to be pursued on the basis of that possibility.

N. was not rehospitalized. He stayed at that day school several more years until he reached its upper age limit, despite the persistence of the symptom (which was only slightly modified by medication). He clearly benefited from the continuity and the excellent social conditioning the school provided even though further academic gains were negligible. It is very likely that his continued growth would have been seriously compromised by expulsion from the school—which was averted by the consultation—since N. was extremely vulnerable to all changes, as is characteristic of autistic children.

At the time of the consultation, the director of the school had spent over thirty years working with retarded and emotionally disturbed children. He had been careful, however, as this vignette illustrates, to screen out those who frightened him. This consultation not only helped N. but it also helped the director to expand his tolerance of deviation somewhat beyond the brittle limits he had previously maintained.

When the consultant perceives adult fear that results in stereotyping a child as impossibly sick or bad, his or her first efforts should be toward restoring to the caretaking adults the lost recognition that they are dealing with a child who has a problem, not simply with a problem to be disposed of.

Developmental Perspective on the Needs of the Psychotic Child

Childhood is the period of life during which survival, growth and development is dependent on the arbitrary authority, ordinary strength and wisdom, obligatory support, and the social modeling and instruction of adults—parents and surrogates.* Because of these inescapable circumstances of childhood, context is always as vital as the content of problems presented to the child psychiatrist.

Quite apart from the concept of universal human interrelatedness, a child (as contrasted to an adult) does not present him or herself alone. Whether or not identified as a family therapist, the child psychiatrist must include in his or her perspective the network of adults in which the child is embedded, and must work to enhance the functioning of the system of essential adults surrounding the child. Viewed in this way, it becomes clear that the child psychiatrist

---

*That there are certain circumstances which define a special group called "emancipated children" only accentuates this truism.

properly functions as a consultant to the child's environment when he or she is the physician of record and the individual psychotherapist for the child.

When a child psychiatrist is called in as a consultant, at least some of the significant adults surrounding the child patient are unsure how to proceed. To this degree, the necessary support of the child by these adults is compromised and every consultation presents a potential crisis. When the child is psychotic, relationships with surrounding people are intrinsically tenuous. Any further attenuation of parental and surrogate structure will, therefore, have an exaggerated impact, exacerbating the illness itself.

This developmental basis for recognizing the desperate need of psychotic children for clarity, confidence, and strength of the surrounding adult structure overlaps with the procedural necessity for a consultant to know who is the responsible person to whom consultative recommendation will be addressed. Sometimes in demanding clarification of this issue the consultant can force a tightening of the parental/surrogate care hierarchy which will be in itself a therapeutic gain for the disorganized child even before the consultation gets under way.

A stark example would be refusal of a potential consultant to proceed when the legal guardian does not wish it. It is not uncommon for social agencies to request consultation against the wishes of a family that is functioning marginally. The consultant's proper refusal to participate in this situation may precipitate action to have custody temporarily removed from the demoralized family so as to allow an assessment to take place. If not a happy circumstance, it may at least establish some stability which is an essential precondition for useful assessment and rational planning and treatment, and may well include family rehabilitation.

DIAGNOSTIC ISSUES IN CHILDHOOD PSYCHOSIS

It is often assumed in consultations and in clinical conferences that all participants mean the same thing when referring to psychosis,* and this assumption has probably operated for most readers up to this point. Marked discrepancies

---

*Adolescents with psychosis present problems largely overlapping those in young adults. To include a full account of relevant clinical situations presented to a consultant by psychotic adolescents would provide relatively little that is the exclusive province of the child psychiatrist. Applicable aspects of assessment, management, and treatment of clinical context with adolescents that are dictated by the patients' immaturity in relationship to family or surrogates will be readily extrapolated from what will be discussed. It will also apply to some degree to adults whose clinical situation result in their being in a markedly dependent relationship to their psychiatrist.

arise with closer scrutiny, however. Therefore, before describing further the consultation process in childhood psychosis the diagnostic problem will now be reviewed.

Diagnosis is essential to rational treatment. The more specific the identification of the phenomena to be treated, the more accurately one can aim a treatment approach and assess the effectiveness of treatment. However, there are many levels in diagnosis. The relatively recent movement for "problem-oriented records" reflects the time-honored medical truth that overall labels are of limited determining value when one is making a specific therapeutic decision about an individual patient. For example, Diabetes Mellitus is a specific medical diagnosis and yet by itself it cannot predict what treatment will be necessary for a given diabetic patient. There are many axes of significant differentiation—severity, age of onset, family history, degree of overweight, other precipitating factors, activity level, general health, special states (such as pregnancy), signs of complications, idiosyncratic response to medications, attitude towards the illness, and competence for self care—with many different combinations that make up what could be called "the universe of diabetes."

Compared to the relatively specific diagnostic label of Diabetes Mellitus, however, the diagnostic label "psychosis," particularly with children, is nonspecific in the extreme. Yet while physicians in general will readily acknowledge a certain clinical vagueness in the label "diabetes," even psychiatrists treat the unqualified label "psychosis" as something quite specific. Some psychiatrists also share the dread that laymen have, discussed above. When a professional has a phobic response to the idea of psychosis it can only exacerbate avoidance mechanisms in parents and impede necessary action. There are cogent arguments for avoiding the use of terms such as "schizophrenic" and "psychotic" in order to prevent further alienation of a child from his or her family. But the reaction referred to here is not one of elective tact but of defensive denial which leads to spurious reassurances such as, "Your child will grow out of it," and consequent unfortunate, even critical, delays of intervention.

There are not yet unequivocal differentiating criteria for all categories of psychosis in adults. However, after centuries of evolution of descriptive categories for adults there is considerable stability within the limits of certainty and clarity. Compared to the long history of development of diagnostic categories of psychosis in adults, the evolution of comparable categories in children has been brief, having begun only in this century. It is understandable, therefore, that the confusion should be greater.

By the 1960s there existed a profusion of diagnostic labels within the universe of childhood psychosis. The bases for categorization were varied, some diagnoses referring to behavioral description, some to underlying pathology, some to theories of causations. The diagnostic labels included childhood schizophrenia, childhood psychosis, infantile psychosis, atypical child, schizophrenic syndrome, Heller's disease, infantile autism, symbiotic psychosis, developmental psychosis, protophrenia, protoschizophrenia, schizophreniform psychosis of childhood, anaclitic depression, among others (Blau, 1962; Laufer and Gair, 1969).

There have been spirited disagreements among various authors and schools of thought and many attempts at syntheses and compromises. The issues and concepts have to do with theories of personality development and pathogenesis which are of fundamental importance and great clinical and theoretical interest. Much of the literature of the past thirty years is still relevant and includes most of the major contributors to child psychiatric and psychoanalytic literature. Even a cursory summary would be beyond the scope and purpose of this chapter.* However, the current status of diagnosis of childhood psychosis including DSM III, will be presented briefly, together with those factors on which there is useful consensus.

Ambiguities of Categories

Despite the admirable success of DSM III in reclassifying psychiatric entities into clear and useful groups of symptomatic descriptions and diagnostic trees, the ambiguity of classification in childhood psychoses remains. The authors of DSM III recognize a range of diagnoses in the field but lack unanimity about their equivalence. Writing about the new DSM III diagnosis "Pervasive Developmental Disorder," the authors say, "The criteria for this disorder describe children who have been described by some clinicians as childhood schizophrenia, childhood psychosis, atypical children, and symbiotic psychosis. It is likely that some children with this disorder will indeed develop schizophrenia as adults. However, there is currently no way of predicting which children will develop schizophrenia as adults." Since DSM III has eliminated the diagnosis of childhood schizophrenia and called for use of the general term, schizophrenia, for children who have the necessary criteria, the quoted statement clearly indicates recognition of diagnostic haziness.

In the past, although childhood schizophrenia connoted a specific entity to some authors, in practice it was the generic term for childhood psychosis (Laufer and Gair, 1969). With DSM III, pervasive developmental disorder will become the generic term. It will be rare for children below the age of 12 to fit the DSM III guidelines for schizophrenia since delusions and hallucinations are not reliable signs in many children. Distinction between obsessions and intense fantasies or delusions may be extremely difficult in children (Despert, 1955), if

---

*This author's bias against the doctrine of parental causation of psychosis and the importance of the issue in consultation has resulted in its discussion later in the text without any review of the literature pro and con.

possible at all, and of increasingly questionable significance as the age is lowered. Hallucinations may exist without serious pathological import, certainly in the absence of what experienced child psychiatrists would call psychosis (Wilking and Paoli, 1966).

The clearest exception to diagnostic ambiguity is infantile autism (although with an incidence of 2 or 3 per 10,000 this is not a huge slice of the diagnostic pie). DSM III has finally established Kanner's (1943) brilliant delineation as an official diagnosis with the following criteria: "Onset before 30 months of age; pervasive lack of responsiveness to other people (autism); gross deficits in language development; if speech is present, peculiar speech patterns such as immediate and delayed echolalia, metaphorical language, pronominal reversal; bizarre respnses to various aspects to the environment, e.g., resistance to change, peculiar interest in or attachments to animate or inanimate objects; absence of delusions, hallucinations, loosening of associations, and incoherence as in schizophrenia" (DSM III, p. 89-90). But here, too, there is an arbitrary end point of onset before 30 months. This only technically obscures the overlap with pervasive developmental disorder. The latter implicitly separate entity has, by definition, an onset beginning no earlier than 30 months but can be descriptively indistinguishable from infantile autism, and, as indicated in the quote earlier, itself overlaps with schizophrenia in the minds of the DSM III authors.

Autism vs. Schizophrenia

DSM III attempts to take the ambiguity out of the term "psychosis" by restricting its meaning to "gross impairment in reality testing," as distinguished from DSM II's standard of "mental functioning sufficiently impaired to interfere grossly with . . . capacity to meet the ordinary demands of life." In childhood, when reality testing and judgment are characteristically weak, the general standard of gross failure of overall adaptation is more useful.

What one is left with are two spectrums. One, the more practical, of disorders ranging from infantile autism on the one hand to fairly clearly delineated schizophrenia on the other. This spectrum roughly parallels ages of children concerned and, as stated above, the majority of latency age children diagnosed as childhood schizophrenia under DSM II will be diagnosed under DSM III as pervasive developmental disorder. The second spectrum is of causative factors which will not be discussed in this chapter because it would lead into the extensive literature referred to above without sufficient relevance to the task at hand.*

Of the younger group of severely disabled youngsters, including those with infantile autism, there has long been wide agreement on the essential features.

---

*See footnote page 337.

In one of the first major studies of psychotic children published in the United States, Potter (1933, p. 1268) epitomized the disorder he had observed as follows: "The outstanding symptomatology is found in the field of behavior and a consistent lack of emotional rapport. The drive for integration with the environment, so characteristic of normal children and so essential for their personality development, is outstandingly absent."

Kanner, who created the diagnosis of early infantile autism with his classic article in 1943, identified, in his group, the same lack of emotional rapport cited by Potter as being present virtually at birth (although he raised the age of onset of infantile autism several times in succeeding years). He described the quality of human relatedness in this group of children as follows:

The outstanding, "pathognomonic," fundamental disorder is the children's *inability to relate themselves* in the ordinary way to people and situations from the beginning of life. . . . There is from the start an *extreme autistic aloneness* that, whenever possible, disregards, ignores, shuts out anything that comes to the child from outside [p. 242] (author's italics).

Three decades after Potter's article, in a report of psychiatric opinion from several countries collected by Creak et al. (1964), the only descriptive characteristic present in virtually all of a group of 155 children who were considered examples of schizophrenic syndrome (the term arbitrarily chosen for the group of severely disturbed children being surveyed) was: "Gross and sustained impairment of emotional relationships with people" (Creak, 1964).

In older children with severe disorders of emotional integration but in whom deficiencies in human relatedness are not as prominent as in the above descriptions, current child psychiatric practice increasingly uses the diagnostic term of borderline psychosis or borderline state. This usage is not compatible with DSM III categories—neither Borderline Personality Disorder nor Schizophrenia will apply to most of the children who would be diagnosed as borderline in child psychiatry settings. Although many will place these children in the category of Pervasive Developmental Disorder (stretching the concept of grossly impaired social relationships), this will not provide nearly enough specificity of diagnosis to guide recommendations and plans. Using the alternate category (299 .8X), Atypical Pervasive Developmental Disorder, will do nothing to facilitate planning.

Mentally retarded children should be most carefully assessed for signs of disordered relatedness. The incidence of severe emotional disorder is much higher than in the general populations and responsiveness to treatment is the same as in nonretarded patients in the great majority of retarded children (Gair, 1980).

Organic Brain Damage

In approaching the diagnostic problem with those children whose severity of disorder places them in the spectrum of psychosis, the index of suspicion of central nervous system damage should be high, and sufficient screening procedures should be used to pick up signs of such defects. Also, deafness, severe learning disorder, intrinsic speech development disorder, all may be present with symptoms of disordered relatedness. Relatively rapid onset of profound regression to psychosis may be produced by encephalitis, which is otherwise asymptomatic or undetected. Fixed damage to the brain, while in itself irreversible, is an important finding since it may influence the emphasis placed on various aspects of treatment. School records may be of help in pinpointing a time of change in cognitive functioning or, conversely, in clarifying that an intellectual deficiency has been consistent from the beginning.

In the area of intrinsic personality functioning it is of most importance to assess areas of overall adjustment and maladjustment, of strengths, weaknesses, complexities, and undeveloped areas. The approach to ego assessment presented in 1956 by Beres has not been improved upon in its essentials and is a most useful format.

Beres (1956) wrote of approaching the problem operationally. He accepted schizophrenia as a generic term but cited marked deviations in specific ego functions as the identifiable problems. He begged the question of calling the deviations he cited psychotic, in essence recognizing the arbitrariness and nonspecificity of the term that is also being emphasized here. The ego functions he listed for appraisal are: reality-testing, impulse control, object relatedness, thought processes, defensive functions of the ego, autonomous functions of the ego, and the synthetic function of the ego. This is a useful format for assessment of children in general and of severely disabled children in particular and is particularly useful in the consultative process, precisely because it defers the question of a specific diagnosis of psychosis, focusing instead on actual problems in the patient.

Semantics

The major reason that the term "psychosis" is such a slender diagnostic reed on which to lean is semantic. Psychosis is a comparative concept masquerading as a concrete entity. In actuality, most people, including psychiatrists, use the terms psychosis and psychotic to designate disturbed patients who present more than a certain (and indeterminate) degree of difficulty or deviation. When symptoms are abstracted from groups of patients with similar psychiatric problems of extreme severity, generally called psychotic, these symptoms will soon be recognized in other patients whom one would not consider sick enough to be called psychotic and later on in the normal population as well. Ambivalence, first used by Bleuler to describe schizophrenia, is an example of a mechanism which is no less normal than psychotic.

It is not enough to say that no single phenomenon will demand the diagnosis of psychosis. No constellation of symptoms will suffice. The issue is always one of severity and the degree of severity is judged by operational impact, which is to say, by the demands the symptom or constellation of symptoms place on a particular environment—in childhood, on the surrounding adults responsible for the care of the children involved. Once again we come to context.

All of the above is not intended as a statement of diagnostic nihilism but rather as an outline of the limits of specificity of the concept of psychosis which remains, nonetheless, both a useful and unavoidable diagnostic term. It is as useful, unfortunately, as it is vague. The unavoidability of the concept is attested to by its persistence through all changes in terminology over the centuries. Its limitations must be kept explicit throughout all consultative activities where it becomes an issue.

In summary: We mean something very intensely when we say a patient is psychotic, but it denotes either a generic universe of severe disturbance or a personal reaction to a particular patient. It does not delimit a specific entity.

THE PRACTICAL DIAGNOSTIC QUESTIONS

All calls for consultation that arise on an emergency basis raise the critical and primary diagnostic question which is fundamentally a clinical management question. This question is central to all consultations about psychosis in children: *can the child remain living and going to school where he or she already is and receive what is necessary to lead to the minimal acceptable outcome?* The answer to this is not simply a matter of discovery by skillful investigation. The situation is almost always initially presented as an unworkable fit between child and family and/or school. Too often this picture is reinforced by labeling the child as impossible or the family/school as inadequate, or both. However, what the consultant does as the first or one of the early figures on the scene can materially influence the situation and subsequent course, as in the following composite clinical account:

The parents of an eight-year-old adopted boy called a children's psychiatric hospital at one o'clock in the morning and spoke with the staff child psychiatrist on duty. Mother and father felt desperate—at the end of their rope. The boy had been found to be epileptic at age three. He had been adopted extralegally at age one following a first year of minimal care and minimal stimulation. The epilepsy was under medical control, but he had been impulsive, had frequent tantrums and functioned at a mildly retarded level in special classes. Lately, he had been wandering about at night waking the family. The night in question was the seventh in a row. This night he was found urinating in a darkened hall and said he was "killing the monsters." The parents reported that a school psychologist had told them two weeks earlier that the boy had "a thought disorder," and the parents were heartsick because they "knew this meant schizophrenia." They wanted and expected an emergency admission to the hospital that night.

The staff psychiatrist maintained the role of consultant. He was genuinely sympathetic and understood how frightened the parents must be. He explained that it was clear the boy was terrified as well, and that a rapid car ride to a strange building in the middle of the night, followed by separation from his parents, would only be likely to increase that terror to an extreme. Tired as the parents were, they would get no more rest in the process of hospitalizing the boy that night than if they followed what was recommended instead.

It was recommended that the parents change their son's pajamas, offer him some food, settle him in his own bed and stay with him the rest of the night, soothing him as best they could. They were reminded that it was understandable that they were frightened but that hospitalization could certainly be put off until the next day at least. An evaluation for admission was scheduled for the next morning.

The boy was never hospitalized. The next day at the hospital, the parents were no longer overwhelmed. They had been able to help their son to get back to sleep for several hours. They elected to have an outpatient psychiatric evaluation. Parents and boy became effectively involved in outpatient psychotherapy with a child psychiatrist who had frequent meetings with parents and kept close liaison with the school. Three years later, the boy is still in public school, now in regular classes but with a special program, progressing well.

This vignette is meant to illustrate the importance of making every effort to revive and support nurturant parental and educative potential in the home and local school setting or in other settings that have been functioning until such a crisis. Because of the self-perpetuating nature of the stereotyping process whereby children become labeled as "impossible" (either sick or bad), anything that will succeed in restoring the child to a position of interactive reality with parents or surrogates will often have a dramatic effect, sharply reducing manifest psychotic symptomatology in the child. It is in this area that the consultant's functioning may make a critical difference.

When suggestions with this potential can be put into effect without the consultant having yet seen (or ever seeing) the child, the impact of success will be optimum, as in the example given. Then the indigenous caregivers know that it was their approach that made the difference. Demonstration interviews in which the consultant makes unprecedented emotional contact with a child run the risk of confirming to consultees their belief that they cannot manage and that the consultant has some rare and alien magic. The more acute the sense of bankruptcy by the consultees, the more vital is this consultation principle. Circumstances will not always allow the opportunity to plan ideally but the principle is central and should always be borne in mind.

When parents or other caretakers are in a panic they are bound by the immediate moment and have limited perspective. Focusing on the fact that survival has been possible up to the present sometimes, as in the example given previously, allows an expansion of the present into a larger time of reflection and evaluation. Decision making can then proceed on an elective, rather than an emergency, basis. Sometimes the parents cannot be reassured sufficiently and will need either outside help or some immediate placement of the child.

Nevertheless, the goal should remain the same—to retain and enhance as much as possible of the parents' (or surrogates') self-possession and reserve capacity to continue as effective adults for the child. When the person calling for the consultation is a professional with clinical responsibility who has not as yet taken the reassuring steps outlined above, the task is to try to help him or her to go through these processes.

Moving beyond the immediate crisis, the clinical management necessities that must be provided for any psychotic child, if there is to be hope of effective treatment, are a school and a home setting that *accept* and respond to and care for the child *as a child*. These are prior conditions to anything specific that may be prescribed or provided as treatment and educational programs required by the child's problems.

The discussion above describes the policy of trying to keep the original home and school involved. If that kind of acceptance cannot be provided there (which is understandably less likely in proportion to the severity of disturbance in the child), then another setting must be found that can. Programs that maintain some involvement with the home are more desirable than those that cannot. For instance, five-day overnight programs allow the parents to contribute necessary support and continuity every weekend (Gair and Salomon, 1962). Day programs or special schools are often suitable for children whose families can manage them at home. However, some children cannot remain at home but can be maintained, with or without special programs, in the local school while living elsewhere—in foster home, group home or hospital.

When the consultant reviews material about (or directly interviews) a child with a previously unrecognized disorder of relatedness or of personality integration gross enough to be considered psychotic, the consultant finds him or herself in the position of having to enlighten parents and others with diagnostic information that most often gives rise to discouragement and fear (as has been discussed at length earlier). In such situations the specific problems suspected should be carefully spelled out without using the heavily charged words psychosis and schizophrenia.

If the parents or referring agents ask, "Do you mean the child is psychotic (or schizophrenic)?" then the meaning of these terms to the person asking the question should first be explored to insure that, in answering, the consultant knows all the underlying fears that must be addressed. It is most important to let it be known that the consultant will answer this question directly after the inquiry about the full meaning of the question to those asking it. In then answering, it is important to clarify the limits of meaning of the terms, outlined earlier in the chapter. Difficult does not mean hopeless.

The reason for consultation for these children is most frequently a failure of the child to improve in current therapeutic programs. The fact should be emphasized that the previous failure to recognize the underlying disorganization of the child has complex meanings and potentials. One is that the child's very adaptability has contributed to obscuring the problem. Another is that the previous lack of improvement largely stemmed from excessive expectations; with new clarity of therapeutic focus based on the new diagnostic understanding, improvement is much more likely to begin.

THE POLITICS OF CONSULTATION

Consultation is political in the sense that all adult human interaction is political, insofar as it involves the identification of complementing and opposing interests and policies and the development of consequent strategies to achieve new goals or to protect existing situations. In this sense the variability of the consultant's role requires that it be defined clearly in each instance so that the effort will not be futile and will not, even worse, miscarry and support mischief. There are also several reasons why child psychiatric consultation is more explicitly political in the colloquial sense of the word.

One major political aspect of child psychiatric consultation is that it often involves a recommendation for expenditure of resources which may be scarce and subject to problematic public policy and related controversy. This is particularly relevant to consultation involving children in that range of the spectrum of disorder which is considered psychotic because these children frequently, if not invariably, require special efforts which are expensive. For instances, child psychiatrists consulting to schools are increasingly familiar with pressures to avoid formulation and recommendations that call for residential placement because of the fear of bankruptcy on the part of the school systems (fears that are not unreasonable). Consultants thus cannot escape involvement in major societal and political problems.

The distinction between consultation and treatment is vital. When a child or family is seen by a consultant, it must be made explicit that the consultant is not undertaking to treat but only to provide expert advice to those who are responsible. That is not to say that the child and family's interests are not of great concern (indeed, they are the ultimate reason for the consultation) but, rather, to clarify the consultant's role and function.

However, a psychiatrist treating one patient may have a consultant role vis-à-vis another family member. In treating children part of the responsibility involves advice to school and family, and in these aspects of clinical work there is not infrequently an overlap with consultative function (as mentioned earlier). For instance, when marital problems appear to call for specific intervention such as therapy for one or both parents, the therapist may be asked for an opinion or may believe it justifiable to volunteer one.

One consultation situation which is immediately political in the colloquial sense is that involving a call to a hierarchical setting such as a hospital. A chief may call in an expert, for instance, confident that what he or she views as re-calcitrance in subordinates will be overriden. Whether or not to use major tranquilizers is a frequent issue of this sort, but the questions may be on any aspect of management or treatment, even on disagreements about diagnosis. Often enough such internal disagreements are candidly presented but the pos-sibility of their existence must always be considered.

In such situations the clinical specifics must take second priority to what amounts to a group process consultation. This can readily be justified as part of (in fact it always overlaps with) the clarification of the general question being asked, "Tell us what's really going on and what to do." Some of the most chal-lenging, rewarding, and valuable consultative work is in this category. Not in-frequently these situations involve clinical management emergencies including scapegoating of a patient (which will be discussed in a separate section below). When a consultant can identify and help reverse tendencies towards staff de-moralization, it ranks with the most important work he or she can do.

Such consultations demand extreme care by the consultant. Remarkably enough, some consultants bring about increased demoralization by harsh criti-cism, didactic arrogance, divisive assessments (singling out one person or group for censure) or any mixture of these. Since the need for consultation implicitly risks exposure to discovery of clinical error, the first step of the consultant ought always to be the establishment of the common ground of universal falli-bility, especially during crises.

Closely related to the politics of consultation are the resistances to con-sultative input. This is most characteristic of consultation called for by other professionals. One of its more obvious bases is the belief that what the con-sultant will present is something the original professional ought to have known in the first place. The defensive tendency, often quite subtle, is to minimize the novelty of the consultant's views—for instance, to see what is recommended as essentially the same as views or programs already considered or tried and proven valueless. This problem is one of the very strong indications of the need for the consultant to express his views specifically and avoid the nondirective interview approach to the consultees. This does *not* mean that the consultee's opinions, diagnostic formulation and ideas for treatment should not be elicited. Quite to the contrary, they must be elicited and understood clearly enough so the consultant can be specific in his or her agreements, disagreements, and additions to the thinking about, understanding, and planning for the child or family. The desirable tact can be prescribed but not specified.

Although the kind of defensiveness just summarized may be most striking with fellow professionals, it is also to be expected with parents and surrogates involved in the consultations and the considerations are invariably important.

It is surprising that in this litigious era, the legal status of consultation has been little defined in the courts. The limits of protection of the consultant's position are mentioned to underscore the importance of clarifying one's role and perceived limits of responsibility at the outset of each consultative relationship. It is equally vital that one's opinion and advice be clearly understood, and to this end it should always be put in writing after verbal presentation. If a consultant assumes too open-ended or nondirective an approach to questions from those inviting an opinion, it may be confusing and irritating at best and at worst taken by the consultee as support for actions or opinions not at all intended by the consultant. These concerns are true of all consultations but here, as with other aspects of the process, the seriousness of the clinical problems and the likelihood of limited progress when the question involves psychosis all intensify the probability of misconceptions and distress related to them.

There are, in fact, legal limits to the inviolability of the consultant's role as one of nonexecutive recommendation only. Child abuse reporting statutes in many states, for instance, mandate that a physician (among others) must intervene on the basis of a clinical impression even if in a consultant status. Even without legal constraint, clinical conviction of the need for treatment of a child may oblige a consultant on ethical grounds to go beyond simple recommendation to those who called for the consultation if the recommendation is clearly not going to be followed. The troublesome problem of consultant intervention in opposition to families' wishes will be discussed in the following section.

Difficulties with Parents

An immeasurable pall of anguish has been gratuitously cast over several generations of parents of psychotic youngsters by explicit accusations of guilt based on theories of parental causation.* This period in the history of child psychiatry, in this author's view, has seriously damaged the credibility of the profession. Unfortunately, *doctrinaire* belief in parental causation of psychosis in children is still held by some groups of psychiatrists and other mental health professionals (with some extending this idea to many other psychiatric problems of children and adolescents).

The bias is now part of conventional wisdom—it is "known" by knowledgeable parents—and this adds to the natural assumption of guilt intrinsic to human parenthood when a child has a failing of any kind. It is therefore essential to address this concern at all times, to assume its presence and to anticipate reactions based on such expectations of psychiatric bias, as much as one possibly can.

The following is an instance of an experienced consultant's failure to anticipate strong parental feelings of guilt with the result that a consultation that might have led to critical intervention was nullified:

N.S., a 12-year-old boy with recurrent school failure and "incorrigible" behavior at home and school was referred, via the mother, for consultation by his pediatrician to a child psychiatrist because the pediatrician feared that the boy might be psychotic.

Although the mother complained that N. was always disobedient and feared he would "grow up to be a criminal" and school reported he had been repeatedly disobedient for years, neither at home nor at school had he ever committed destructive or dangerous acts. He alienated many peers and adults but had friends among other rebels. He almost certainly had a moderately severe Attention Deficit Disorder together with a learning disability. In interviews, N. was well organized, related well and seemed accessible to help. He had self-critical capacity. The consultant asked the parents if the question of hyperactivity and its treatment had ever come up, and the mother answered that it had but that the pediatrician had discouraged trials of medication because it might lead to drug abuse.

The consultant believed that rapport with the parents at this point was good enough to allow an outline of the probability that untreated Attention Deficit Disorder with learning disability was likely to be a large part of the problem, although he did not at the time know the pediatrician's account of this aspect of the case. The consultant outlined a plan for extensive psychological testing (which was performed, supporting the diagnostic impression already outlined, and with no indication of psychosis), a conference with the school, and discussion with the pediatrician to overcome his reluctance to prescribe

---

*See footnote page 337.

medication for hyperactivity. The question of psychotherapy was deferred until later.

When the consultant spoke to the pediatrician he learned that it had been the mother's serious misgivings about giving N. "speed" that had prevented treatment of his presumed hyperactivity. By this time, however, although she had followed through on the recommended psychological testing, the mother had withdrawn from the consultative procedure without notifying the consultant. In a conference with the school the consultant learned that the mother had tearfully told the school that the consultant had declared her an unfit mother and was going to have N. removed from her care. She refused to speak to the consultant nor did she answer a long and carefully written letter. The father did not fully share her views and did talk with the consultant but said he was unable to modify his wife's reaction.

The pediatrician was glad to learn that the boy was not considered psychotic, but was no further ahead, otherwise, in helping him.

Precisely because this mother's reaction was extreme and with little explicit warning, is this a good example of the need to maintain a high level of alertness to the possibility of parental feelings of guilt? The mother's strong expressions of negative feelings toward her son should have been some indication of her vulnerability. In addition, the consultant should have resisted the urge to try to be helpful when the lack of data from the pediatrician made any definitive comment premature. In retrospect, this family might have been better handled by following a more limited consultation role at first, rather than the extensive one outlined and embarked upon, with the threat of "finding out everything" which may have tended to undermine the mother's defenses against her own convictions of guilt. A baseline set of interviews without conclusions with child, parents, school and pediatrician with a planned follow-up later in the year might have allowed maintenance of contact and salvaged an opportunity for effective intervention for this referral.

Some parents can become deeply, even suicidally, depressed when a psychotic child who has been impossible to manage at home is hospitalized with evidence of improvement. Such depressions are not simple to explain. They include elements of guilt exaggerated by the implication that the good effect of separation means the parent(s) was (were) bad; reactions to the loss of a symbiotic tie; or reactions to other changes in family dynamics. All of these possibilities are aspects of parental vulnerability that consultants must bear in mind whenever the presenting problem, its explication, or recommended remedy is or might be perceived by the parents as being grave.

Effective neutralization of such parental fears requires their clear identification (and again, anticipation must be stressed as the best aid to identification) by the consultant; fostering of trust in the consultant; and reassurance which should be as explicit as the identification of the fears allows.

Parents' feelings, attitudes, and behavior can contribute significantly to a psychotic child's problems, either in their beginning or continuation. To be alert for signs of parental involvement in psychotic (or other) children's problems is in no way to endorse the doctrine of parental causation of psychosis. The task of being a parent of a child with the kinds of difficulties presented by childhood psychosis is extremely draining of emotional reserves. It is in itself a situational predisposition to interpersonal difficulties from which few would be exempt. To attribute infallibility to parents is to overlook many opportunities for helping parents and children.

Sometimes children can be helped only over the objections of their parents. In those circumstances, conflict over who shall determine what is best for a child involves thorny and extremely controversial issues. Child care statutes vary from state to state in the extent to which concepts of parental abandonment justifying state custody are extrapolated from basic physical neglect or overt physical abuse. Failure to provide proper medical treatment is one ground for intervention by the State of Massachusetts. The model is the refusal of parents to give permission for surgery that is presumptively life-saving. Judges are on 24-hour call to come to hospitals to grant temporary injunctions allowing life-saving procedures over parental objection. In more long-standing situations with prolonged treatment needs, such as psychosis or other psychiatric conditions requiring 24-hour care outside of the home, more prolonged shift of custody and guardianship away from the parents may be the only way that treatment will be provided.*

Child psychiatrists consulting to courts are often involved in such questions. There follow two vignettes illustrative of the problem.

F.N. was a five-year-old girl whose parents died in an accident when she was two. She lived with an aunt and uncle and grandmother. In kindergarten, her first school experience, she quickly became assaultive to other children, explosively scratching, hitting, and even choking her peers. When the teachers

---

*The principle of obligation to oppose parental objection to vital medical recommendation was dramatically endorsed in the case of Chad Green, a four year old boy whose parents withdrew permission for continuation of the chemotherapeutic treatment of his leukemia by physicians at the Massachusetts General Hospital. The physicians brought the matter to a court and the judge ultimately appointed a guardian to implement his mandate that treatment should continue over the parents' objections. The parents defied the court order and moved to Mexico where Chad received alternative treatment (including Laetrile). The child died there. As of June of 1981 there was still an outstanding warrant for the parents' arrest for contempt of the Massachusetts court.

reported their concern to the family the relatives minimized the problem and refused to do anything about her aggressiveness. In fact, the teachers learned that F. had set several fires at home which the family had ignored. Since the child was below the age of delinquency responsibility (seven years in Massachusetts) she could not be brought to court and charged with her delinquent assaultive acts, which would have allowed court-mandated intervention. The teachers called a child psychiatry clinic and arranged a consultation for learning difficulties which the family allowed. Apprised of the situation, the psychiatrist at the clinic recommended hospital admission for psychiatric evaluation, which the relatives refused. The clinic brought this matter to court. Following the strong recommendation of the consultant child psychiatrist the judge ordered psychiatric hospital admission. The judge appointed a guardian to insure that proper medical (in this instance psychiatric) attention be provided. With the maintenance of a guardian outside of the family, family involvement was nonetheless maintained. The child, eventually not considered psychotic, is being treated in a combination of special school setting, foster care and family treatment.

P.L. an adopted boy, was 13 when he was referred to a psychiatric hospital from court where he had set a fire in a residential treatment center as part of a suicide plan. He believed that "God would take him, because he was bad." His sense of worthlessness was often conscious and approached the delusory extreme expressed in this account of his fire setting. At other times he was impulsively aggressive in league with other similar boys. The only adopted child in the family, he had an older brother and three younger sisters. Both parents were intolerant of aggressiveness and had seen their first son as a problem but "not as bad as P." They prided themselves on being good parents. They sensed that P. was "evil" as soon as he was adopted. They "could see it in his eye." Their view of his problems—extreme school recalcitrance which led to his residential treatment center placement—was that his inner badness had been resistant even to their best efforts. The parents were clearly in conflict for, despite their obvious projection, they had genuine affection for P.

P. initially continued the picture of behavior described above while in the psychiatric hospital but over an 18 month period of treatment he developed consistent positive relationships with peers and adults and related positive feelings about himself. Family meetings crystallized around the issue of his being bad in his parents' eyes.

A critical issue arose when P. was ready for discharge in the minds of the hospital staff but not in the minds of the parents. Despite a succession of successful weekends at home the parents insisted that P. was still dangerous and clearly needed continued, even indefinite hospitalization. Despite his history of fire setting, he was accepted at a residential school, but the parents refused their *permission for the transfer. At this point the hospital physicians appealed to the court. The child psychiatrist consultant to the court concurred with the hospital's assessment and recommendations, and the judge agreed. Guardianship was shifted by the court from the parents to the Department of Social Service to allow the boy to be discharged to the residential school. The parents' rejecting stance was explicit in their acceptance of this arrangement, which included demands for guarantees that they "would no longer be responsible for anything about P." Although understandably shaken, P. was nonetheless able to maintain his gains and made a successful transition to the school**

SCAPEGOATING

A major role of a consultant (or of a primary therapist who is functioning as a consultant to the interlocking groups of people and systems involved with a psychotic child) is identifying and neutralizing scapegoating. The more difficult a patient is (and psychotic patients are often the most difficult) the more prone he or she is to scapegoating. In a seeming paradox, the intense interaction inescapable in being the target of scapegoating makes the position attractive to some psychotic children as they become more organized. To children in that situation, being a scapegoat sometimes offers the reassuring feeling of a clear and stable place in the social world.

The fear felt by so many about psychotic children is basically scapegoating of a general kind, with the projection of fear of losing control onto the deviant child. The scapegoating may shift from the patient to others. What is projected onto the child initially is then displaced. With understanding and acceptance of the child, the feeling of frustration in helping the child may become part of the scapegoating of other staff members or agencies, or of family by staff and conversely of professionals by family. Schools may see parents as sinister and causing schizophrenia, so may many psychiatric professionals who should know better (see earlier section on difficulties with parents). Parents may see teachers or hospital staff as cruel and the cause of the child's problem or too rigid and unsympathetic to themselves. In hospitals or residential treatment centers, nurses or counselors may blame psychiatrists or administrators and vice versa.

It is almost inevitable that clinical effort frustrated by a child's difficult and unyielding behavior gives rise to scapegoating among staff and family members. Ekstein commented on the narcissistic threat to therapists from the implicit rejection by unresponsive, severely ill child patients and saw this as necessitating the scapegoating of such children's parents as "regression in the service

---

*The hospital social worker was extremely supportive to the parents during this entire process, mindful of the parents' vulnerability to emergence of feelings of guilt.

of the therapist's ego" (Ekstein, 1964). Consultants who have had experience with these problems can readily convey empathic understanding and may have the opportunity to relieve a great deal of tension when they come upon this phenomenon. Recognition of the intrinsic treatment difficulty and acceptance of limited goals are two major areas of useful focus.

The more intolerable or dangerous the patient's behavior, the more likely it is that this phenomenon will arise and will interfere with a helpful clinical process. Suicidal risk, firesetting, assaultiveness, and persistent running away, as well as more flagrant psychotic symptoms, such as tearing off clothes or smearing, are intrinsically dangerous or anxiety-provoking to an extreme degree and are the kinds of problems that one finds in the scapegoating situation. Many of the interagency struggles and doctrinaire disputes between advocacy groups and professional groups represent self-perpetuating, institutionalized efforts at scapegoating. Sometimes aroused advocates succeed in blocking professional recommendations. The only effective route to preserving reasonable therapeutic programs in the face of these obstacles is reaching a common agreement on the child's needs and problems and focusing on specific areas of both the problems and the programs designed to address them.

Violent delinquents with episodes of disorganization give rise to classic tugs of war between juvenile court services designed for delinquents and mental health departments. The former emphasize that the child's mental health problems make him or her impossible to handle with ordinary delinquents. The mental health department points to the destructive potential as beyond the scope of facilities which are equipped to handle more helplessly disorganized youngsters, even if that population may also be quite violent at times. This general argument can never be settled by a consultant. However, the consultant can help all concerned to focus on the particular child and the particular facilities available and determine the most workable placement to try. He or she can also offer follow-up consultation to assist with the program development.

If a psychotic child in crisis gives evidence of control in one setting and not another or if, in an interview, he or she comes quickly into control, the problematic setting should be scrutinized for scapegoating issues. Bolstering the environment may suffice to allow the child to stay. If this cannot be done promptly enough to forestall a dangerous situation, a short-term placement is the next arrangement to seek while the home or school is provided with help in changing responses to the child. Even long-term placements, in hospitals or residential schools, are properly regarded as temporary with efforts made to help the home or its equivalent accept the child after adequate changes may have taken place. Clearly, since the problem is in the balance between parent/surrogates and the psychotic child, the change does not have to be all in the child.

SUMMARY

When the child psychiatrist consults in a problem involving psychosis, he or she must be prepared to deal with confusion and intense anxiety in all parameters of the clinical situation: interpersonal, political, diagnostic, prognostic, theoretical, clinical management, and treatment.

The utmost in sensitivity, tact, and clarity is called for so that those in the field—parents, surrogates, referring professionals and/or agency representatives—are supported and enabled to cooperate in what are often complex arrangements, with frustrating delays and disagreements at every step along the road to full assessment and implementation of treatment plans.

The range of the diagnostic spectrum in psychiatry called psychosis includes the most serious problems. The overall task of the consultant may be epitomized as helping all concerned maintain realistic recognition of the difficulties without slipping into the ready stereotyping of the problems as impossible.

In no other area of consultative work is there more demand for a creative blend of advocacy, education, demonstration, and diplomacy.

REFERENCES

Beres D: Ego deviation and the concept of schizophrenia. *Psychoanal Stud Child* 2:164–235, 1956.

Blau A: Nature of childhood schizophrenia. *J Amer Acad Child Psych* 1: 225–230, 1962.

Creak M: Schizophrenic syndrome in childhood, further progress report of a working party. *Dev Med Child Neurol* 6:530–535, 1964.

Despert JL. Differential diagnosis between obsessive-compulsive neurosis and schizophrenia in children. *Proc Amer Psychanal Assn* 44:240–253, 1955.

DSM III, Washington, DC, American Psychiatric Association, 1980.

Ekstein R: On the acquisition of speech in the autistic child. *The Reiss–Davis Clinic Bull* 1:63–79, 1964.

Gair D and Salomon A: Diagnostic aspects of psychiatric hospitalization of children. *Am J Orthopsych* 32:445–461, 1962.

Gair D, Hersch C, and Weisenfeld S: Successful psychotherapy of severe emotional disturbance in a young retarded boy. *J Am Acad Child Psych* 19:257–269, 1980.

Kanner L: Autistic disturbances of affective contact. *The Nerv Child* 2:217–250, 1943.

Laufer M and Gair D: Childhood schizophrenia. *The Schizophrenic Syndrome*, Bellak L and Loeb L (eds.) (Grune & Stratton: New York) 1969, pp 378–461.

Potter H: Schizophrenia in children. *Am J Psych* 12:1253–1270, 1935.

Wilking V and Paoli C: The hallucinatory experience. *J Amer Acad Child Psych* 5:431–440, 1966.

22

Child Abuse: Role of the Child Psychologist in Abuse and Neglect

John B. Reinhart

A child psychiatrist recently said his current advice to pediatric colleagues who consult him about the management of children suspected of having been abused was as follows, "I do not urge them to report these cases since the child welfare system is not able to handle them and I have concerns about these children in foster care." It is not difficult to understand the frustration of the child psychiatrist who deals with problems of neglect and abuse of children, but one cannot condone this passive attitude and unwillingness to act as a child advocate. There are no simple answers to complicated problems, and child abuse and neglect may be one of the most profound and disturbing matters with which pediatricians or child psychiatrists have to deal.

Child abuse and neglect are only the tip of the iceberg and beneath its surface is society's apathy toward adequate child care, the lack of conviction that childrens' interests are equal to parents' interests, and the wish for rather simple answers, such as "hotlines," for these difficult problems. In addition, the problems of child abuse do not belong to any one discipline. There is a tremendous need for increased communication among the child welfare system, the juvenile courts, pediatric care facilities, police systems, and educational systems. Collaboration by all of the professionals who deal with children and the development of mutual respect is absolutely necessary.

The child psychiatrist who becomes a consultant about child abuse must be certain of his or her definition of the problem. One can see abuse as a range of inadequate to hostile child-care practices: (1) allowing a child to be un-immunized; (2) using the bottle as a pacifier at bedtime, leading to dental caries and iron deficiency anemia; (3) putting a three-month-old child on a dressing table without protection from falling; (4) keeping caustic agents in soda bottles that two- and three-year-olds may drink from; (5) the impulsive lashing-out of an angry parent leading to physical injury and even to the murder. There are varying viewpoints among teachers, physicians, policemen, neighbors, parents, and other adults about when discipline becomes abuse. Many parents feel it is appropriate to discipline, even an infant, by spanking at an age when the child has no cognitive awareness of his misdeeds.

Like pediatrics and child psychiatry, juvenile law has only slowly developed out of adult-oriented legal systems. Dichotomies of adult or parent versus child exist, and child welfare systems theoretically must encourage justice for both parent and child. Often what seems fair to a parent can be seen as unjust or not in the best interests of the child. The child psychiatrist as a consultant becomes involved in adversary systems, parent vs. child, and punitive vs. therapeutic philosophies, and will find no easy solutions.

THE EVALUATION OF THE ABUSED CHILD
AND HIS OR HER FAMILY

The child psychiatrist, because of his training in both general and child psychiatry, because of his background in child development, and because of his medical training, particularly if he has had some pediatric experience, is the ideal professional to evaluate the abused child or to be the leader of a multidisciplinary team. It is imperative that not only the child be evaluated but also those adults who may be given the responsibility for his care after the abusive incident. The capacity of the adult to care for a child cannot be adequately evaluated through psychiatric interview alone. The child should be seen in his interaction with the adult caretakers. If in the initial evaluation of the abusive situation, it is deemed not in the best interests of the child to return him to his natural parents, alternative caretaking situations must be considered. This is particularly true for the abused infant because of the likelihood of more serious physical injury to the less ambulatory and less developed child if the child is returned to an abusive environment. The following two case histories demonstrate the dilemma for the professional.

A young, middle-class, white couple in their mid-20s brought their four-month infant, a twin, to the hospital because she had gone into coma. Not only did the child have retinal hemorrhages and evidence of a subdural hematoma, but also evidence of an old fracture of a femur with callus formation. They denied knowledge of any trauma whatever, and the admitting physician in his notes on the case wrote, "doubt abuse as a cause." An ophthalmological consultant made a brief reference to trauma but said the findings were more probably due to another cause. It was only when a more suspicious social worker asked a chaplain to talk to this young couple that the father confessed, not only to the incident causing the fractured leg, but also to shaking the baby, the probable cause of the subdural hematoma. In this particular case the young man did not have a history of severe abuse in his own growing up. It was, indeed, a family of high moral standards and overcontrolled rather than the opposite. This young man in his childhood had been admonished about any kind of aggressive play because of the possible upset to his invalid mother. He was not a person who had ever been able to lose his temper or was ever out of control. Only the stress of the crying infant, and his inability to relieve the baby's distress, seemed to tip the scales, as he himself described it, "from discipline to abuse."

More commonly parents do not admit abuse and profess ignorance about the cause of injury. The identification of the abusive parent is often based on circumstantial evidence, and a confession may be some indication of a psychological strength. In this case, the young parents demonstrated psychological strengths. Their own childhood histories were healthy ones and their family support systems were strong. Additionally, it was the judgment of the district attorney that prosecution of the family was not warranted and the responsibility for management of this case should rest with the child welfare system. Those of us who evaluated the family felt that it was reasonable to leave both children with their parents provided the mother and father received psychiatric help. The father's admission, an unusual occurrence, was an indication of the parents' willingness to admit deficits in parenting and to improve their parenting capacities. The prognosis in this situation seemed good for the marriage and for the caretaking of the babies, but the family would be changed and the question of whether the parents would adapt to the damaged twin was one that only time would answer.

Another case with a longer follow-up may also illustrate the dilemma.

Twin girls, Wilma and Karen, were born to a young couple who were married in 1973 and who had two sons, Eugene, born in 1974, and Steven, born in 1975. The marriage had been a stormy one. The parents had separated, but had reunited and late in 1975 the young mother found herself again pregnant. Wilma and Karen were born in March 1976, Karen weighing not quite four pounds and Wilma weighing less than three pounds. They were healthy premature twins, but did have persistent abnormal cardiac vessel (patent ductus arteriosis). Karen was discharged from the hospital in a month and Wilma was discharged after six weeks, but Wilma was readmitted at age five months for a surgical correction.

From the beginning this was seen as a high-risk family and several agencies offered services, but these were resisted. In the summer of 1976, the young mother again left her husband and took the children with her to live with a girl-friend. During this time, Wilma, then six months old, was brought to the hospital for being given a medication for one of the other children by accident. Also at this time the twins were failing to thrive, and a report of suspected abuse and neglect was made. As a result of examinations of the two older siblings, as well as the twins, legal action was taken. In this case, there was a very real danger that all the children could continue to be seriously neglected. Because of their age and because there were no residential placements where the family could be involved in treatment while the child was in protected care, foster home place-ment seemed the only viable alternative for the twins. However, the older children were returned to the natural parents and supportive services were recommended for the family.

At the time of placement in foster care, the young parents began in coun-seling. Pediatric cardiologists gave the opinion that the twins should be in foster care until they were at least a few years old. When the twins were four, their parents—who had profited greatly from their counseling experience—petitioned the court to have the children returned to them. Lawyers representing the foster parents who were resisting the twins' removal, lawyers for the natural parents, and lawyers for the state agency for children and youth services agreed to a total evaluation of the children, the foster family, and the natural parents. This was done.

Karen initially was seen as a small, developmentally delayed little girl who didn't begin to walk until she was nineteen-months old. Then she did well and, though petite, became active and verbal and behaved more aggressively than her sister. Wilma was brought into the foster home at age ten months, and weighed ten pounds. She also was developmentally delayed, began to walk at about twenty months and was seen as "more self-assured." In the fall of 1979 both twins started in a preschool and were doing well. The twins were seen separately and Wilma was found to be the more talkative and outgoing. However, in the interview during her observation as well as in observations with her biological parents, her speech deteriorated markedly. Karen was seen as a more shy and anxious child. Her speech deteriorated in these situations even more than her sister's and her play was much less structured.

Observations of the twins with their natural parents showed that the mother was a pleasant woman, but the father tended to be aloof. Again, Wilma was quite open but Karen kept to herself, preferring to involve herself in home-making play. After observing the children with both their natural and foster parents, the child psychiatrist attempted to get the children to talk about their preferences for living situations, and both had great difficulty in talking about leaving their current living situations with their foster families. In the play sessions with the foster parents, the children did quite well, and both foster parents were very supportive and sensitive in their interaction with the children.

Both the natural parents were seen for psychological evaluation as well. The mother was viewed as an outspoken, assertive young woman with some tendency to mood swings greater than normal and a tendency to immature behavior. The father was seen as a quiet young man, anxious and very defensive.

People who had worked with this couple reported on the great progress they had made since the time when the twins were placed in foster care. The older boy was in kindergarten and the younger in a preschool. The family moved into a well-kept apartment and the father, who had had a problem with alcoholism, had not been drinking for some time. The only negatives were that, at the time of the evaluation, he was out of work and both the boys had missed over thirty days of school during the year.

It was the feeling of a team of evaluators that in spite of the great efforts and progress on the part of these natural parents, the twins were not psychologically strong enough to be moved from their foster home where they had been doing well. And, of course, they viewed their foster parents as their psychological parents. It was recommended that the children be continued in their current placement until they completed at least one full year of primary school, which would given them an additional three years of placement and, it was hoped, help them stabilize psychologically. At that time another evaluation could be done.

It was appreciated that the natural parents had performed in a maximum capacity in rehabilitation efforts but the stress of a move at this time for the twins was hazardous. In addition, this would put an additional stress on the natural parents who had two little children, ages six and five, who had not yet demonstrated their stabilities.

Obviously, this judgment met with agreement from the foster parents and their lawyers. At the same time, the natural parents and their lawyer were disappointed. However, the ultimate resolution of such judgments is not in the hands of the psychiatrist, either lawyer, or the children and youth services agency. The ultimate disposition of such cases rests with the judge, who is the final arbitrator. His or her abilities to make a fair decision will then be based on previous experience, understanding of the psychological development of children, and judgments as to the best interests of the child which may not necessarily be in the best interests of the parents. Theoretically, what is best for children should be welcomed by their parents. However, it is not reasonable to expect natural parents to agree with decisions which may not appear to be in their own best interests.

In the legal system there is a growing awareness of the complexities of these decisions and, it is hoped over time judges and lawyers will look to other professionals who have competencies in the areas of family dynamics and child development to assist them in making these very serious dispositions.

In the investigation of the abusive incident provisions should be made, particularly in the case of an infant, for the baby's protection while the family is evaluated. Because of the need for such a program, a pilot project, the Parental Stress Center, was instituted as a collaborative venture on the part of the Children's Hospital, the Children and Youth Services, the Juvenile Court, and the Child Guidance Center in Pittsburgh. There the residential program provided a child care facility on a 24-hour basis with additional programs in infant stimulation so that optimum child development was provided outside of the care of the natural parents. In addition, the natural parents were involved in an evaluation and a therapeutic program over several months to determine their capacities to have the child returned to their care. A case history will illustrate this type of program.

Josie, age six months, was admitted to a residential placement following a hospitalization for multiple parietal bone fractures and subdural hematomas. Her father, Joe, age nineteen, had initially called a hotline, admitting that he had struck his daughter and that her head had swollen. He and Josie's mother, Cathy, age 18, had been living in a common-law marriage since shortly after the baby's birth and were in the process of moving to an apartment on the day of the injury.

Josie's mother was the oldest of five children, the first of three girls. Though her family was a relatively stable one, her father was an impatient man and abusive to his children, particularly his sons. The parents quarreled about discipline of the children and on one occasion Cathy had run away from home. She had appeared in Juvenile Court at age 16. She also was in Juvenile Court for shoplifting on one occasion but was returned to her family after some counseling. It was after she returned home that she became pregnant.

Joe, the father, was the youngest of six children in a dysfunctional family. When he was two years old the family moved from West Virginia to Pittsburgh. Because of the father's abusiveness, Joe spent some time in a juvenile shelter and eventually was returned with his siblings to his mother's care. She had a liaison with an alcoholic man. Joe was involved with the court and placed in a youth group when he was almost twelve years old. Soon after, his mother was critically injured in a car accident, suffering brain damage. Older brothers were involved in robberies, shootings and other violent behaviors, and Joe was also in and out of juvenile court. In May of 1977 he suffered a motorcycle accident with serious head injuries but signed out of the hospital against medical advice.

In the residential program this baby seemed to recover from her skull fractures and to make appropriate developmental progress. The mother showed good parenting skills but the father seemed to compete with the baby for the mother's attention.

When Josie was a year old, Joe left the city and was thought to have gone to another state. The baby was transferred to a day care program. Cathy passed her GED and started community college courses part-time. After being discharged from the day care program, Cathy and Josie moved to the maternal great grandparents' home. There was some concern that Josie's father had returned to the Pittsburgh area, but Cathy denied any contact with him. A few months later Cathy rejoined Joe, taking Josie to another state in defiance of a court order. Cathy's mother reported the absence and her feeling that Cathy had been talking with Joe over the phone and making arrangements to join him.

Subsequently, it was learned that Joe was in jail on a traffic violation. By this time Josie was 21 months old and Cathy 5 months pregnant. At a hearing before a judge, mother and child were placed in the custody of maternal grandparents and Joe was forbidden to contact them.

Cathy delivered of a baby girl when Josie was two years old, and this child was placed directly from the hospital into a children and youth services preadoption home when Cathy voluntarily released the baby for adoption, a decision she had come to during her pregnancy.

Early in the program it was possible to see that this young father had little potential for a deep investment in others. He cared about his wife and children as much as he could, but he had little ability to control his feelings or to stay at a job for any length of time. He was an appealing young man, but had almost no ability to tolerate frustration.

Josie's mother also was an appealing and attractive young woman, but immature; unable to see any negatives in her husband's behavior, she rationalized everything. Her return to her own parents was only temporary until she could rejoin Joe, and she jeopardized Josie's life by so doing. It was only by accident that children and youth services learned that Joe was in jail and of Cathy and Josie's whereabouts. In giving up her second child for adoption, Cathy may have shown some evidence of maturation.

A program such as that at the Parental Stress Center is successful, we feel, in evaluating the parental capacity to care for a child. We must admit that there are many adults who are unable to adequately parent, but obtaining hard data to justify removing children from the care of natural parents or terminating parental rights is mandatory.

Such a program as illustrated is not usually available but could be developed in any communities. There are experimental programs using foster homes, where more intensive involvement of the natural parents with their children may be possible, and the Parental Stress Center has been involved in such programs. These are difficult and require a great deal from foster parents as well as from staff involved in being with both foster parents and natural parents. They do give an opportunity to make evaluations of natural parents' abilities to care for their children over several weeks or months, and afford a much more accurate evaluation of the children's behavior as well as the natural parents' behaviors. Such data is absolutely necessary for any consultant to make a judgment about return of a child.

EVALUATION OF ABUSED CHILDREN

Obviously an evaluation will depend on several factors including the age of the child, his previous experience with his family, and his neurological status at the time of the evaluation in relation to the abusive incident. It has been observed that the neglected child, even as a tiny infant, tends to relate better to objects than he does to human beings. This has been observed and seems to be a way of differentiating the organic failure-to-thrive child who relates to humans from the nonorganic failure-to-thrive child who relates better to objects. If hospitalized, unlike normal children who turn to parents for nurturance, the abused child tends to not distinguish parents from others and may be apathetic and withdrawn, turning to no one. Additionally, these children show much more anxiety about their hospital environment than one would expect.

Early in the work with abused children and their parents, it was noted that some children seem to feel it necessary to parent the parent. These children tend to be more compliant than one would expect and to constantly search the faces of adults to gain cues on how they may behave. In interacting with their parents, who usually are emotionally unavailable to the children, they make repeated attempts to become engaged. Sometimes they are aggressive in their behavior and said to be hyperactive.

The verbal child, usually near age three or older, may be able to talk about the abusive incident. He may say, "Daddy hurt me," or "Mommy hit me with a shoe," and particularly in the investigation of sexual abuse, may be quite frank and descriptive in recounting the incident. It is important to remember that children in these clinical situations usually report matters about which it is difficult to fantasize and a rule of thumb is that the child should be believed rather than disbelieved.

The older child who has been living in an abusive environment, when examined in an interview or in psychological testing, will be quite alert to the examiner's behavior. He tends to be more anxious and easily distracted by noise or movement. These older children are concerned about doing well and behaving properly and this anxiety tends to make them appear to have difficulty in listening and paying attention. They often are inhibited in their speech, as well, and have delays in their development of language. During the exam they will answer impulsively rather than take the time to think through possible alternatives. And often they are skilled in avoiding interrogation about themselves and their families. They can be frustrating children to examine, and one may gain some empathy for the parents that have been caring for them.

Whether children can provoke abuse is not clear. However, studies by Chess, Birch and Thomas (1979), and their identification of congenital activity types and the difficult child—coupled with Brazelton's (1973) observations on infants and their abilities to give feedback to parents—may lead to the conclusion that there are, indeed, infants who are more difficult to manage, even for relatively well adjusted and psychologically healthy parents. However, in a study (1969) of children who had accidents, some of whom later turned out to have been abused (25 percent), we were unable to identify any difference in the congenital activity type between children who were abused and a control population, though the accident children were significantly higher in activity, both as infants and as latency age children (Gregg and Elmer, 1969).

EVALUATION OF THE ABUSIVE PARENT

The identification of the abusive parent, in legal terminology, is often based on circumstantial evidence. Rarely do parents admit to abuse and a confession may be an indication of a psychological strength (although in the last case cited above this was not true). More commonly parents deny and profess ignorance about the abusive episode.

Past histories of these parents often show that they were expected to meet excessive demands by their parents or that they lived in an emotionally unstable family where they were not able to have reasonable security and could not depend on their parents for consistent care. They may be found to be people who look for their children to care for them rather than vice versa. They often seem unconcerned about the child or see the child as "bad" or "out to get me." They are emotionally isolated, have little regard for themselves, and expect to be rejected by others. They are usually without friends and have little support from family and spouse. In talking about the child's injuries, they tend to give multiple and contradictory explanations or no explanations at all for the injuries of the child.

Abusive parents sometimes have histories of hyperactivity or convulsive episodes in early childhood, other symptoms of impulsive behavior, poor school performance and school drop-out, multiple types of employment and frequent moves. Alcoholism and drug addiction are not uncommon among them, as well. In themselves none of these characteristics is uniquely present in abuse cases, but when one gathers a profile in such situations with a history of the family and the physical injuries of the child, almost inevitably the conclusion must be that the child has been living in an abusive environment. From the medical standpoint, it is not necessary to identify the abusive parent, though that may be the legal aim. Rather the goal of medical professionals is to identify the family as needing help with parenting and the child as needing protection. That is the manner in which the physician should attack the problem.

CHILD PSYCHIATRIC CONSULTATION IN MEDICAL SETTINGS IN REGARD TO ABUSE AND NEGLECT

The impetus for the recognition of child abuse and neglect came out of pediatric settings from pediatricians such as John Caffey, the father of pediatric radiology, Paul Woolley at the Children's Hospital of Michigan, and Henry Kempe and his colleagues at the University of Colorado Medical Center. Ironically, however, the private practitioners of pediatrics or family medicine, as well as surgical specialists dealing with trauma—(orthopedists and neurosurgeons) have not been an important source of identification or referral—this in spite of efforts at educating and encouraging suspicion of possibly abusive incidents. Many more reports come out of hospitals where groups of professionals or Suspected Child Abuse/Neglect (SCAN) teams are involved in providing support and programs of identification and reporting.

Unlike in the solo practitioner's office, in the hospital setting other professionals are available to offer each other mutual support and consultation so that the burden of reporting can be shared. Dealing with the angry, upset parent who must be told, even if obliquely, of the suspicion of trauma as a cause of a child's injuries is not easy. Practitioners who do report should be commended.

George, age thirteen months, was seen by his pediatrician, a woman, for a complaint of a chest cold. On examination he was found to have bruises of various ages over his lower face, trunk, and arms. There was no explanation for the bruises and the pediatrician told the mother of her concern. She had cared for the baby after his birth until George was only a few months old, when his mother left her parents' home to join her husband in the service. The father was known as an impulsive and somewhat aggressive young man in the community. The mother was asked to bring George back for reexamination in a few days. Five days later George was seen again with a mild ear infection, but also with new bruises on his abdomen.

The physician thereupon told the mother of her suspicions of possible abuse, the need for investigation, and the legal requirement for her to make a report to Children and Youth Services. This was done by telephone and a parent aide was sent to the doctor's office to pick up the child. In the meantime, a skeletal survey showed a questionable fracture of a clavicle. The boy's father then came to the physician's office and was quite aggressive and threatening.

Telephone consultation by the pediatrician with the child psychiatrist was directed toward her concern about the correctness of her action. She was reassured that reporting was legally required and proof of abuse was not her mandate. Additionally, she was reminded of the high mortality rate (three to four percent) and morbidity rate (25 percent of victims suffering permanent injury) associated with such syndromes, and of the need for immediate action. Also she was complimented on her firm, though kind and empathetic, stand with both parents.

The father behaved in much the same way in future contacts with children and youth service personnel as he did with the reporting physician. He had a long history of difficulty in controlling his aggressive behavior as a child as well as in adolescent years, and had been involved in court procedures previously.

Aggressive behavior is anxiety-provoking, and the best of professionals can be made to feel uncomfortable and uncertain. Child psychiatrists consulting in medical settings, because of their interest in behavior, may be helpful by stimulating the organization of multidisciplinary teams to help physicians and other professionals to understand their feelings about abusive adults, about reporting, and about dealing with another person's aggression. These are functions which the child psychiatric consultant should be able to do well.

THE CHILD PSYCHIATRIST AS CONSULTANT TO THE SCHOOL

Most of the severe cases of physical injury involve the young child before he enters school. Because he is physically less vulnerable and can better avoid an adult's aggression, the school age child is safer from serious physical danger. But it is probable that the incidence of abuse in school age children is as high as it is at any age.

Before attending school, children are not available for public inspection and, unless they are seen in the medical setting for physical exams, immunizations and the like, signs of abuse may not be identified. Schools, like children's hospitals, can be thought of as "disguised mental health centers." In the school, as in the hospital, there are a wide range of differences in children and their families, in families' attention to children's needs and in their disciplinary

attitudes. Because of their close daily contact with children and their opportunities to compare children with their peers, teachers are in a unique position
to identify and report abuse early and to intervene directly with the children
as well as their families.

Like the public in general, schools have been reluctant to accept the fact
that child abuse can and does occur. There are few teachers who are unaware
that some of the children who enter their classrooms are poorly cared for, are
developmentally delayed, and have unexplained bruises and other marks which
may be caused by cigarette burns and the like. There is the human tendency to
deny and rationalize, to say "active children do get bruised," but as public
awareness increases, there has been growing attention to child abuse in school
systems.

As with all professionals, among teachers there is a range of behaviors and
attitudes regarding this responsibility for identifying abusive situations. Some
teachers do not see this as part of their professional responsibility, while others
are very sensitive to it and interested in involving other professionals in providing the best possible protection of children. In some states, teachers are required to report suspected abuse; but in all states, teachers are encouraged as
private citizens to report suspected child abuse and neglect. In some states, such
as Hawaii, schools are actively involved in the identification of abuse and neglect
and, accordingly, a greater proportion of reports involve school age children.

The in-service training opportunities and knowledge about child abuse and
neglect vary, but all teachers should be familiar with their states' reporting laws,
particularly with the definition of reportable conditions, reporting procedures,
and their own specific obligations and legal protections in regard to reporting.

The child psychiatrist who would be involved with the school system as
consultant might play a number of roles. Certainly he could be an educator of
the school system about the problem of child abuse and neglect, and he might
be a motivating force to establish school committees whose tasks would be to
facilitate identification, help with reporting procedures, and even develop some
treatment programs.

Parent–teacher associations might hold meetings devoted to discussions of
child abuse and neglect with members of the child protective service agency in
the community and other professionals such as social workers, pediatricians, and
child psychiatrists who would talk about these matters.

Another area in which the consultant can help a school system is in
helping add to a curriculum material to teach child rearing. Schools should
develop curricula including child growth and development, sex education,
family life education and, perhaps, even programs in which the adolescent can
care for children and learn about the stress of being a child caretaker. It is even
conceivable that schools could be persuaded to develop day care nurseries for
young infants which would serve as community support systems for young

families who need to have children cared for while they shop, keep medical appointments and the like, or just need respite from the demands of a child. Nursery school teachers could become members of junior high school faculties, with child psychiatric consultation, and create innovative programs.

Yet another rule for the consultant is as a school's adviser on discipline. Spanking in the schools is supported by the Supreme Court. Though all states have child abuse reporting laws, few prohibit spanking in the school. The child psychiatrist, acting as a psychiatric consultant to the school, would have an opportunity to attempt to influence the thinking and philosophy of principals and teacher regarding the entire matter of the discipline of children.

Child psychiatrists who are consultants to school systems should keep in mind that the prevalence of child abuse is high and abuse may be one of the major causes of or contributing factors to developmental delays and learning disabilities. Child psychiatrists are in a position to stimulate in-service training programs regarding these matters. As consultants to the schools, they can stimulate the development of SCAN teams within the schools. It is much easier for a group of professionals than an individual teacher to consider the matter of whether to report. The team of a school nurse and principal or senior teacher can be of great consultative help to the individual teacher who suspects abuse.

CHILD PROTECTIVE SERVICE AGENCIES

Child protective service agencies are usually the agencies with the responsibility of receiving abuse reports and making plans for the care of the abused child and his family. The need for adequate child caretaking services in the United States far exceeds the capabilities of the child welfare system. For the most part, child welfare systems are inadequately funded and inadequately staffed. Their staff turnover, even in the best of agencies, is great, and continuity of services is difficult. For all of these reasons, other systems, such as health care, judicial, and school, as well as the public, are critical of them. Everyone is slow to accept the fact that, in the United States, we do not have a national policy for child care. Therefore, there is a great deal of frustration and anger to be dealt with by the child psychiatrist who functions as a consultant.

Child welfare systems have a schizophrenic charge in the sense that they have a responsibility for adequate care and protection of the child at the same time that they are given the responsibility for the care and just treatment of parents. They are often dealing with advocates for the "sanctity of the family" at all costs, and it sometimes seems as if there is no way of making decisions which will seem equitable to both the child and the parents.

On receiving reports of suspected abuse, child welfare systems are required to make an investigation. Obviously, the investigation of these reports depends on multiple factors: the training and experience of the child welfare worker, the amount of time available for the investigation, and the availability of others to assist in the investigation. In the case of the infant who is suspected of being subjected to abuse, of primary importance is the protection of the infant from further injury because of the high incidence of repeated episodes of abuse and the fact that the young child is more susceptible to serious injury. In these instances, it is necessary to lean over backwards to protect the child, which also means separating the child from his natural environment and placing him in either temporary foster homes, hospitals, or institutions. Because of the child's attachment to his caretakers and the fact that prolonged separation may also be abusive in effect, it is essential that judgments about the child's caretaking situation be made as soon as possible. Once the infant begins to develop attachments to another caretaker, one is faced with the dilemma of taking that child away from a second caretaker to return to his first.

For these reasons, child welfare systems often request consultation from professionals who are skilled in child development, developmental and neurological assessment of infants and children, and the psychiatric assessment of adult caretakers. The child psychiatrist should be able to attend to these matters, and certainly should be able to be the head of a team of multiple disciplines for such evaluations.

Those child psychiatrists who become consultants to child protective agencies and other public agencies must be aware of the fact that their examinations and opinions often will have to come to the attention of the juvenile court. Here they will be subjected to interrogation and crossexamination by attorneys for the child welfare system, attorneys for parents, and attorneys for the child or the guardian ad litem.

THE ROLE OF THE POLICE OFFICER IN CHILD ABUSE

At a SCAN meeting, a police officer said, "I'm only here to see if you'll do anything, because if you really are able to do something, I will refer a lot of cases to you; on my beat there is a lot of abuse of children." Police officers are in a unique position to identify and protect the abused child. They usually know the community in which they work and sometimes have a history of involvement with many families in a way that no other public servant does. They have opportunities while walking their beat, while involved in making arrests or conducting searches and investigations, to observe families and the way they care for their children. Police have a wide range of responsibilities and their responsibilities in the area of child abuse vary, depending on the nature of state laws regarding identification and reporting, their local communities and the responsibilities of other agencies such as child protective services agencies, and the reporting by other professionals such as physicians and teachers. The Los Angeles Police Department has a specialized unit, the Abused and Battered Child Unit, and the police in California have a far more active role in case management than is typical in other states. In California, the Central Register of Reports is maintained by the Department of Justice, Bureau of Criminal Identification and Investigation, the only statewide register in the country maintained by a police authority. Such specialized units often have responsibility for the education or other police officers and arrange for interdisciplinary workshops. The Honolulu Police Department has a woman sergeant who is especially adept in the interviewing and management of sexual abuse problems, as well as other types of abuse.

Traditionally, personnel in law enforcement have attempted to avoid becoming involved in family disputes. They have felt that family matters are privileged, that one cannot intervene unless an absolute emergency occurs, and that their role is to preserve the sanctity of the home. These are delicate matters, and the edge between abuse and discipline is sometimes ill-defined.

Police officers brought an eight-year-old boy to the hospital emergency room. An officer, in talking with the boy at the school playground, had noted a black eye and learned that his father had beaten him. On examination in the emergency room the boy had parallel bruising marks such as inflicted with a whip or electric cord across his back and upper thighs. The officers brought in his father who clearly stated that he had given the boy a beating as a disciplinary measure. These officers knew this family, knew the father's propensity for abusive discipline, and correctly brought him to the emergency room where physicians made official reports to the child welfare system. The officers, though firm with the father, did not act in a punitive fashion and viewed him and the family as needing some type of psychologic help.

Traditionally, the police have two general functions: criminal law enforcement and emergency aid. However, as Flammang (1970) points out, the function of modern police in reality is to be involved in more activities unrelated to crime control than police or the public recognize. In their role as law enforcers, police are usually viewed as authority figures and a threat. As providers of emergency care or protection, they are viewed as supportive. In child abuse cases, a policeman may function in either role, depending on how he views the situation.

Experienced police officers can often get admissions of abusive behavior without being threatening because they are viewed as people of authority. It may also be that because they are less naive than many professionals and have had more experience with abusive situations, they can interrogate more comfortably.

Ideally, when police become involved in an abusive case they should focus on the condition and welfare of the child. Attention to the criminal aspects of abuse tends to be punitive and not particularly helpful to the family, the parent, or the child.

Police should be responsible in several ways. In those jurisdictions where cases of suspected abuse or neglect are reported to them, they should immediately investigate the reports. In jurisdictions where the law requires reports to be filed with some other agency, such as the child protective service agencies, police should promptly report to that agency. When children require medical care, then officers should take them to the nearest hospital that cares for children or, possibly, to the child protective agency. In addition, police officers should observe whatever is relevant about the incidents they report. Such information will be valuable in the ultimate disposition of these cases, either by the child protective service agency or in the juvenile court.

Child psychiatrists could be used as consultants to the police in regard to the management of individual cases, and in the development of training programs for police personnel. This will not develop until child psychiatrists have more involvement with police in their work, a hope for the future.

THE CHILD PSYCHIATRIST AS A CONSULTANT IN THE JUVENILE COURT IN MATTERS OF ABUSE AND NEGLECT

Child abuse or neglect cases may be dealt with in either or both the criminal and civil courts. The criminal court is involved in the prosecution of the abuser and detention or rehabilitation of the defendant, but has no role in protecting the victim of abuse.

It is in the juvenile court that there is jurisdiction and authority to deal with children who are abused, dependent, or neglected. This jurisdiction continues until the age of majority, 18 years in most states.

The juvenile court did not exist prior to the turn of the century, and the first courts in Denver and Chicago were a tribute to the growing awareness on the part of law and the courts that the problems of children were family problems and needed to be dealt with in a special manner. With the Gault decision in 1968 a movement to a recognition of the rights of children gained momentum and has led to the courts' obligation to ensure that a child's safety and interests are protected. Now almost all states have statutes which provide that a guardian ad litem be appointed for the child. The guardian ad litem is a third party, usually a lawyer, whose responsibility is to provide independent legal representation apart from that of the children and youth services system or the parents.

The child psychiatrist may be asked to be a consultant in regard to matters of abuse and neglect by the children and youth services system, by a guardian ad litem, or by a lawyer representing either a foster parent or the natural parents. Ideally, the child psychiatrist can attempt to get agreement by lawyers for the child welfare agency, the parents, and the child for a single evaluation or a team of evaluators who would see all of the parties involved. Such an evaluation could then be given to all of the concerned parties as well as to the court. The child psychiatrist then could appear in court to present the findings of the evaluation and be available for cross-examination.

The philosophy of the legal system is somewhat different from the traditional medical system in that it is adversarial. There is presentation of evidence and opinion from both sides, that of parents and that of child advocates, and the ultimate decision is that of the judge.

Consultants should have the consent of those they evaluate to share information with the court; this is implied in the request for consultation. Obviously discussion is needed of the fees for the time necessary to do the evaluation, to prepare a report, and to appear in court.

If the child psychiatrist is a consultant to only one of the parties, to the child or to the child welfare agency, it is worthwhile to seek a conference with the attorney to discuss the lines of questioning and review the data he wishes to present. It is wise to submit a written report with recommendations and supporting data which can be submitted to the court.

From the standpoint of the child psychiatrist, it would be ideal to be a consultant to a court which would use a team of behavioral scientists to make assessments and give opinions to the court. This has been suggested in family courts in matters of custody but still is not a common way for the child psychiatrist to be used.

Occasionally, a child psychiatrist may be asked to be an expert witness to offer opinions, based on training and experience, without examining the child or parents. This can be viewed as the kind of consultation which is defined as "the act of seeking information or advice; meeting to exchange ideas and talk things over." As in all dialogues, there needs to be appreciation and respect for each other's position in law and medicine. The child psychiatrist's role as a consultant in legal matters related to child abuse will depend on his or her availability, adaptability, and ability, and on the court and lawyer's perception of the child psychiatrist as helpful to them in their work.

REFERENCES

Brazelton TB: Neonatal behavioral assessment search. *Clin Dev Med* 50, 1973.

Flammang CJ: *The Police and the Underprotected Child* (Charles C Thomas: Springfield, IL) 1970.

Gregg GS and Elmer E: Infant injuries: Accident or abuse? *Pediatr* 44:434–439, 1969.

Swanson LD: Role of the police in the protection of children from neglect and abuse. In *The Battered Child: Selected Readings*, Leavitt JE (ed.). General Learning Corp, 1974.

Thomas A and Chess S: *Temperament and Development* (Brunner/Mazel: New York) 1977.

ADDITIONAL RECOMMENDED READING

Child Abuse and Neglect: *The Problem and Its Management*. Three volumes: (1) An Overview of the Problem, (2) The Roles and Responsibilities of Professionals, (3) The Community Team: An Approach to Case Management and Prevention. DHEW publication no (OHD) 75-30073, 75-30074, and 75-30075.

Kempe CH and Helfer RE: *The Battered Child*, 3d ed. (University of Chicago Press: Chicago and London).

Mrazek PB and Kempe CH: *Sexually Abused Children and Their Families* (Pergamon Press, Ltd) 1981.

23

The Treatment of Cult Victims

John G. Clark and Michael D. Lanzone

In recent years, thousands of parents and former cult members have warned the nation that the current proliferation of destructive cults, both religious and political-terrorist, threatens not only individuals but fundamental religious, political, economic, and social values of our society as well. Speaking from personal experience, these witnesses have contended that such organizations use deceptive recruitment and coercive persuasion (popularly called mind control or brainwashing) to assemble armies of converts who proselytize and solicit money for the cult.

Regularly denigrating the family, established religions, and existing social-government institutions, destructive cults purportedly aspire toward lofty spiritual goals. But, critics say, close examination of cult activities—which include illegal economic practices, infiltration of governmental agencies, and vicious harassment of critics and former members—clearly shows that many seek temporal, rather than spiritual, power and influence. Furthermore, in their grasp for money and power, such cults have seriously damaged the psychological well-being of hundreds of thousands of converts and their families.

TREATMENT GUIDELINES

Former destructive cult members and their parents experience much emotional turmoil. Parents are frequently alarmed and angry at the cults, hungry for advice on how to get their child out of the cult, or worried about their capacity

Copyright © 1984 by Spectrum Publications, Inc. Handbook of Psychiatric Consultation with Children and Youth. Edited by N. R. Bernstein and J. N. Sussex.

to provide a constructive environment for a child recently returned from a cult. Ex-cult members usually exhibit such symptoms as depression, guilt, serious deficiencies in decision making and information processing in general, volatile emotions, anger toward the cult, and a tendency to slip into dissociative states in which they often "float" between their cult and reawakening pre-cult personality. Guilt is frequently burdensome, particularly among those who have behaved contrary to their pre-cult moral standards, such as Children of God members who commit prostitution in order to win converts through "flirty fishing." Medical illnesses or serious dietary deficiencies are also common, especially in those who belonged to cults that shunned the medical establishment or followed unhealthy dietary regimens.

According to psychiatrists and other clinicians who have worked closely with ex-cultists, these symptoms, which seem to suggest the existence of deep-rooted psychopathology, are, on the contrary, often a consequence of the patient's cult experience and the shock of returning to the mainstream environment. Thus, even though many exmembers have lengthy histories of psychological disturbance, clinicians should show extra care in diagnosing former cultists. A majority of the more than two hundred cases of the senior author, for example, were relatively normal adolescents experiencing standard developmental crises at the time of conversion.

There are several reasons why individuals and families affected by destructive cults seek treatment from mental health professionals. First of all, the ex-cultist and/or family may need counseling or therapy (sometimes including medication) in order to cope with the post-cult problems mentioned above. Second, parents may seek advice about how to extricate their child from a cult. And third, parents may wish to have a professional involved in the deprogramming of their child. Although guidelines for responding to the first two treatment needs constitute the focus of this chapter, a word on deprogramming is in order.

The practice of deprogramming appears essentially to involve a sometimes forced reawakening of the convert's old personality and an evaluation of his cult experience. Basically, the process consists of two steps. First, the convert is separated from the cult environment, whether by legal conservatorship, by his voluntary cooperation, or by parent-sponsored abductions. The deprogrammers then spend several intense days discussing the cult's doctrines and practices, especially its coercively manipulative methods of bringing about and maintaining conversion to the cult's way. The goal of deprogramming is to put the convert back in touch with his pre-cult beliefs, values, and goals and to help him re-establish the capacity to think independently and critically. (Cults, on the other hand, strive to enhance dependency and obedience.) Generally speaking, successful deprogrammings involve participation by former members of the cult, for their personal experience with its manipulative techniques gives their criticisms and advice a special credibility to the convert.

Clinicians should show great care before recommending any type of deprogramming. Even responsible and skilled programmers can fail and thereby further alienate the convert from his parents. Moreover, psychological damage may result, particularly if the deprogrammer is not sensitive to long-standing psychological problems which the convert may have.

Deprogramming should be considered only when the parents are fully informed about the procedure and are prepared to take full responsibility for all eventualities. Parents should become knowledgeable about the cult phenomenon and the psychological and legal risks of deprogramming. They should be prepared to shoulder the high cost (often more than $10 thousand) of deprogrammers, detectives, security, lodging, travel, and legal and mental health consultation. They should realize that many problems will remain after the convert leaves the cult. And they should be prepared to provide the level and types of support that he will require upon his return to the mainstream society.

Deprogramming is controversial within professional circles because it is a much more directive procedure than is usually considered acceptable, save for the severely disturbed or retarded. Many exmembers, however, contend that cultists are so "brainwashed" that they are, for all intents and purposes, sufficiently disturbed psychologically (in the sense of their capacity to make informed, voluntary decisions) as to warrant treatment in the highly controlled environment of deprogramming.

In addition to these ethical considerations, mental health professionals should realize that they, as well as parents and deprogrammers, are frequently the targets of lawsuits. Although judges and juries have generally been sympathetic to the cultist's families and to clinicians, the legal costs of winning can be crushing. This is especially so in cases involving members of wealthy cults that sometimes view lawsuits as a means of harassing and impoverishing opponents, even when the opponent's ultimate legal victory is likely.

For these reasons, psychiatrists and other professionals should deliberate very carefully before participating in a deprogramming. Even when treating excultists, whether they left the cult voluntarily or through deprogramming, caution is in order, for exmembers have been known to return to their cults and sue those who have tried to deprogram or counsel them.

Assessment of Cultists

As with any clinical problems, the treatment of cult converts begins with a thorough assessment. First, the clinician should evaluate the convert's current mental status. Second, attention should be paid to the strengths and weaknesses of current and past family relationships. Third, the clinician should study the convert's history, paying particular attention to the possible existence of pre-cult psychopathology, the convert's behavior during developmental crisis periods, and his circumstances and state of mind in the six months preceding conversion. Fourth, the clinician should inquire into the nature of the convert's cult environment. Finally, a medical doctor should perform a thorough examination in order to rule out or begin treatment for dietary and other medical problems.

To speed up the assessment process and ensure that it is comprehensive, various instruments may be used, although care should be taken so as not to overwhelm the ex-cultist. The California Medical Survey is a useful screening device that can alert clinicians and physicians to the existence of medical issues that should be examined. The Mooney Problem Checklist can help the clinician understand how the exconvert or his parents perceive his problem. The Symptom Checklist-90 aids in evaluating the nature and severity of psychiatric symptoms such as depression, anxiety, and psychoticism. And finally, questionnaires specifically designed for parents as well as exconverts may be used in order to collect and organize information concerning the client's experience within the cult (e.g., with regard to methods of proselytizing, guilt and terror, living circumstances).

Treatment of Former Cult Members

The difficulties of former cult members reflect an impaired capacity to exhibit an adaptive autonomy in their daily functioning. They are deficient in the capacity to make independent decisions, to test beliefs and perceptions in consensual reality, to tolerate the inevitable ambiguities and uncertainties of life, and to respond constructively to the demands of social living.

The reason ex-cultists are not autonomous is that they are still very much under the influence of the cult's values, belief-attitude systems, and mode of conceptualizing experience. The cult demands obedience to superiors, regulates closely the activities of daily living, isolates the convert from the social demands of the mainstream culture, propounds doctrines that admit no ambiguity or uncertainty, and denies the authority of traditional methods of validating assertions. In essence, the returnee carries within him a cult personality that both competes with and obscures the pre-cult personality which, to a large extent, was suppressed by the cult experience. Consequently, in his day-to-day life the former member will tend to vacillate, to float, between the cult and noncult ways of experiencing and responding to the world.

As he vacillates between two modes of conceptualizing and responding to the world, the former cultist must cope with daily tasks, reconnect to old memories, examine the nature and implications of the cult experience, and be prepared to meet the developmental demands of our culture. Helping him deal with these issues in an integrative way that enhances his achieving an adaptive autonomy is the ultimate goal of treatment.

Coping with Daily Tasks. The confusion and indecisiveness associated with the experience of floating between two personalities greatly impedes the returnee's capacity to manage the daily tasks of life. This is an ongoing source of stress that must be regularly addressed in therapy. For exmembers, life is a series of mini-crises (such as what to say to an uncle who visits), which, despite their apparent insignificance to others, generate substantial anxiety. During such emergencies the clinician should be rather directive and should make liberal use of other resources available to the ex-cultist, such as parents, siblings, friends, and other professionals. However, in the interests of promoting decision making skills, he should encourage the former member to do as much for himself as possible.

In helping the returnee cope with daily tasks the clinician should not lose sight of a fundamental problem of the exmember: integrating his experiences in two radically different cultures in such a way that he can behave adaptively in one culture without disassociating himself from the experiences—both good and bad—of the other culture. Unlike some workers in this field, who try merely to bring back the returnee's old personality and bury the cult one, the authors maintain that proper treatment calls not only for an awakening of the old personality, but for an intelligent confrontation with and analysis of the cult personality as well.

Before discussing these issues it should be noted that establishing a therapeutic rapport with exmembers necessitates, contrary to the practices of some schools of therapy, an active, directive, and sometimes even conversational approach by the clinician. Because his flow of consciousness is disturbed, the exmember has great difficulty with certain mental operations, including synthesizing ideas, remembering past events, articulating the logical implications of a train of thought, or even recalling what has just been said in a conversation. For this reason the returnee needs much more from the clinician than reflection, paraphrasing, and interpretation. He also seeks and needs information about the cult phenomenon, concrete advice concerning day-to-day as well as long-term problems, and someone to demonstrate commonsense analytical processes (modes of conceptualizing experience) which he must rediscover and further develop in order to cope with his many problems. Of course, since building and strengthening a rapport is not an independent phase of therapy, the clinician must remain alert to the need for this while dealing with developmental tasks, confronting the cult experience, and reconnecting to the past.

Reconnecting. The most efficient way to facilitate reconnecting is to talk about the exmember's past. The clinician should especially ask specific questions about events involving family, intimates, school, work, and friends. Such conversations: a) awaken old memories; b) bring to the fore, while providing useful information about, developmental tasks that were "placed on hold" during the person's time in the cult; and c) alert the clinician to possible longstanding psychological difficulties that require attention. (The questionnaire mentioned earlier can also be useful in this regard.) Because parents generally have special knowledge about the returnee, family interviews (with and without the exmember) can also contribute to the reconnecting process. While helping the exmember reconnect to his past, however, the clinician must take care that neither he nor the family overwhelm the returnee. Old memories often generate anxiety which, if not managed properly, can induce the returneee to seek relief by going back to the cult ways or even to the cult itself.

Confronting Cult Experiences. Although our clinical experience clearly suggests that the tasks of reconnecting to the past and dealing with day-to-day crises should be addressed very early in therapy, we cannot offer clearcut guidelines as to when to elicit and confront the returnee's cult experiences. There is simply too much diversity in the backgrounds and coping skills of former cult members. Naturally, some discussion of the client's cult experiences will occur during the first clinical contact, but the extent to which the cult experience can be explored and analyzed will vary greatly among clients. We suggest that the clinician proceed as though he were dealing with a case of trauma, which in many ways is what the cult experience has been for the convert, but it must be dealt with in managed stages, at a pace and intensity that the exmember can handle.

Although the timing and intensity with which cult experiences are confronted in a particular case is a matter for the clinician to decide, we do feel confident in making several recommendations regarding topics to be explored. First of all, it is important that the exmember learn about the process of cult conversion in general and analyze, with the clinician's guidance, the specific factors that brought about his own conversion. Doing this will a) help the returnee better understand his current difficulties, such as inability to make decisions; b) decrease his guilt and tendency to blame himself for his conversion, because he will become aware of the potency of the cult milieu in the conversion process; c) serve as an exercise in common-sense analysis of events; and d) help the exmember identify pre-cult psychological disturbances or developmental needs that may have influenced his conversion and may be contributing to current distress.

A former member can examine his conversion in various ways. Naturally, individual counseling is one method. But the clinician can also give the exmember reading material, ask him to write about his experiences, and arrange for him to meet with other former cult members in professionally led groups.

The returnee's experience of love, friendship, and a sense of purpose while in the cult are also issues that should be explored. The clinician should help the exmember analyze these feelings objectively, for they were frequently much less solid than they seemed when first experienced. Like a lover who has been deceived, the exmember becomes acutely disillusioned as he recognizes the extent to which these prized feelings were regulated, manipulated, and exploited by the cult. A positive aspect of this disillusionment, however, is that it helps to diminish the apostate's guilt regarding the abandonment of cult friends and helps him realize that even the important sentiments of love, friendship, and a sense of purpose involve much ambiguity and uncertainty. Upon achieving such a perspective, the former member will be better able to experience these valued feelings in the relative freedom of the mainstream culture.

Such an objective analysis elicits strong emotional reactions. Disillusioned that he is not really among the spiritual elect, the exmember feels both anger and grief. Indignation about being duped results in crushed self-esteem and sometimes a maddeningly persistent frustration over his inability to destroy the evil that the cult now represents to him. And an intense concern for the well-being of his friends still in the cult arouses strong desires to fight the organization and rescue them from it.

The clinician should help the exmember identify and respond constructively to the various aspects of this intense, volatile mixture of emotions. For example, the returnee can be helped to see that in his disillusionment lie many lessons regarding how to evaluate events and belief systems, that his indignation reveals the underlying moral fiber that will give him the courage to create a coherent world view for himself, and that his concern for cult members demonstrates that his capacity to experience genuine fellowship is very much alive.

Managing Developmental Demands. In confronting the cult experience, the returnee painfully realizes that he was fooled. This realization renders him unsure of his capacity to manage the developmental demands that society places on individuals: getting a job, deciding on or preparing for a career, getting an education, having intimate relationships, interacting effectively with people.

Besides being formidable challenges in their own right, these developmental tasks, because of their constant, implicit presence, may spawn a variety of day-to-day crises, such as when Uncle Harry asks whether the returnee plans to go back to college. Exploring such crises can reveal much about the exmember's evaluation of his ability to cope with the various developmental tasks and can be a first step in assisting him to respond effectively to them.

The clinician, however, should do much more than explore. He should help the returnee identify the specific developmental challenges that confront him, accept their unavoidable pressures, assess his skill levels relative to each, and establish a strategy for responding to them in an adaptive manner (seeking information, setting priorities, improving skills, examining alternatives). Standard therapeutic procedures may be used in order to work with the client in these areas, especially after the issues of reconnecting to the past and confronting the cult experience have been substantially resolved. However, if these issues are still active (as evidenced, for instance, by a high frequency of floating), it is important that the clinician subordinate developmental goals to the more pressing objective of decreasing the degree of fragmentation within the returnee's mind.

Treatment of Current Cult Members

The near-total lack of adaptive autonomy in current cult members makes their treatment even more difficult than that of former converts. And since the current member's willingness to talk to a professional is usually highly conditional, if not a mere concession to parental pleas, the clinician—who should be knowledgeable about the member's cult milieu—must be very careful in his interactions.

Because the clinical relationship in such cases is so delicate, rapport building is especially important. The clinician should scrupulously avoid theological debates and other actions that are likely to result in an emotional confrontation. Respectful listening and very gentle probing may be all he can do at first.

As trust and respect build, the clinician may gradually become more directive and more open about his opinions, but in a way that does not obviously assault the convert's beliefs. Rather, the clinician should try to persuade the convert to listen to another view of events, another—the commonsense—way of thinking. By modeling, so to speak, a more critical way of thinking, the clinician helps to awaken the convert's own dormant critical capacities which, once operating, lead him to question the cult's beliefs and practices. The clinician treating a Moonie, for example, may in passing talk about how working late the other night made him so tired that he almost fell asleep while visiting friends. To the Moonie who has become accustomed to thinking that fatigue is caused by sleep spirits, rather than overwork, such a statement may serve as a jolting reminder that there are ways in which to conceptualize experience other than that propounded by Reverend Moon.

In addition to teaching the commonsense way of thinking, the clinician can stimulate the convert's critical faculties by asking for specifics from his past, inquiring into his opinions about current events, gently exploring his doubts regarding the cult, using "what if" questions to induce abstract thinking and unrehearsed answers, and especially by exploring his preconversion circumstances and state of mind.

The clinician may also meet with the cult member along with his family in order to demonstrate how greatly people (even members of the same family) can differ in their interpretations of the same or similar events. In recognizing the existence of conflicting interpretations of an event, the convert will begin to compare interpretations and apply criteria of validity in order to assess their relative merits. By subtly injecting common-sense criteria of validity into the conversation, the clinician can gradually reactivate the convert's critical capacities.

A convert, for example, may interpret the Russian invasion of Afghanistan as a sign of the coming apocalypse. Since everybody in his cult shares the same interpretation, the convert will have had little opportunity to consider alternative viewpoints. In a family interview, however, the convert may find that his mother senses no danger at all, while his father feels that firm and prudent action by the United States can contain the danger. The clinician, whose goal is to promote critical thinking, may encourage the convert to consider the pros and cons of each point of view and to speculate on how various hypotheses may be discounted or conditionally accepted. By doing this, the clinician helps to re-awaken the cultist's dormant analytical capacities.

Once the cult member begins to reconnect to past mental experiences and to think critically, doubts about the cult will arise spontaneously. The powerful emotion often accompanying such doubts, however, will inevitably threaten the therapeutic rapport and the convert's willingness to talk to the clinician and to his parents. The clinician's ability to be supportive, to discuss the positive aspects of cult life, and to show a good sense of timing may be critical in determining whether or not the convert will keep lines of communication open with the non-cult world during these times of doubt or respond to his stress in ways sanctioned by the cult, such as chanting, meditation, and seeking cult fellowship.

So long as the convert keeps in touch with the non-cult world and with his past, there is hope that he may be persuaded to leave the cult, at least temporarily, or to reconsider his relationship to it. As the convert begins to verbalize his doubts, the clinician may judiciously begin to challenge cult doctrines, proselytizing methods, money-making activities, and day-to-day life-style. If all goes well, the member's doubts will at least increase to a point where he will want a respite from cult life in order to reconsider his commitment. Unpressured support from the clinician and the family can be invaluable during such a respite, which is often a period of lonely soul searching. Although the convert may not immediately choose to renounce the cult, his doubt will certainly be continuously rekindled so long as he maintains close contact with the clinician and his parents. Naturally, if the convert does choose to renounce the cult, then clinical goals change somewhat, with much more emphasis being placed on educating him to the mind-control techniques of the cults, integrating pre-cult and in-cult experiences, coping with daily stress, and managing developmental tasks.

Obviously, none of these therapeutic goals can be achieved unless lines of communication with the convert are maintained. This, then, must be the first priority of all who try to help the convert. Unfortunately, the uncooperativeness of cult leaders and the convert's anxiety regarding an open discussion of his feelings and thoughts greatly limit the influence of outsiders. For this reason, parents and clinicians must proceed circumspectly and prepare themselves psychologically for a sudden closing off of communication, something that happens all too often.

Should communication be severed (when, for instance, the cult sends the member to an out-of-the way place) some alternatives, however unappealing, are still open to the parents. Rescuing and deprogramming the convert, for example, remains an option, although the risks are great. Legal proceedings, such as those leading to conservatorships, may also be a viable course of action, although this strategy also involves much risk and expense. Clearly, the preferred means is to persuade the convert to leave the cult voluntarily. Although this course is often difficult, it appears that a fairly large proportion (one-third being the best current estimate for one of the more coercively manipulative cults) of cult members do in fact leave cults voluntarily. Distraught parents may receive some consolation from this tentative finding.

Treatment of Parents

Parents of cult members need to come to terms with a variety of emotions, which they have usually stifled for fear of alienating or harming their child. The parents need to reflect upon their cult-related experiences, articulate more accurately their thoughts and emotions about these experiences, assess the validity of their insights into the cult phenomenon, deal constructively with the caretaker urge, promote the child's psychological development, and cope effectively with any of their own personal and marital problems, whether of recent or remote origin. Clinicians can take a variety of steps to help parents meet these needs.

Creating an Atmosphere of Safety. Most importantly, of course, the clinician should create a supportive, though not merely reassuring, atmosphere in which parents feel safe expressing emotions and perceptions or beliefs that may seem in conflict with the world around them. A first step in creating such a climate is to reassure the parents that the striking and sometimes very sudden changes observed in their child are most likely attributable to the cult environment, that their fears concerning the child's psychological well-being are well-founded, and that many other parents of converts have had experiences similar to their own. Professionally led discussion groups made up of parents of cult members and/or exmembers can be very useful in driving home this latter point and in enhancing a constructive expression of attitudes toward the cult phenomenon.

Examining Feelings, Perceptions, and Beliefs. After parents begin to feel safe expressing themselves, the clinician should devote more attention to helping them examine and more accurately articulate their feelings, perceptions, and beliefs. This task, a prerequisite to constructive family communication, is crucial to the healthy resolution of the convert's and parents' difficulties. Paraphrasing the parents' responses, asking direct questions, providing information that bears upon particular cult-related experiences, having the parents paraphrase each other in order to ensure that they are communicating accurately, and asking questions or making statements that stimulate them to think about and describe the implications of many of their experiences may all contribute to a clear and full articulation of their perspectives.

Verifying Perceptions and Beliefs. In addition to helping parents better express their points of view, the clinician should teach them how to test the validity of their perspectives on various matters. Learning how to subject beliefs and perceptions about their child, their own behavior, the cult, and so forth, to empirical analysis and how to evaluate their diverse feelings will help parents deal with, rather than deny, the ambivalence and conflict that is unavoidable when a child enters or returns from a cult.

Dealing with the Caretaker Urge. Identifying and critically evaluating ambivalent feelings is extremely important when the parents feel the urge to take on a caretaker role towards their child. Since this urge directly contradicts their desire to give the child more autonomy, something that most parents deem essential to normal development, much familial conflict may occur. Some members of the family may be more inclined to resist challenging the child's autonomy; other members may feel compelled to protect the convert; and still others in the family may be paralyzed with indecision. In such situations the clinician should help each family member become aware of both his own and his relatives' feelings and opinions. The family must examine all conflicting perspectives and arrive at an informed decision, preferably one agreeable to all, regarding what to do about the problems posed by the former convert's return or how to recover a child who still belongs to the cult.

Promoting the Returnee's Psychological Development. When the clinician begins to help the family formulate such a strategy he is beginning the most difficult part of the counseling process, that of teaching them how to promote the convert's psychological development. Most family members want, and sometimes demand, dependable advice. They want to know how to help the ex-member recover his old personality, deal with the challenges of everyday living, and reestablish or establish vocational and educational goals. Further, they want to learn how the family can deal with the psychopathological reactions often exhibited by former cult members. Unfortunately, however, not enough is known about the varied individual responses to cult conversion and deconversion to provide parents with reliable or exact formulae that address their concerns. Nevertheless, the clinician can inform the parents about the cult phenomenon, examine with them the pros and cons of alternative courses of action, and help them accept the uncertainties and ambivalence that inevitably accompany the decisions they must make.

Problems of Family Members. The complications involved in helping parents promote a convert's psychological development are compounded when serious marital, family, or personal problems trouble family members. In such cases the clinician should be very careful not to set inappropriate priorities. Unsually the convert's psychological state is much more vulnerable than that of other family members and, consequently, should be the first priority; long-standing family, marital, and personal problems should be dealt with (at least initially) only insofar as they impinge on the convert's difficulties.

The clinician should resist "diversions," that is, the temptation to work on an "interesting" marital conflict, or the desire to escape the ambiguity of the cult counseling process by focusing on a problem with which he feels comfortable. Nevertheless, he should realize that personal, marital, or family conflicts may sometimes be so severe as to sabotage any therapeutic strategy aimed at assisting the convert.

Thus, from time to time it may be necessary to place a convert's problems "on the back burner," however risky this may be, in order to concentrate on serious problems within the family. Occasionally, in fact, a convert's potential or actual return may be so disruptive to the family equilibrium that the clinician is faced with the prospect of breaking up the family while trying to save the convert from the cult. As with so many aspects of the cult phenomenon, no clear-cut guidelines can be given for such situations.

Indications and Contraindications of Drugs

In deciding whether or not to prescribe medication for former cult members, the physician should keep in mind that it is difficult to determine the extent to which the ex-cultist's symptomatology is a function of the cult experience rather than a function of a true psychiatric illness. Therefore, the physician should be more cautious than usual in making the decision to prescribe and follow the patient's progress very closely when medications are given.

This latter point is especially important, for the clinical evidence suggests that exmembers respond to medications more rapidly (and sometimes more adversely) than one would normally expect. This appears to be the case whether the symptomatology is psychotic or nonpsychotic or whether or not a history of psychiatric disorder exists. Consequently, when prescribing medications for ex-cultists, the physician should be prepared to decrease dosages or discontinue the medication sooner than customary practice would suggest.

Although somewhat more deliberation than usual is called for in deciding to prescribe, the physician, once he makes this decision, can use standard clinical criteria in determining what to prescribe and at what dosage. In evaluating psychotic symptomatology, however, the physician should be careful to distinguish between idiosyncratic delusions and bizarre beliefs that the exmember adopted as a result of his conversion. Similarly, in evaluating the degree of functional impairment, the physician should realize that the ex-cultist has experienced a culture shock that may make him appear to be psychiatrically ill when, instead, he is experiencing a severe adjustment reaction.

BIBLIOGRAPHY

The Advisor (bimonthly) (American Family Foundation: Lexington, MA) 1978–1981.

Boettcher RB: *Gifts of Deceit* (Holt Rinehart Winston: New York), 1980.

Clark JG: Investigating the effects of some religious cults on the health and welfare of their converts. Paper submitted to the Vermont Legislature, 1977.

Clark JG: Problems in referral of cult members. *J Nat Assoc Pri Psych Hosp* 9: 17, 1978.

Clark JG: Cults. *J Am Med Assoc* 242:179–181, 1979.

Conway F and Siegleman X: *Snapping: America's Epidemic of Sudden Personality Change* (Lippincott: New York) 1978.

Cooper P: *The Scandal of Scientology* (Tower: New York) 1971.

Delgado R: Religious totalism: Gentle and ungentle persuasion under the First Amendment. *Southern California Law Review* 51:1–97, 1977.

Derogatis LR: *SCL-90R, Manual-1* (Clinical Psychometric Research Unit, Johns Hopkins University School of Medicine: Baltimore) 1977.

Edwards C: *Crazy for God: The Nightmare of Cult Life* (Prentice-Hall: Englewood Cliffs, NJ) 1979.

Enroth R: *Youth, Brainwashing, and the Extremist Cults* (Zondervan: Grand Rapids, MI) 1977.

Information meeting on the cult phenomenon in the United States (transcript). Senator Robert Dole, chairman. Washington, DC, February 5, 1977.

Langone MD: *Cult Family Questionnaire* (Center on Destructive Cultism: Boston) 1980.

Langone MD: *Cult Involvement Questionnaire* (Center on Destructive Cultism: Boston) 1980.

Massachusetts State Senate: *Public hearing on solicitation utilized by religious and charitable groups* (transcript). Senator John G King, chairman, March 21, 1979.

Mooney RL and Gordon LV: *The Mooney Problem Check List: Manual* (The Psychological Corporation: New York) 19oo.

New York State Assembly: *Public hearing on treatment of children by cults* (transcript). Assemblyman Howard Lasher, chairman, August 9–10, 1979.

Rudin AJ and Rudin MR: *Prison or Paradise? The New Religious Cults* (Fortress: Philadelphia) 1980.

Singer M: Coming out of the cults. *Psychology Today* 72–82, 1979.

Snow HL and Manson MP: *The California Medical Survey Manual* (Western Psychological Services: Los Angeles) 1962.

Subcommittee on International Organizations of the Committee on International Relations, US House of Representatives: *Investigation of Korean-American relations* (transcript). Representative Donald Fraser, chairman, October 31, 1978.

Index